DEATH ON THE NILE

MNEMOSYNE
SUPPLEMENTS

SUBSERIES

HISTORY AND ARCHAEOLOGY OF CLASSICAL ANTIQUITY

EDITORS

WILLEM M. JONGMAN · IAN MORRIS

VOLUME CCXXVIII

WALTER SCHEIDEL

DEATH ON THE NILE

DEATH ON THE NILE

DISEASE AND THE DEMOGRAPHY OF ROMAN EGYPT

BY

WALTER SCHEIDEL

BRILL
LEIDEN · BOSTON · KÖLN
2001

This book is printed on acid-free paper.

Library of Congress Cataloging-in-Publication Data

Scheidel, Walter, 1966-
Death on the Nile : disease and the demography of Roman Egypt / by Walter Scheidel.
p. cm. — (Mnemosyne, bibliotheca classica Batava. Supplementum, ISSN 0169-8958; 228)
Includes bibliographical references.
ISBN 900412323 7 (alk. paper)
1. Diseases—Egypt—History. 2. Demography—Egypt—History. 3. Medicine, Ancient. I. Title. II. Series.

R653.E4 S36 2001
614.4'232—dc21 2001043185

Die Deutsche Bibliothek - CIP-Einheitsaufnahme

Scheidel, Walter:
Death on the Nile : disease and the demography of Roman Egypt / by Walter Scheidel. – Leiden ; Boston ; Köln : Brill, 2001
(Mnemosyne : Supplementum ; Vol. 228)
ISBN 90–04–12323–7

ISSN 0169-8958
ISBN 90 04 12323 7

PRINTED IN THE NETHERLANDS

For my Cambridge friends

CONTENTS

Abbreviations ix
List of maps, figures, and tables xi
Maps xviii
Introduction xxi

1. Mortality patterns and causes of death 1
2. Age structure and life expectancy 118
3. Population size and demographic change 181

Appendix One Months of death in epitaphs from ancient and medieval Egypt and Nubia 251
Appendix Two Persons with exact ages in the census returns 256

Bibliography 259
Index 281

ABBREVIATIONS

References to ancient authors and modern periodicals have not been abbreviated. The following abbreviations have been used for modern editions of papyrological, epigraphic and literary sources:

CEML	*Corpus des etiquettes des momies* [Boyaval (1976)]
CMG	*Corpus medicorum graecorum*
FGrHist	*Fragmente der griechischen Historiker*
I.Fay.	*Recueil des inscriptions grecques du Fayoum* [Bernand (1975, 1981)]
KSB	*Koptisches Sammelbuch* [Hasitzka (1993)]
O.Claud.	*Mons Claudianus: ostraca graeca et latina*
P.Berol.	*Catalogue of Greek and Roman literary papyri in Berlin*
P.Carlsberg	*Papyrus Carlsberg*
P.Ebers	*Papyrus Ebers*
P.Erlangen	*Die Papyri der Universitätsbibliothek Erlangen*
PGM	*Papyri graecae magicae*
P.Harris	*The Rendel Harris papyri of Woodbrooke College*
P.Lond.	*Greek papyri in the British Museum*
P.Mich.	*Michigan papyri*
P.Mil.	*Papiri milanesi*
P.Oxy.	*The Oxyrhynchus papyri*
P.Prag.	*Papyri Wessely Pragenses*
P.Princ.	*Papyri in the Princeton University collection*
P.Tebt.	*The Tebtunis papyri*
P.Wisc.	*The Wisconsin papyri*
SB	*Sammelbuch griechischer Urkunden aus Ägypten*
SEG	*Supplementum epigraphicum graecum*
SFK	*Stèles funéraires de Kom Abu Bellou* [Abd el-Hafeez abd el-Al, Grenier and Wagner (1985)]

LIST OF MAPS, FIGURES, AND TABLES

Maps

1 Roman Egypt xviii
2 Roman Fayum xix

Figures

1.1 Seasonal mortality in Upper Egypt and Nubia according to Greek and Coptic funerary inscriptions (raw data) 6
1.2 Seasonal mortality in Upper Egypt and Nubia according to Greek and Coptic funerary inscriptions (smoothed data) 7
1.3 Seasonal mortality in three Coptic monasteries (smoothed data) 8
1.4 Seasonal mortality in the Monastery of St Simeon, Aswan (smoothed data) 9
1.5 Seasonal mortality in Upper Egypt and Nubia according to Greek and Coptic funerary inscriptions, excluding the Coptic texts of Sakinya (smoothed data) 11
1.6 Seasonal mortality in Upper Egypt north of Aswan according to Greek and Coptic funerary inscriptions (smoothed data) 11
1.7 Seasonal mortality in Upper Egypt according to Greek and Coptic funerary inscriptions and monthly incidence of dates on mummy labels (raw data) 14
1.8 Seasonal mortality in Upper Egypt according to Greek and Coptic funerary inscriptions and monthly incidence of dates on mummy labels (smoothed data) 14
1.9 Seasonal mortality in Upper Egypt according to Greek and Coptic funerary inscriptions and adjusted monthly incidence of dates on mummy labels (smoothed data) 15

1.10 Monthly incidence of dates on mummy labels of known and unknown provenance (smoothed data) 16
1.11 Seasonal mortality in the Fayum according to Greek and Coptic funerary inscriptions 18
1.12 Seasonal mortality in the Nile Valley and in the Fayum according to Greek and Coptic funerary inscriptions (smoothed data) 18
1.13 Seasonal mortality in Alexandria according to Greek funerary inscriptions 21
1.14 Seasonal mortality in Carthage according to Latin funerary inscriptions 22
1.15 Seasonal mortality in Terenouthis according to Greek funerary inscriptions 23
1.16 Seasonal mortality in Lower Egypt outside Alexandria and Terenouthis according to Greek funerary inscriptions 24
1.17 Seasonal mortality in Lower Egypt outside Alexandria, according to Greek funerary inscriptions (smoothed data) 25
1.18 Seasonal mortality in Egypt and Nubia (smoothed data) 26
1.19 Seasonal mortality at specific ages in Terenouthis (1) (smoothed data) 29
1.20 Seasonal mortality at specific ages in Terenouthis (2) (smoothed data) 29
1.21 Seasonal mortality at specific ages according to mummy labels (smoothed data) 30
1.22 Seasonal mortality according to specific samples of the funerary inscriptions of Terenouthis (smoothed data) 33
1.23 Monthly incidence of unadjusted dates in specific samples of mummy labels (smoothed data) 33
1.24 Seasonal mortality in Palestine according to Greek funerary inscriptions 37
1.25 Seasonal mortality in ancient Upper Egypt and Italy 38
1.26 Seasonal mortality in ancient and modern Egypt 39
1.27 Seasonal mortality in the ancient and modern Fayum 41
1.28 Seasonal mortality in specific age groups in modern Egypt, 1961 to 1970 42

1.29 Seasonal mortality in Cairo, December 1798 to January 1800 ... 43
1.30 Seasonal mortality in Cairo, June 1800 to February 1801 ... 43
1.31 Seasonal mortality in Cairo, August 1859 to July 1860 ... 44
1.32 Seasonal mortality in Alexandria, August 1859 to July 1860 ... 44
1.33 Seasonal mortality in Cairo and Alexandria, 1859/60 and 1926 ... 45
1.34 Seasonal mortality at specific ages in Italy, 1869 ... 46
1.35 Seasonal mortality at specific ages in late antique Rome ... 47
1.36 Seasonal mortality in the Mediterranean in the nineteenth and early twentieth centuries ... 48
1.37 Regional seasonal mortality in ancient and modern Egypt ... 50
1.38 Seasonal mortality in Japan, 1921 to 1955 ... 52
1.39 Seasonal incidence of causes of death in Cairo, July 1859 to June 1860 ... 73
1.40 Seasonal incidence of causes of death in Alexandria, July 1859 to June 1860 ... 74
1.41 Seasonal mortality in Geneva, 1617 to 1649 ... 95
1.42 Monthly mortality figures in Cairo, May 1800 to May 1801 ... 99
2.1 Ages in the census returns of Roman Egypt (raw data) 119
2.2 Comparison of proportions surviving by age in 'good' and 'bad' decades, United Provinces (North India), Females, 1881 to 1891 and 1911 to 1921 ... 127
2.3 Age-specific survivorship according to different model life tables ... 129
2.4 Age-specific probability of dying for Mino villages, 1751 to 1869, compared to model life table schedules ... 130
2.5 Age-specific life expectancy among the Qing of Beijing in 1800 and according to model life tables (Model West) ... 135
2.6 Age-specific male mortality rates in rural Liaoning, Manchuria, from 1792 to 1867, and according to model life tables (Model North Males) ... 136

2.7 Age-specific female mortality rates in rural Liaoning, Manchuria, from 1792 to 1867, and according to model life tables (Model North Females) 136
2.8 Probability of dying between ages x and $x + n$ according to Weiss's model life tables 138
2.9 Age-specific life expectancy in the cemetery population of Kulubnarti, Nubia 139
2.10 Weighted age distribution in the census returns of Roman Egypt 143
2.11 Age composition of the census population of Roman Egypt 146
2.12 Female age composition of the metropolitan census population of Roman Egypt 147
2.13 Male age composition of the metropolitan census population of Roman Egypt 148
2.14 Age composition of the 'core' metropolitan census population of Roman Egypt (1) 151
2.15 Age composition of the 'core' metropolitan census population of Roman Egypt (2) 152
2.16 Female age composition of the 'core' metropolitan census population of Roman Egypt 152
2.17 Male age composition of the 'core' metropolitan census population of Roman Egypt 153
2.18 Age composition in two urban census populations of Roman Egypt 154
2.19 Age composition of the 'core' metropolitan census population of Roman Egypt fitted to a model life table 155
2.20 Age composition of the village census population of Roman Egypt 157
2.21 Male age structure in the village census returns and tax lists of Roman Egypt 159
2.22 Male age structure in the village census returns and tax lists of Roman Egypt 159
2.23 Male age structure in the village census returns and tax lists of Roman Egypt 161
2.24 Female age composition of the village census population of Roman Egypt fitted to a model life table 161
2.25 Age composition of the census population of Roman Egypt before and after 166 CE 163

2.26 Age composition of the census population of Roman Egypt before and after 166 CE ... 163
2.27 Age-specific sex ratios in two census populations of Roman Egypt ... 169
3.1 The earliest European statistics of Egyptian plague mortality: monthly incidence of deaths, Cairo, 1799 to 1801 ... 191
3.2 Incidence of plague and mortality peaks in Egypt, 1601 to 1870 ... 192
3.3 Mortality crises and the endemicity of plague in Egypt, 1780 to 1890 ... 192
3.4 The probable size of the population of Egypt (excluding foreigners), 1805 to 1907 ... 212
3.5 Value of Egyptian exports of wheat, maize and beans ... 238
3.6 Value of Egyptian imports of wheat, maize and beans ... 238
3.7 Value of Egyptian trade in cereals and flour ... 239

Tables

1.1 Monthly distribution of deaths in Upper Egypt and Nubia according to Greek and Coptic funerary inscriptions ... 5
1.2 Monthly distribution of deaths in three Coptic monasteries ... 7
1.3 Monthly distribution of deaths according to mummy labels ... 13
1.4 Monthly distribution of deaths in Lower Egypt according to Greek funerary inscriptions ... 20
1.5 Age-specific seasonal mortality according to the funerary inscriptions of Terenouthis (1) ... 27
1.6 Age-specific seasonal mortality according to the funerary inscriptions of Terenouthis (2) ... 27
1.7 Age-specific seasonal mortality according to mummy labels ... 28
1.8 Age-specific incidence of deaths according to funerary inscriptions and mummy labels ... 31
1.9 Age-specific incidence of deaths according to the funerary inscriptions of Terenouthis ... 32

1.10 Age-specific incidence of deaths according to mummy labels 32
1.11 Monthly distribution of reported raindays at Alexandria according to Ptolemy and al-Biruni, and at present 55
1.12 Seasonal incidence of plague in early modern Egypt 97
1.13 Principal causes of death in the Egyptian population of Cairo and Alexandria, July 1859 to June 1860 105
1.14 Reported cases of disease and causes of death in the European Hospital in Cairo, 1844 to 1861 106
1.15 Principal causes of death in Cairo and Alexandria, 1859/60, 1871 and 1920/25 107
1.16 Causes of death from ages one to five in Cairo and Alexandria, 1889, expressed as a share of all causes 107
1.17 Principal causes of death in Cairo, 1920 to 1925, expressed as a share of all causes 108
1.18 Principal and unknown causes of death in Cairo, 1922, expressed as a share of all deaths 108
1.19 Seasonal contours of infectious disease in Egypt from the sixteenth to the early twentieth centuries 110
2.1 Probability of dying (${}_nq_x$) between ages x and $x + n$ and life expectancy at birth ($e(0)$) in Grosseto, Italy, in the 1840s, and according to model life tables 132
2.2 Incidence of deaths per person-years lived between ages x and $x + n$ (m_x) for four Essex marsh parishes, 1780s to 1812 133
2.3 Proportion of individuals aged twenty dying between ages twenty and x in four Essex marsh parishes, 1780s to 1812, and according to model life tables 133
2.4 Age structure of discrete subsamples of the census population of Roman Egypt 145
2.5 Proportional representation of age cohorts in different subsamples of the census returns of Roman Egypt 165
2.6 A speculative simple model of annual demographic change in Roman Egypt from Augustus to the Antonines 170
3.1 Contemporary assessments and modern estimates of the population of Egypt 205
3.2 Intercensal growth rates of the population of Egypt 206
3.3 Baer's estimates of the population of Egypt 206

3.4 Scenarios of population growth in Egypt 212
3.5 Cultivated area in Egypt 221
3.6 Area devoted to major crops in Egypt 222
3.7 Total area devoted to the production of basic foodstuffs in Egypt 223
3.8 Average yields on state domains in Egypt 224
3.9 Agricultural production in Egypt according to contemporary statistics 229
3.10 Volume and indices of production of six staple crops in Egypt 230
3.11 Exports of foodstuffs from Egypt 236

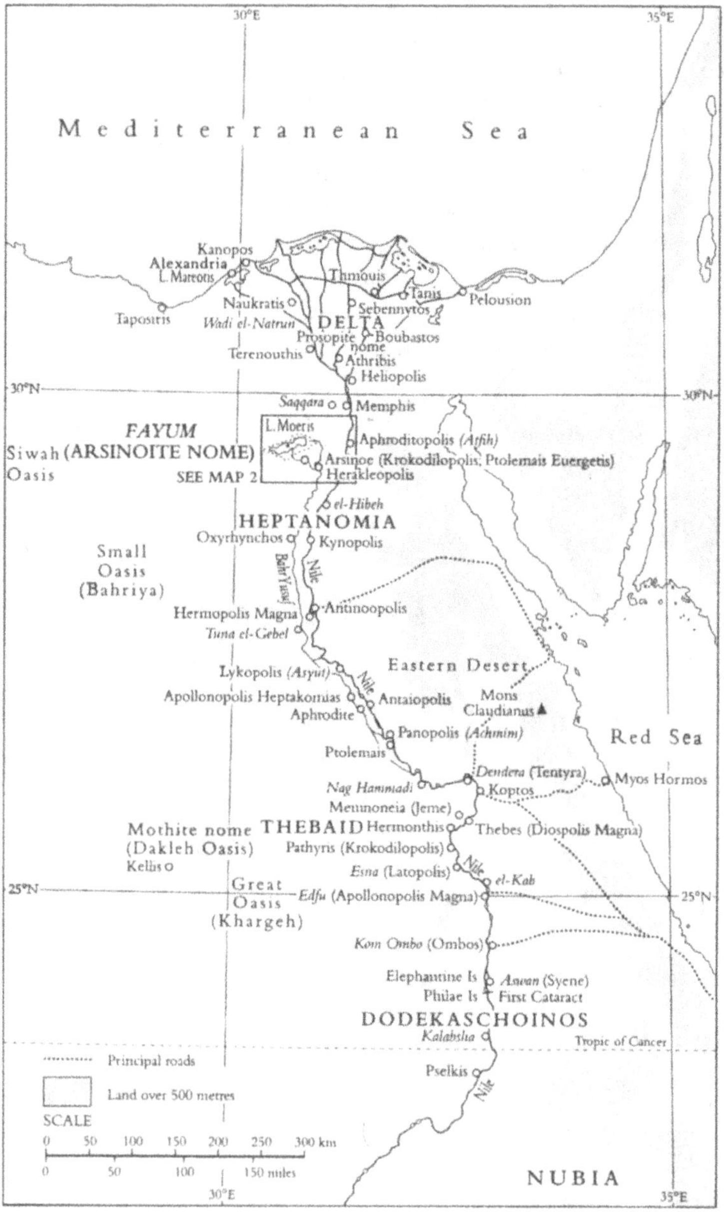

Map 1 Roman Egypt
(Reproduced with permission from: J. Rowlandson, ed., *Women and society in Greek and Roman Egypt: a sourcebook*, Cambridge: Cambridge University Press, 1998, XIX)

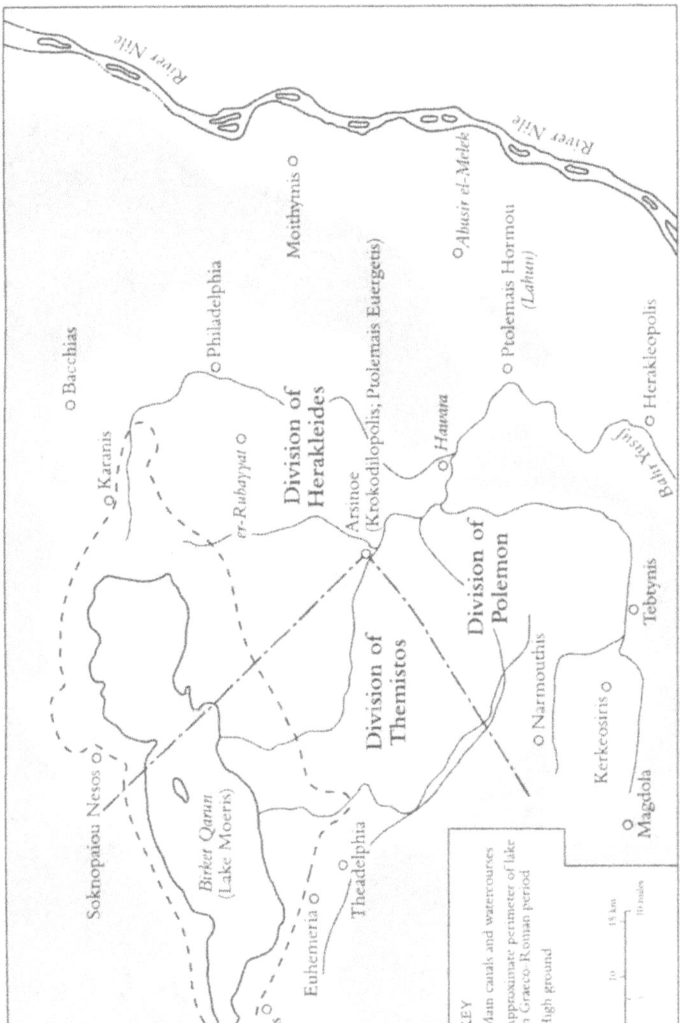

Map 2 Roman Fayum
(Reproduced with permission from: J. Rowlandson, ed., *Women and society in Greek and Roman Egypt: a sourcebook*, Cambridge: Cambridge University Press, 1998, XX)

INTRODUCTION

Demography is one of many ways of attempting to capture the essence of life: its transmission, and its end. Historical demography, by extending this process of measurement and analysis into the past, helps situate and define the properties of the present in the context of a dynamic model of continuity and change. In all this, perhaps paradoxically, death comes first. As the demographic transition has shown, mortality is ultimately the principal determinant of reproductive performance: in the long run, fertility responds to the survival rates of progeny. Mortality, in turn, is largely a function of disease, rather than—but interacting with—nutrition or other factors. The prevalence of endemic infectious disease, the main cause of morbidity and mortality in pre-modern populations, has itself been influenced by the most fundamental subsistence choices of the human species, its break with its ancestral hunting-gathering existence, the resulting multiplication of population density and its attendant sanitary and epidemiologic consequences. As a result, life in pre-industrial societies was shaped by pervasive illness and death. Death was a common occurrence across the life cycle to an extent that has become barely imaginable to denizens of the modern West. The true nature of 'the world we have lost' is worth remembering.

At first sight, it might seem that students of the Greco-Roman world have begun to take proper account of the harsh environment that bore their traditional 'classics'. Over the past few decades, the study of ancient population history, and of Roman demography in particular, at long last waking up to the concepts and methods of professional historical demography, has made considerable headway. Though still the preserve of a mere handful of practitioners, its claims and suggestions have been widely incorporated into recent research on other issues from political participation to economic institutions (Scheidel (2001)). At the same time, the medical history of antiquity has always been a well-established field, long confined to a community of specialists but now gradually opened up through its discovery by gender studies.

Even so, it soon becomes apparent that all is not well. Demography and disease are almost invariably studied separately. The leading contributors to our emerging vision of Roman population structure, such as Keith Hopkins, Bruce Frier, Richard Saller, Brent Shaw and Tim Parkin, have been exclusively concerned with aspects of the formal demography of the Roman world and its impact on social structure and cultural practice. The underlying causes of the demographic regime have failed to attract any attention. At the same time, ancient disease is explored not only separately from demography but in two completely different ways, as an element of Greek and Roman intellectual history as embodied in the Hippocratic tradition and other medical texts, and from the perspective of physical anthropology, centred on the increasingly sophisticated scientific investigation of human remains. There is hardly any overlap between these two spheres of medical history, let alone between them and historical demography. Even the outstanding work of Mirko Grmek that seeks to synthesise textual and scientific evidence betrays little interest in its demographic implications.

This mutual isolation makes it impossible to proceed from description to explanation. Reconstructions of ancient population structure that ignore the determinants of mortality are reduced to describing observable phenomena or speculating about their precise qualities. So are studies of manifestations of disease that fail to enquire into their repercussions for the affected populations. It would be easy and not entirely unjustified to blame this unsatisfying state of affairs on the lack of reliable, 'hard' data. Causation is particularly hard to study if the variables that form the object of the analysis are themselves not particularly well known. Analogous reasoning from comparative data and theoretical models opens new paths but may also obscure genuine diversity and encourage unhistorical projection and aprioristic or circular arguments.

Nevertheless, the situation is not completely hopeless. So far, the debate among ancient historians has revolved around the question of whether certain samples of ancient data are usable for the demographic analysis of mortality patterns or whether we ought to abandon the primary evidence in favour of models and analogy. The former position, unfashionable since Hopkins' work in the 1960s (Hopkins (1966, 1987)), has recently been reinvigorated by the pathbreaking study of the demographic information contained in the surviving census returns of Roman Egypt undertaken by Roger Bagnall and Bruce Frier (Bagnall and Frier (1994)). However, there is no comparable controversy concerning the study of the underlying causes:

is it possible to derive at least corroborative evidence from ancient sources, or are we reduced to mere guesswork? With the exception of some of my own earlier work (Scheidel (1994, 1996a)), potential proxy data for causes of death, such as seasonal mortality patterns, have so far been studied without more than token reference to their epidemiologic implications, most recently by Brent Shaw (Shaw (1996)). Usually firmly set apart from these studies, the discussion of the numerical size of ancient populations has also regained momentum, thanks largely to the revisionist efforts of Elio Lo Cascio. These studies, even when they are not exclusively concerned with the exegesis of statements gleaned from literary texts, are still characterised by a fairly cavalier attitude towards comparative data, which are selectively deployed as required to support a particular claim, and by superficial probabilistic reasoning from carrying capacity and sustainability.

This state of affairs is highly unsatisfying. Population history is embedded in a much wider ecological context, and cannot be understood without it. It requires a holistic, interdisciplinary approach that aims to take full account of both written and archaeological data from antiquity, of comparative evidence from other periods and locations, and of the expanding armoury of scientific analysis and modelling. It is true that even in this scenario, the primary evidence needs to meet certain minimal standards in order to permit any meaningful attempt at reconstruction and explanation. It is also true that in Roman history, this is rarely the case. Egypt is the main exception. Owing in the first instance to the survival of primary documentary population data, and also to the sheer time span of continuously documented history that facilitates comparative assessments, Roman Egypt serves as a unique window to demographic conditions in the very distant past.

Thus, the demography of Roman Egypt is of interest perhaps not so much for its own sake as for this rare chance to glimpse *la longue durée* of mortality, fertility and population structure. The population history of ancient China, the only other region that offers similar opportunities, has already begun to be drawn into the ambit of historical demography, and it will be the lasting merit of Bagnall and Frier to have endeavoured to accomplish the same for Roman Egypt. For all that ancient historians stand to profit from their growing acquaintance with the concerns and techniques of the demographic study of more recent periods, this exchange need not be entirely one-sided. The study of the formal demography of Roman Egypt greatly expands the scope of historical demography, which is largely confined to the post-medieval period, and affords much-needed background to our appreciation of the population dynamics of recent centuries.

Yet Bagnall and Frier would be the first to admit that their contribution was only a first (if huge) step. Of course no-one will ever be able to write a *Population history of Roman Egypt* along the lines of Wrigley and Schofield's seminal *Population history of England* (Wrigley and Schofield (1981)), given the inevitably vast gulf between such projects created by the very different quality of the available data. Despite its general title, *The demography of Roman Egypt* is a study of one particular type of demographic evidence from that region, namely those census returns (and some tax lists derived therefrom) which happen to survive on scraps of papyrus. In conjunction with demographic models, these texts can be used to reconstruct likely patterns of mortality and household formation. Other types of sources yield information on other aspects. Some are of little practical value, such as death certificates on papyri, while others are more promising. Dates of death recorded in epitaphs on tombstones and mummy labels document seasonal variation in the death rate. Osteological remains hint at causes of death. Bureaucratic lists record the number of inhabitants of some cities and villages, sometimes even over time; others allow us to calculate the average size of households. Excavations and field surveys give us an idea of the size of individual settlements. And there is a wealth of comparative data waiting to be brought into the debate.

In the following chapters, I will turn to some of these other sources in the hope of contributing to a better understanding of the co-evolution of the disease environment and the demographic conditions in Egypt in the Roman period and beyond, in a sense up to the twentieth century. My results have also encouraged me to take a fresh look at the documents studied by Bagnall and Frier, and to propose an alternative model of mortality and life expectancy in Roman Egypt. This brings me to an important point. The scrutiny and re-evaluation of existing findings and interpretations is the daily trade of historians. Not so in ancient demography: studies appear, their results are accepted or ignored, and that is it. What little debate has been generated in recent years has centred on very traditional methods and concerns—the unending quest for the number of Athenian citizens is the most notorious example—, while more novel approaches to the study of mortality, fertility and family structure have failed to arouse much controversy. Only a very few critiques have so far been published in this area, sometimes with a decade's delay or more (Scheidel (2001)). Newly discovered census documents merely enabled Bagnall and Frier to discuss their previous work with themselves (Frier (1997)). This curious reluctance to engage in real debate seems hard to reconcile with the widespread willingness to acknowledge the valuable and useful contribution of demographic enquiries to our understanding of Roman history. In any event, this shows how much work there is still to be done in introducing population studies to the mainstream of classical scholarship.

The demography of Roman Egypt—both the subject and the book—provides a suitable starting point. In earlier studies, I have explored the physiological and psychological implications of sibling marriage in the Roman Fayum (Scheidel (1995, 1996a, b, 1997a)), an institution which is of interest and significance far beyond the study of ancient history. Here, the study of Roman Egyptian census returns has made a unique contribution to other fields, from social, cultural and physical anthropology to grand debates about nature, nurture and human nature. I have also attempted a more wide-ranging and detailed examination of the biases of the population data from Roman Egypt than provided by Bagnall and Frier (Scheidel (1996a, d, 1997b)), and assessed the demographic value of the Egyptian death declarations (Scheidel (1999b)). In a major forthcoming publication and discussion of population lists from early Ptolemaic Egypt, Willy Clarysse and Dorothy Thompson will furnish us with invaluable information on family and household structure several centuries prior to the period of the Roman census documents, facilitating comparative analysis and extending our horizons farther backwards in time. Robert Sallares has embarked on the first full-scale study of the spread of leprosy in and from Greco-Roman Egypt. His forthcoming book on the demographic impact of malaria on the population history of Roman Italy will highlight local and regional variation and invite comparisons with conditions in Egypt.

As a result, the study of ancient demography is set to move from the contemplation of decontextualised samples of data and simple umbrella models to an increasing awareness and appreciation of actual complexity and interconnectivity. On a previous occasion, I predicted that owing to the rarity of demographic features in antiquity that permit more than an impressionist appraisal, 'as far as quantitative analysis is concerned, the end of ancient demography is already in sight' (Scheidel (1996a) 165). Though the present volume might be taken to give the lie to my apparent pessimism, I stand by my conclusion: 'in sight' is not yet 'here'. But I also pointed out that demography is 'firmly embedded in a vast and tremendously intricate ecological framework'. The following chapters can be no more than a feeble attempt to act on this weighty premise. Robert Sallares, in his pioneering work on the ecology of the ancient Greek world, more than half of which is taken up by a discussion of demography (Sallares (1991)), as well as in his forthcoming monograph on the demography and epidemiology of malaria in Roman Italy, has made more forceful strides in this direction. Ideally, and notwithstanding insuperable constraints imposed by the character of the sources for ancient history, an interdisciplinary and ecological approach to ancient demography will help bridge the chasm between ancient history and population history in general, and likewise between historical demography and medical history. In this regard, Mary Dobson's recent work on the ecological context of English population history shows the way (Dobson (1997)). It is also the best way to combat the pervasive parochialism of much of ancient history: for this is not just a question of finding out more about antiquity, but also of making non-specialists want to take it into account, of benefiting from the expertise of specialists in other areas, of negotiating artificial disciplinary boundaries—in short, of introducing (or rather re-introducing) classical antiquity to mainstream historiography. Text-oriented students of classical antiquity have been quick to embrace messages and concerns from outside their own profession, from Foucault to Derrida. It is high time ancient historians displayed a comparable openness to the approaches of contemporary social science history.

* * *

This is a book about Roman Egypt, but it does not seek to address only those with a professional interest in that province. Rather, it is intended as a contribution to the study of the ecological dynamics and living conditions in complex pre-modern societies. As I hope to show, Roman Egypt is an appropriate object for case studies to this end.

My first chapter draws on one of the most substantial samples of quantifiable demographic evidence from the ancient world. Dates of death, recorded in Greek and Coptic epitaphs on tombstones and wooden mummy labels preserved in Egypt, range over the entire first millennium of the Christian Era. In terms of volume, this sample is second only to the mass of corresponding records provided by the early Christian funerary commemorations from the late antique city of Rome. These data can be used to reconstruct the seasonal distribution of deaths in the represented population, above all among adolescents and adults, who dominate the record, and to delineate regional and age-specific differentiation. Comparison with analogous evidence from the last two centuries highlights the specific properties of the ancient mortality patterns, which are characterised by conspicuously high levels of seasonal variation at mature ages, a phenomenon which elsewhere is usually limited to early childhood. This finding has significant implications for our understanding of the nature of the underlying disease environment. Juxtaposing written and physical medical evidence from Roman Egypt with comparative evidence from the Middle Ages to the present, the principal diseases of the region are related to the observed seasonality pattern. In the absence of proper statistics of causes of death, these proxy data offer the only opportunity to elucidate, however tentatively, the relative incidence of endemic disease. The results of this analysis are consistent with high levels of exposure to a variety of infectious disorders from diarrhoeal diseases to malaria and tuberculosis. It also becomes apparent that during the first millennium, seasonal mortality patterns—while reassuringly consistent across large parts of the region—did not only vary within Egypt but were also different from those recorded for the nineteenth and early twentieth centuries. This raises the possibility that far from being static, the structure of overall mortality, and its impact on the age distribution, may have undergone significant changes throughout the pre-modern period.

This theme is pursued further in the second chapter, in which I attempt a re-appraisal of the demographic evidence preserved in the census returns from Roman Egypt. These documents, tax registration records which list the members of individual households with their ages and other specifics, have long been regarded as the best textual evidence for ancient population history. In their recent work, Bagnall and Frier used them not only to study household structure and fertility but also to reconstruct the average age distribution of the Egyptian population and mean levels of life expectancy. Their results were supported by a close match between standard model life tables for high-mortality populations and the attested age distribution. Here I argue that this fit is probably spurious. The census age data reveal different patterns when disaggregated according to provenance: while the urban sample suggests higher adult mortality than predicted by standard models, the rural records are vitiated by reporting biases that render them largely unusable for demographic purposes. As a consequence, I suggest an alternative way of interpreting these texts that gives due weight to their cultural and environmental background. Thus, urban texts point to excess mortality in large cities, an interpretation that tallies well with comparative information on the demographic burden of urbanism and with the evidence of the seasonality data discussed in the previous chapter, whereas the rural texts betray the limits of administrative efficiency in the countryside. When viewed from that perspective, the census returns of Roman Egypt cannot be used to reconstruct average rates of life expectancy, the age distribution or sex ratios in Egypt as whole, let alone extrapolate from them to the entire Roman empire. Instead, these texts document diversity at the local level, emphasising the often intractable complexity of demographic conditions in the past.

The final chapter moves on to an issue that was not considered at any length by Bagnall and Frier, namely the likely size of the population of Roman Egypt under the early empire. Side-stepping the well-trodden paths of inductivist analysis of isolated claims in ancient sources, I probe this issue from a comparative perspective, drawing primarily on documentation from the nineteenth century. Not unlike ancient texts, the modern data pose serious difficulties of their own which call for detailed scrutiny. I argue that the epidemiologic and economic specifics of Egypt during the early nineteenth century complicate analogising comparisons with the conditions of the Roman period. Instead, it is suggested that the population of Egypt may have peaked at a higher level than suggested in recent studies, approaching an average population density that Egypt was to re-attain only after the middle of the nineteenth century. Once more, I hope that the gain will be in method as much as in substance, and that this comparativist endeavour, to my knowledge the first detailed study of its kind, will encourage future research along similar lines.

* * *

In 1997, Robert Sallares and I decided to collaborate on a book about the relationship between disease and demographic structures in the Roman world. Sallares at first concentrated on ancient and comparative evidence for the impact of malaria on the population of Latium and Tuscany, and subsequently considered the spread of leprosy in the Roman period, while I turned to the issues addressed in the present volume. Over the following three years, as the range of our comparative investigations kept expanding, the aggregate bulk of our case studies grew to an extent that eventually persuaded us to present the results of our researches in two (or more) separate monographs. For this reason, this volume will shortly be followed by a comparative and interdisciplinary study of the role of malaria in shaping the demography of Roman Italy. While each of our books offers clearly delimited and self-contained case-studies, they should be seen as complementary in terms of subject-matter, method and approach. We will measure the success of our combined efforts by our ability to persuade our readers to accept, or at least to consider in earnest, the integration of ancient sources, more recent comparative evidence and scientific data as a viable model for future work in this and related areas. In our view, a cross-disciplinary approach, though demanding and by nature risky and open to expert criticism, is the most promising—and ultimately the only—way forward.

* * *

In the course of preparing my chapters, I have greatly benefited from the inspiring if daunting breadth of multidisciplinary expertise of my original collaborator, Robert Sallares. Everyone familiar with the scope of his landmark study of the ecology of the ancient Greek world will appreciate what a privilege it has been to work with him. Peter Garnsey, Brent Shaw and Dorothy Thompson very kindly read earlier versions of all three chapters and provided helpful comments. I am also indebted to Richard Duncan-Jones, Richard Saller and Laurens Tacoma, who read drafts of the second chapter. Bruce Frier has always been available for discussion: I should like to thank him for saving me from some slips in the representation of views held by others and for his readiness to set me straight on a number of issues (though sometimes to little effect). His interest and critical encouragement have been much appreciated. Laurens Tacoma,

Günther Thüry and Yan Zelener very helpfully provided me with samples of their work, in most cases prior to publication. Once again, I am indebted to Willem Jongman for his suggestion to publish my work in this series. I would also like to thank my editor Michiel Swormink for his support. Most of this book was prepared during my tenure of the Moses and Mary Finley Research Fellowship in Ancient History at Darwin College, Cambridge. It is a particular pleasure for me to acknowledge the support and intellectual stimulation I have received from my friends and colleagues at Cambridge, and to dedicate this work to them as a modest token of my gratitude.

CHAPTER ONE

MORTALITY PATTERNS AND CAUSES OF DEATH

1. *Introduction*

Modern research in ancient demography has been hamstrung by the scarcity of evidence that is both quantifiable and relevant.[1] Some types of source material that invite quantification yield results that are either downright misleading, such as records of ages at death in tombstone inscriptions, or extremely difficult to interpret, such as skeletal remains.[2] Figures and other observations proffered by ancient literary texts pose a whole range of different problems, many of which ultimately stem from the inevitable ignorance of their authors.[3] Thus, our hopes rest on a handful of somewhat more promising samples of evidence. The census returns of Roman Egypt, which afford unique insight into crucial demographic features such as age distribution, reproductive behaviour and household structure, have recently been studied by Bagnall and Frier, and will be reconsidered in the second chapter.[4]

Epigraphic records of seasonal mortality provide quantitative information on an important issue that cannot be approached through

---

[1] For a critical survey of recent scholarship on the formal demography of the Roman world, see Scheidel (2001).

[2] The various biases inherent in ancient epitaphs are discussed by Hopkins (1966); Ery (1969); Clauss (1973); Frier (1983) 336–41; Hopkins (1987); van der Horst (1991) 73–84; Scheidel (1991/92); Parkin (1992) 5–19; Saller (1994) 15–18; and below, section 2.5. For changing patterns of distortion, see Shaw (1991). On paleodemography, see below, Chapter 2, n. 17 and pp. 135–40.

[3] The intrinsic limitations of these sources have lured generations of modern scholars into interminable and increasingly repetitive debates that cannot be resolved on the basis of ancient evidence alone. The most testing polemics have revolved around the questions of the size of the population of classical Athens (see Scheidel's survey of recent studies in Garnsey (1998) 197–8) and the number of Roman citizens in Italy (from Beloch (1886) and Frank (1924) to Brunt (1971) and Lo Cascio (1994a, b); cf. Morley (1996) 46–50; Scheidel (1996a) 167–8); and see below, Chapter 3.1. Suder (1988) and Corvisier and Suder (1996) provide a full bibliography of these and related issues. See Scheidel (2001) 49–72 for a critical overview.

[4] Bagnall and Frier (1994); Frier (1994), Bagnall (1997a); Bagnall, Frier and Rutherford (1997). See also Scheidel (1995), (1996a) 9–51, (1996b, d, 1997a, b).

the census texts. Unlike the Greeks and Romans of 'pagan' times, Christians, for whom the end of their earthly existence marked the beginning of eternal life, frequently adorned their epitaphs with references to the date of death.[5] Wherever such dates are present in sufficient numbers it becomes possible to reconstruct the profiles of seasonal mortality. The very few studies that have dealt with this material have mainly focused on the city of Rome. In the early 1960s, Nordberg gleaned over two thousand pertinent references from Christian funerary records dating from the third to the sixth centuries CE, most of which had been recovered from the vast catacombs surrounding the city. Despite this wealth of new data, it was only thirty years later that the underlying causes of the documented seasonal pattern began to attract scholarly attention.[6] In a study published in 1996, Shaw replaced Nordberg's sample with a larger collection of almost four thousand references from the same location which he considered in conjunction with corresponding evidence from other parts of the late Roman world.[7] In most cases, however, local or regional samples from outside Rome itself have proven too small in size or too wide in scope to generate reliable distribution patterns.[8] Even so, at least with regard to the city of Rome, this recent research represents significant progress: 'It is difficult, sometimes very difficult, for modern historical demographers to elucidate seasonality of mortality for populations of even three or four centuries ago. To have been able to track the seasonal mortality of the population of a large urban centre over one and a half thousand years ago (. . .) is still an achievement of sorts and a real contribution to the demographic history of the period'.[9]

[5] Shaw (1996) 101–05, discusses the novel character of this Christian custom.

[6] Nordberg (1963) 55–7 tabs. 12a–c (2,125 data). The first and only book-length introduction to Roman demography, Parkin (1992), completely ignores this material. Scheidel (1994) and (1996a) 139–53 addresses the relationship between seasonal mortality and disease based on the Nordberg sample.

[7] Shaw (1996), esp. 115–21 on Rome (3,938 data). Although this sample is almost twice as large as the previous version, both sets produce identical seasonal patterns. In this respect, a comparison between studies that are based on either the Nordberg or the Shaw sample would not be as 'instructive' as Bagnall (1997c) 877 n. 1 suspects: it merely illustrates the law of diminishing returns.

[8] Scheidel (1996a) 155–7, on Altava in North Africa (n = 172), and 157–61, on Carthage (n = 159); Shaw (1996) 123–31, on Roman North Italy (n = 533), South Italy (n = 244), Spain (n = 161), Gaul and Germany (n = 427), and North Africa (n = 620). For Egypt, see below.

[9] Shaw (1996) 134. His paper forms part of a series of studies of seasonal aspects of Roman demography: Shaw (1997, 2001).

Egypt has been the source of a greater number of published references to the month of death than any other region of the Roman world outside Rome itself. Whilst also largely drawn from a Christian background, some of this evidence extends even farther back in time. Unfortunately, the study of seasonal mortality in ancient Egypt got off to a slow start. Bernard Boyaval's attempt to construct a monthly mortality profile from unspecified dates on mummy labels is invalidated by the fact that these dates refer to the completion of the mummification process rather than the moment of death.[10] When in a subsequent study he conflated these misinterpreted data with epigraphic references, the resulting aggregate samples produced flawed patterns which Shaw later considered implausible.[11] In his own analysis, Shaw added to the existing confusion by introducing mortality data from death declarations of the Roman period that have survived on papyrus. The monthly incidence of deaths reported in these documents, which were used to report the deaths of taxpayers and other individuals to the local authorities, can be shown to be governed by factors that are extrinsic to the demographic regime, such as bureaucratic requirements, and therefore fail to reflect actual mortality patterns.[12] At the same time, more than half of the pertinent evidence is missing from these earlier studies. Many of the data in the Greek epitaphs from Terenouthis in Lower Egypt have yet to be considered, while the copious Coptic evidence of seasonal mortality in the early Middle Ages has so far gone virtually unnoticed.[13]

In the following, I will aim to combine a comprehensive survey and comparative evaluation of the available documentation with a discussion of the underlying causes of death. In their study of seasonal mortality in early modern London, Landers and Mouzas emphasise that 'proximate explanations of levels and trends in mortality must be couched in terms of disease patterns'.[14] However, Landers

[10] Boyaval (1975) 62 (but cf. 62 n. 29), 68 n. 36; followed by Scheidel (1996a) 153–5, whose discussion is fully superseded by the present study. On the meaning of dates on mummy labels, see below, section 2.2, and Scheidel (1998).

[11] Boyaval (1981); Shaw (1996) 121–3.

[12] Shaw (1996) 122–3. For a re-appraisal of the dates on death declarations (gathered and discussed by Casarico (1985)), see Scheidel (1999b).

[13] Bagnall (1997c) 877 rightly draws attention to the publication of numerous inscriptions from Terenouthis subsequent to Boyaval's studies. Wietheger (1992) 154–5, 514 fig. 4, calculates the monthly incidence of deaths according to the funerary inscriptions at the Coptic monastery of St Jeremiah near Saqqara but refrains from further discussion.

[14] Landers and Mouzas (1988) 59. Cf. Alter and Carmichael (1996) 47: 'Since

opens his more extended discussion of the same issue with the observation that 'the importance of cause of death patterns for the understanding of mortality in the past has been widely acknowledged, but has not generated a corresponding body of demographic literature on the subject.'[15] What is true for the study of early modern populations is even more true for ancient history.[16] This book hopes to contribute to a better understanding of the causes of death in ancient societies, or at the very least to define a problem of historical interpretation that is commonly ignored by scholars in the field.

2. *Evidence of seasonal mortality*

2.1. *Upper Egypt and Nubia: funerary inscriptions*

Egypt can be divided into two regions, the Nile valley, or Upper Egypt, and the Delta, or Lower Egypt.[17] Most of the pertinent evidence comes from Upper Egypt and Nubia, a territory that is relatively homogeneous in terms of climate and ecology. The Fayum, a large quasi-oasis centred on a lake (Birket Qarun) to the west of modern Cairo, is not part of the Nile valley proper. This region, however, yields only a small number of epigraphic testimonies which have been included in the sample for Upper Egypt.[18]

---

many diseases follow distinct seasonal patterns, seasonality can often be used to identify the causes of epidemics and the major components of mortality.'

[15] Landers (1993) 201. See now Alter and Carmichael (1996), and the contributions to Alter and Carmichael, eds. (1997), esp. Risse (1997).

[16] In his study of Roman seasonal mortality, Shaw (1996), esp. 133, notes the problem but takes a sceptical stance. For earlier attempts to shed light on causes of death in antiquity, see Scheidel (1994), (1996a) 141–53, 163, and more generally Grmek (1989); Sallares (1991).

[17] In keeping with the epigraphic evidence of seasonal mortality that points to a split between two distinct parts of the region, the terms 'Lower Egypt' and 'Delta (region)' are here applied to Egypt north of Memphis, while the terms 'Upper Egypt', or 'Upper Egypt and Nubia', and 'Nile valley' are used to describe the region between Meroe (south of the fifth Nile cataract) and Memphis. (In this chapter, to avoid confusion, I will not normally refer to the division of Egypt south of the Delta into Upper and Middle Egypt.) Unless specified otherwise, the terms 'Upper Egypt(ian)' and 'Nile valley' will be used as shorthand for Egypt south of the Delta and Nubia (Sudan). Moreover, for the sake of simplicity, the whole period covered by the texts studied in sections 2.1–3 will be defined as 'ancient', even though it extends into the Middle Ages.

[18] Although they differ from the evidence from the Nile valley, thanks to their small number they do not affect the overall seasonal mortality distribution (see

The first set of data to be investigated here consists of tombstone inscriptions written in ancient Greek and set up in Upper Egypt and Nubia. While some of them come from the pre-Christian period, the majority are Christian texts dating from the fourth to the seventh centuries CE. For the purposes of this study, I have been able to gather 353 data from this region (Table 1.1). This sample is complemented by epitaphs written in Coptic, most of which were produced in the eighth, ninth and tenth centuries. Only a small number of texts, especially from Nubia, extend this sample into the following two centuries. 585 data could be culled from the Coptic material (Table 1.1). The months of the Egyptian calendar largely coincide with the modern western months.[19]

Table 1.1 Monthly distribution of deaths in Upper Egypt and Nubia according to Greek and Coptic funerary inscriptions[20]

	Greek	Coptic	Total
Tybi	38	37	75
Mecheir	22	47	69
Phamenoth	44	46	90
Pharmouthi	44	75	119
Pachon	33	67	100
Pauni	31	69	100
Epeiph	26	55	81
Mesore	20	49	69
Added days	4	–	4
Thoth	12	42	54
Phaophi	18	24	42
Hathyr	26	32	58
Choiak	35	42	77
Total	353	585	938

below, n. 39, and Fig. 1.12). These differences between the Nile valley and the Fayum, which hint at significant variation in ecological conditions and the disease environment, will be discussed in sections 2.3 and 3.5.

[19] Tybi runs from 27/28 December to 25/26 January, etc. Thoth (~September) is the first month of the Egyptian year; the added days cover only a few days from to 24 to 28/29 August. In the text below, I use modern months as approximations for the corresponding Egyptian months.

[20] The individual source references for this and the subsequent samples are collected in Appendix 1. The present sample does not include data from Coptic epitaphs of unknown regional provenance, for which see Kamel (1987); Brunsch (1991, 1992, 1993). See Krause (1991) 1293–6 for a concise survey of Coptic funerary epigraphy.

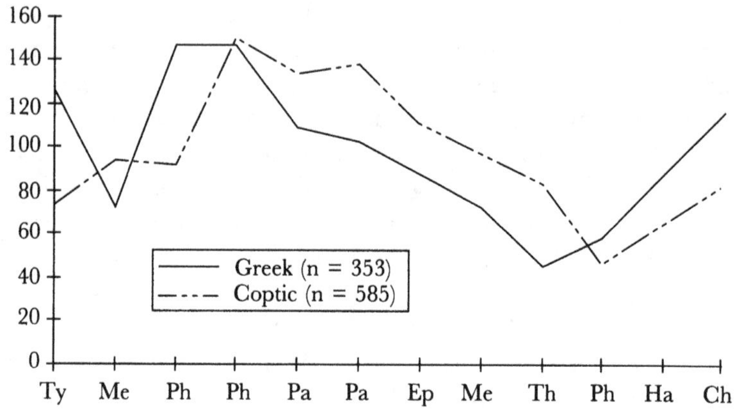

Figure 1.1 Seasonal mortality in Upper Egypt and Nubia according to Greek and Coptic funerary inscriptions (raw data)

Figure 1.1 shows the monthly distribution of the raw data. Converted into three-month moving averages, the smoothed data highlight the principal patterns of seasonal variation (Fig. 1.2). The two curves are very similar in shape but appear to be slightly dissociated by the fact that according to the Coptic data, mortality rises and falls one month earlier than in the Greek texts.

However, this picture conceals a considerable amount of local variation (Table 1.2 and Fig. 1.3). Whereas the findspots of the Greek epitaphs are scattered across the Nile valley, the Coptic texts show a very uneven geographical distribution. 460 of the latter, or more than three-quarters of the total, were preserved at three locations, namely, the Coptic monasteries of Saqqara (Dayr Apa Jeremiah) south of Memphis, Aswan, and Sakinya in Nubia. Since the first of these places sits right at the border to Lower Egypt and the other two are in the far south of the region, most of the Egyptian Nile valley in between is rather poorly represented in the Coptic record.

The seasonal mortality distributions generated by the data from Saqqara in the north (127 references mostly from the eighth and ninth centuries) and from Sakinya in the south (210 references mostly from the tenth century) resemble the shape of the 'Greek pattern' but differ in terms of timing: in Saqqara, the death rate apparently peaked about two months earlier than in Nubia, in April and May as opposed to May, June and July. The pattern for Aswan is altogether more erratic. These texts (123 references mostly from the

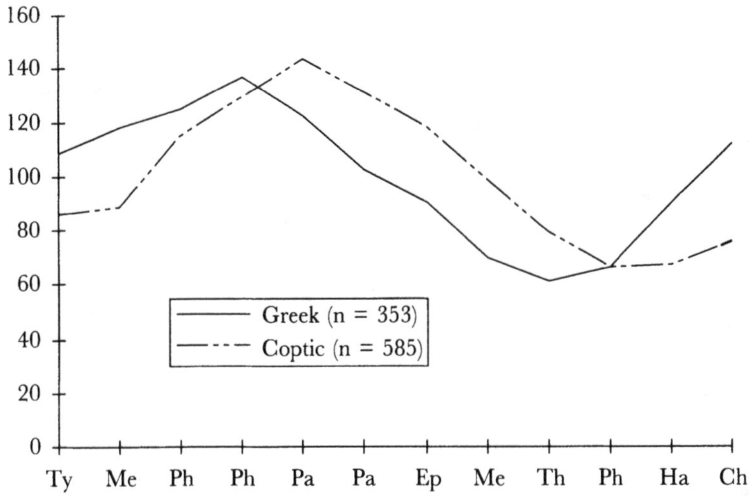

Figure 1.2 Seasonal mortality in Upper Egypt and Nubia according to Greek and Coptic funerary inscriptions (smoothed data)

eighth and to a smaller extent from the ninth centuries) do not reveal any concentration of deaths in the spring or early summer but instead a moderate increase in August.

Table 1.2 Monthly distribution of deaths in three Coptic monasteries

	Saqqara	Aswan	Sakinya
Tybi	6	6	15
Mecheir	14	15	14
Phamenoth	12 or 13	11	11
Pharmouthi	19 or 20	10	21
Pachon	20	8	24
Pauni	13	9	37
Epeiph	10	12	24
Mesore	9	12	21
Added days	–	–	–
Thoth	4	17	15
Phaophi	7	4	8
Hathyr	6	11	8
Choiak	6	8	12
Total	127	123	210

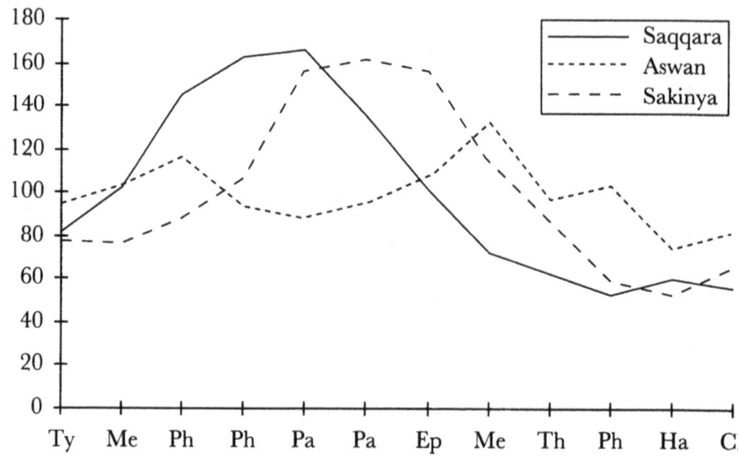

Figure 1.3 Seasonal mortality in three Coptic monasteries (smoothed data)

Most or all of the tombstones from Aswan belong to the monastery of St Simeon. Only part of these 123 texts contain precise dates or may reliably be assigned to a single century. Even so, it seems possible to hazard some differential analysis of this body of evidence. Those fifty-five epitaphs that have been dated to the eighth century (with a concentration in its second quarter) produce a seasonal mortality pattern that is much closer to the general distribution for Upper Egypt than that derived from the complete Aswan sample.[21] This group of texts suggests that mortality peaked in the late winter, somewhat earlier than in other locations in the Nile Valley (cf. Fig. 1.3), and decreased during the second half of the year in much the same way as elsewhere (Fig. 1.4). Thus, the shape of the curve is consistent with other samples from Upper Egypt and Nubia. By contrast, inscriptions that have been taken to predate that particular subsample, and therefore probably originate from the seventh and the beginning of the eighth centuries, invert this pattern through an atypical peak in the late summer and early fall.[22] It is only the combi-

[21] *KSB* I 551–61, 563–4, 567–73, 575–82, 584–5, 587–92, 594, 596–7, 599–603, based on Munier (1930–31). The precisely dated texts range from 716 to 799 CE. Two of these texts come from the first quarter of the century, fifteen from the second, seven from the third, and nine from the fourth.

[22] *KSB* I 498–550, if dated, are dated by indiction only, which leads Munier (1930–31) 263 to believe that they were set up earlier than the remaining texts. Cf. also Krause (1991) 1293. References to the month of death are found in *KSB* I 499–507, 510–20, 522–39, 541–2, 544–50.

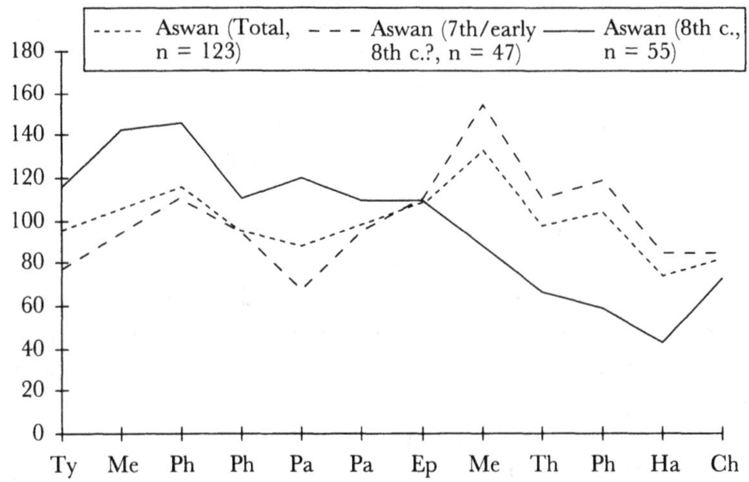

Figure 1.4 Seasonal mortality in the Monastery of St Simeon, Aswan (smoothed data)

nation of these two very different samples that creates the seemingly aseasonal distribution for Aswan in general.[23]

It is true that the small numbers involved forestall firm conclusions. Nevertheless, the peculiarities of the 'early' Aswan data are put into perspective by considering the proportion of all cases of death during the first half of the year documented in different samples. 62.3 per cent of the Aswan epitaphs from the eighth century refer to these six months, compared to 58.1 per cent of the Coptic texts from Sakinya, 58.3 per cent of all Coptic texts, 60.1 per cent of all Greek inscriptions, and 66.9 per cent of the Coptic texts from Saqqara.[24] Thus, the 'late' Aswan data clearly follow the general trend of mortality in Upper Egypt and Nubia to be concentrated in the first half of the year, whereas the 'early' Aswan data, only 40.4 per cent of which refer to these months, fail to do so.[25] It is possible that this discrepancy stems from the chronological provenance

[23] The number of texts that can be dated to the ninth century are too few in number to permit a meaningful analysis: see *KSB* I 604–14, 616–18, 620, 622. *KSB* I 498–550 and 623–75 are not dated.

[24] The same is true for 67.4 per cent of adjusted mummy labels: see below, section 2.2.

[25] If we quite cautiously assume that in the Nile valley, sixty per cent of all deaths occurred during the first half of the year, the 'early' Aswan data deviate very significantly from this norm ($p < 0.0062$).

of the latter. Mortality data for the seventh century are rare. Greek epigraphy flourished in the preceding centuries. The dated Coptic inscriptions from Saqqara range from 695 to 831/49 CE and most of the texts come from the eighth and ninth centuries; many of the dated inscriptions from Sakinya were set up in the tenth.[26] During the seventh century and especially in the decades close to the year 700, Egypt was repeatedly ravaged by bubonic plague and probably also by smallpox: it is therefore at least conceivable that the 'early' Aswan inscriptions reflect an atypical disease environment. Pandemics aside, occasional mortality crises in individual communities may well have been sufficiently frequent to explain temporary local anomalies such as those observed in Aswan.

Local deviations account for the apparent 'shift' between the Greek and the Coptic data. If we exclude the evidence from Sakinya in Nubia with its peak in the late spring and early summer from the Coptic sample, the remaining 375 references produce a monthly distribution that very closes follows that of the 353 Greek data (Fig. 1.5).

In a second step, the focus may be narrowed to Egypt proper by excluding any Greek and Coptic texts from south of the Thebaid. This leaves 314 Greek and 228 Coptic references. The two distributions are now very well synchronised, although the Coptic material indicates a stronger seasonal maximum in the spring than the Greek data (Fig. 1.6).

2.2. *Upper Egypt: mummy labels*

Further evidence is provided by mummy labels.[27] These tags, attached to mummified corpses to confirm their identity, usually give the name of the deceased and often the names of close relatives but on occasion also supply further details, such as age at death, occupation and geographical location. In about five per cent of all cases, the labels record a date, giving either day and month or, more rarely, merely the month with or without reference to a specific year. 132 such

[26] Saqqara: Wietheger (1992) 154; Sakinya: Monneret de Villard (1933) V.

[27] This section draws on Scheidel (1998). For a general discussion of mummy labels, see Quaegebeur (1978); cf. also Boyaval (1991). They mostly date from the mid-second to the mid-third centuries CE; see Boyaval (1981) 116: three dated tags come from the first century, four from the first half of the second century, seventeen from the period from 150 to 212 CE, and fifty-four from after 212. The last precisely dated text belongs to the year 272 CE (111).

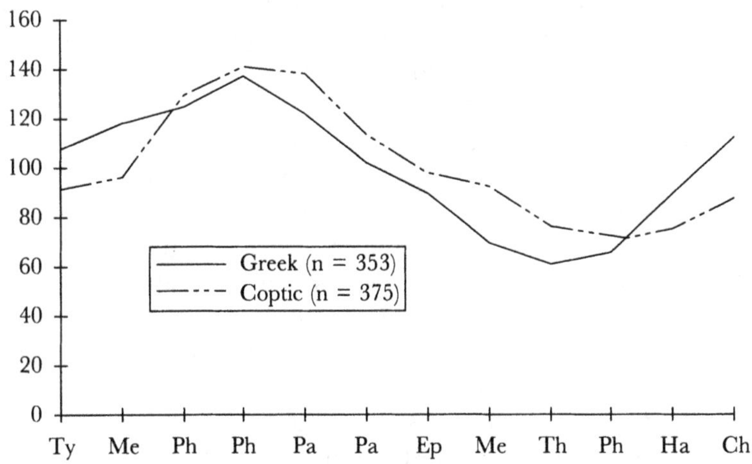

Figure 1.5 Seasonal mortality in Upper Egypt and Nubia according to Greek and Coptic funerary inscriptions, excluding the Coptic texts of Sakinya (smoothed data)

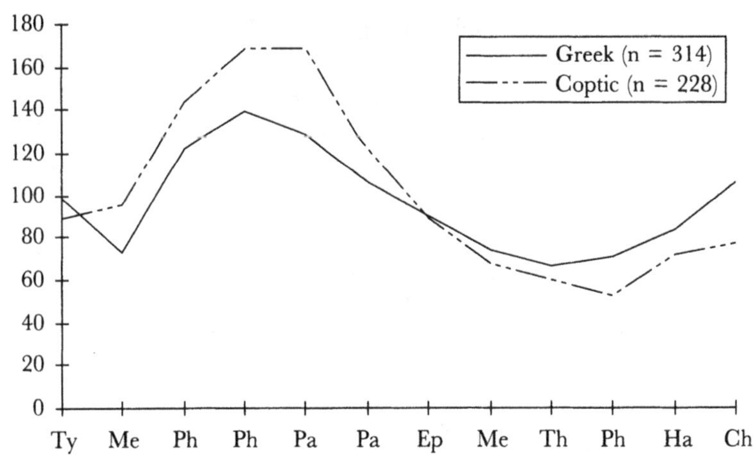

Figure 1.6 Seasonal mortality in Upper Egypt north of Aswan according to Greek and Coptic funerary inscriptions (smoothed data)

data have been collected here (Table 1.3, col. 1).[28] The meaning of these dates is not normally specified and must therefore have been considered self-evident by the authors of these texts. In the light of comparative evidence from tombstone inscriptions, such dates have usually been taken to refer to the day and/or month of death of the embalmed individual.[29] As a result, these dates have been subsumed under the epigraphic evidence from Upper Egypt.[30] However, this traditional interpretation is highly unlikely to be correct. Rather, unspecified chronological references on mummy tags generally record an event that occurred some time after death, namely, the formal completion of mummification some seventy days later.[31]

As Figures 1.7 and 1.8 show, the seasonal distribution of dates on the mummy labels (n = 132) is greatly at variance with the monthly distribution of deaths documented by the tombstone inscriptions from Upper Egypt. There is no linear association between these two samples in terms of the seasonal distribution of dates: Pearson's r is 0.034 for the raw data and 0.069 for the smoothed data. However, if each date recorded on a mummy label is moved back in time by seventy days,[32] both curves rise and fall in tandem: r = 0.771 for the raw data and 0.953 for the smoothed data (Fig. 1.9). This is true irrespective of whether we use only the 113 precise dates (consisting of day and month) or all 132 dates including those which give only the month.[33] Given that the sample of mummy label data is rather small in size and therefore more likely to be affected by some amount of random fluctuation than the epigraphic evidence, the observed degree of association is indeed extremely high. Both samples appear to mirror a

[28] For references, see Appendix 1. All published mummy labels come from the Nile valley from the Thebaid to the northern confines of Upper Egypt. Only twenty-one texts in this sample can be assigned to a particular location. The provenance of the majority of the texts may be established indirectly through an interpretation of the dates: see below, Fig. 1.10.

[29] E.g., Boyaval (1975) 62 (but cf. 62 n. 29), 68 n. 36, (1980) 282; Quaegebeur (1978) 236, 238; Montserrat (1997) 38. Cf. also Schmidt (1894) 62; Thieme and Pestman (1978a) 132 n. 8. This standard view was accepted by Scheidel (1996a) 153–5 and Shaw (1996) 121–3.

[30] Boyaval (1980) 282–3, whence Shaw (1996) 122 fig. 14.

[31] This interpretation was first advanced by Scheidel (1998).

[32] So that, for instance, 11 Mecheir becomes 1 Choiak.

[33] In these nineteen cases, on the simplifying but hardly wildly inaccurate assumption that on average, any given reference to a month is equally likely to pertain to any given day of that month, a reference to, e.g., Tybi is converted into one-third of a reference to Phaophi and two-thirds of a reference to Hathyr. The text gives the correlation coefficients for the complete sample. For the 542 inscriptions and the 113 adjusted precise mummy labels, r = 0.955.

Table 1.3 Monthly distribution of deaths according to mummy labels

	Recorded dates	Adjusted dates (rounded)	Adjusted dates (days and months only)
Tybi	5	6	6
Mecheir	11	11	10
Phamenoth	5	13.3	10
Pharmouthi	12	19	15
Pachon	15	22.3	18
Pauni	17	17.3	14
Epeiph	14	6.3	6
Mesore	23	6.7	6
Added days	1	–	–
Thoth	10	6.3	6
Phaophi	7	5.7	5
Hathyr	4	7.3	7
Choiak	8	10.7	10
Total	132	132	113

single seasonal distribution pattern that characterised the underlying base population. All or virtually all of the individuals recorded in dated mummy labels must have died approximately seventy days (or at any rate two to three months) prior to the unspecified occasion these dates refer to.

This occasion may be identified as the moment when a mummy was released, or ready to be released, for burial. A substantial body of sources ranging from the early New Kingdom to the Roman period shows that the interval between death and the completion of embalmment traditionally lasted seventy days.[34] The notion that some mummy labels record the latter tallies well with modern views of their origin.

[34] See Shore (1992) 228 (Eighteenth Dynasty); Habachi (1947) 278–9 (Twenty-first Dynasty); id., 279 and Griffith (1909) 85 no. 9.10.9–10 (Twenty-sixth Dynasty); Griffith (1900) 30 n. and Smith (1987) 27, on the 'Story of Khaemwese'; Erichsen (1956) 61, col. 3, ll. 4–7 (and cf. 50 n. 3) (demotic tale). On the Ptolemaic period, see Griffith (1900) 29 n.; Spiegelberg (1923) 421; Habachi (1947) 279; Vercoutter (1962) 39, Text E 5–6, 50, Text G 6–8 (and see 41 n. O–P, 42–3); de Cenival (1972) 187–9; Quaegebeur (1972) 86, 92; Reymond (1981) 143 no. 18 § 13; Shore (1992) 229. Roman period: *P.Carlsberg* 1.5.38–9, with Neugebauer and Parker (1960) 37, 73, 78. For non-Egyptian accounts, see *Genesis* 50.3, with Vergote (1959) 199; Herodotus 2.86, with Lloyd (1976) 361; cf. also Diodorus 1.19.6, with Shore and Smith (1960) 291; Shore (1992) 229. This evidence is presented in greater detail in Scheidel (1998).

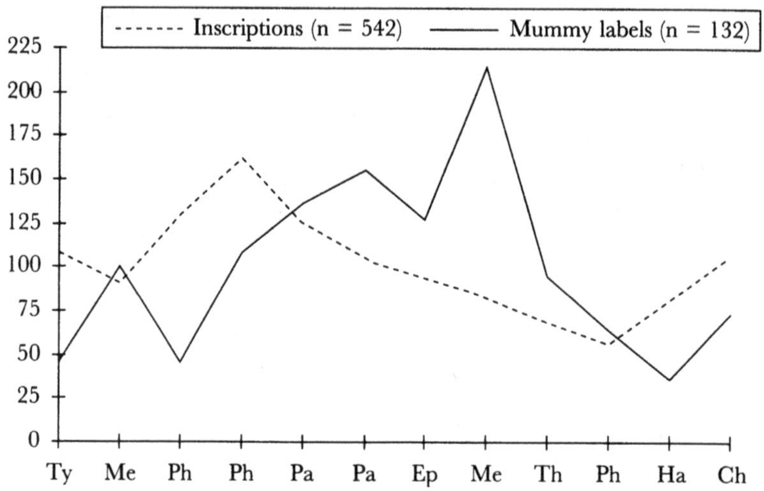

Figure 1.7 Seasonal mortality in Upper Egypt according to Greek and Coptic funerary inscriptions and monthly incidence of dates on mummy labels (raw data)

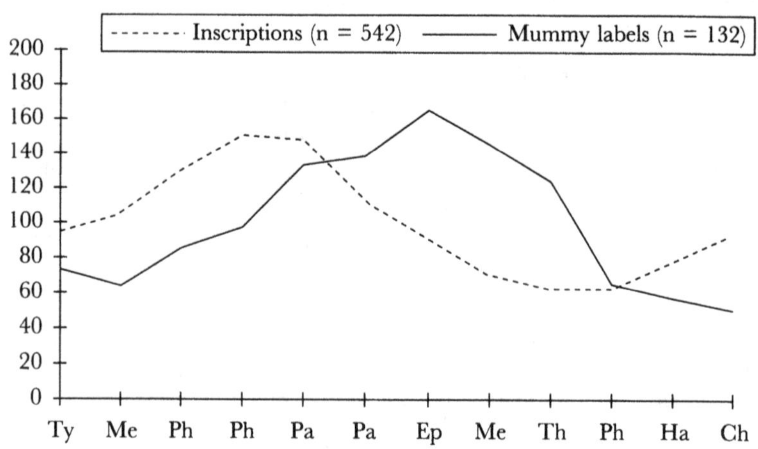

Figure 1.8 Seasonal mortality in Upper Egypt according to Greek and Coptic funerary inscriptions and monthly incidence of dates on mummy labels (smoothed data)

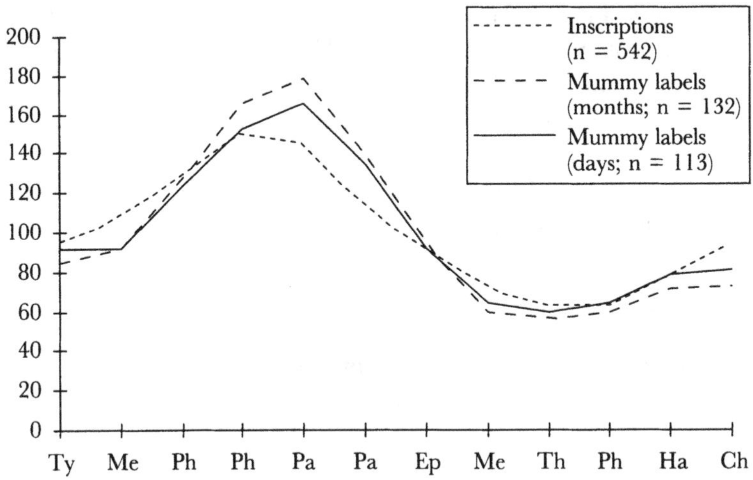

Figure 1.9 Seasonal mortality in Upper Egypt according to Greek and Coptic funerary inscriptions and adjusted monthly incidence of dates on mummy labels (smoothed data)

It has been argued that these documents were prepared in the context of mummification rather than of burial, probably by the embalmer-priests or their staff. In this context, the meaning of unspecified dates would have been self-evident.[35] The paucity of such references suggests that they were not considered particularly important and presumably added at the discretion of the embalmer in charge.

The attested rigidity of the seventy-day interval, presumably modelled on the seventy-day period of the invisibility of the star Sirius associated with the myth of Osiris, justifies the adjustment that harmonises the seasonal patterns of inscriptions and mummy labels from Upper Egypt.[36] This fit also supports the idea that by and large, the

[35] Quaegebeur (1978) 246. Compare a small group of demotic mummy tags authorising the interment of a completed mummy (Nur el-Din and Pestman (1978) 171–89). Four of these texts record dates which mark the day of their composition, which coincided with the completion of mummification.

[36] Neugebauer and Parker (1960) 73. The possible alternative interpretation that the dates on mummy labels refer to the day of burial is invalidated by the fact that once embalmment had been completed, interment could safely be delayed for a considerable amount of time. This practice is frequently attested: see, e.g., Quaegebeur (1972) 101, and (1978) 238 n. 54; Montserrat (1997) 38. Compare evidence of the shipping of mummies to other locations that would also result in delays: Quaegebeur (1978) 237–8; Drexhage (1994); Boyaval (1995). Only in exceptional cases did mummy labels refer to the date of death: on such occasions, the original

seasonal mortality regime was quite homogeneous across different parts of the Nile valley from Nubia and the Thebaid up to Memphis.[37] The assumption that all or most mummy labels come from Upper Egypt proper receives support by the fit of the seasonal mortality pattern generated by the texts of known geographical provenance (all of which come from Upper Egypt)[38] with the pattern derived from all other documents (Fig. 1.10).

2.3. *The Fayum: a special case?*

Before we move on to Lower Egypt, the epigraphic evidence from the Fayum deserves closer scrutiny.[39] At first sight, the difference

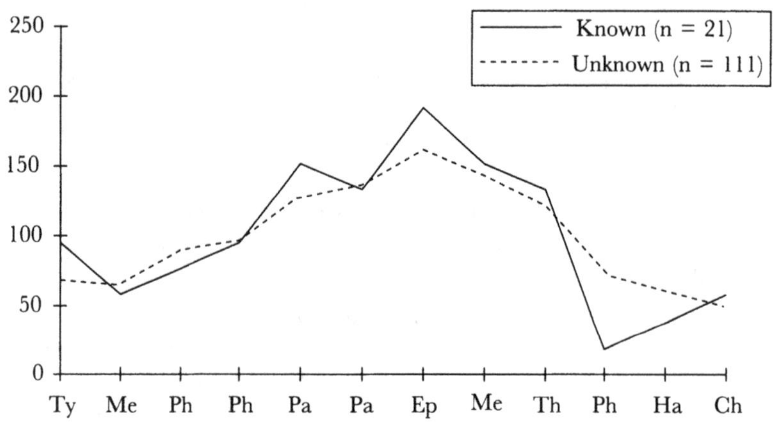

Figure 1.10 Monthly incidence of dates on mummy labels of known and unknown provenance (smoothed data)

tag had been replaced by a new one at the burial, usually after some substantial delay: see Scheidel (1998) on the texts in Thieme and Pestman (1978b) 229; Quirke (1988) 229 no. 184a. Such replacement tags could also record the date of the burial: *SB* I 776, 1195, 3580.

[37] This adjustment removes the summer-time irregularities in the rise and fall of the mortality curve caused by the conflation of unadjusted mummy label data with epigraphic data that are discernible in the graphs of Boyaval (1980) 285 and Shaw (1996) 122 fig. 14.

[38] *SB* I 1196–7, 1201–2, 3553, 4185, 4238, 5372, 5467, 5470, 5487, 5623, 5699, III 7079, 7124, V 7731, X 10477, XIV 11990, Wilfong (1995) nos. 1, 21, 25.

[39] Greek inscriptions: Tybi: Lefebvre (1907) no. 80, *SB* 5758; Mecheir: Lefebvre (1907) nos. 97, 100, 103–104, 795; Phamenoth: Lefebvre (1907) nos. 88, 101, *SB* 4013 = *I.Fay.* I 51, *SB* 7883, 10515, 10705; Pharmouthi: Lefebvre (1907) nos. 76, 81, 85, 95, 107, 112, 786, SB 726 = *I.Fay.* I 36, *SB* 10517; Pachon: *SB* 10516;

between the monthly mortality distributions of the Nile valley and the Fayum is quite striking (Figs. 1.11–12). Unlike the 'early' Aswan material, the Fayum pattern is consistent with but overemphasises the central characteristics of the general distribution for the Nile valley. This discrepancy cannot be explained away with reference to the small size of the Fayum sample. In the latter, deaths are strongly concentrated in a three-month period from February to April: twenty of the thirty-seven Greek epitaphs, or 54.1 per cent, refer to these months, compared to 110 of all 353 Greek data, or 31.2 per cent, from Upper Egypt and Nubia. The additional six Coptic texts from the Fayum do not change this picture: twenty-three of forty-three, or 53.5 per cent, of all persons commemorated in the Fayum died between February and April, against 278 out of 938 cases in Greek and Coptic epitaphs, or 29.6 per cent. By any measure, the difference between the Fayum and the entire sample is statistically highly significant: $p < 0.0016$ if n(Fayum) = 37 and n_{pop}(Upper Egypt/Nubia: Greek) = 353, and $p < 0.0004$ if n(Fayum) = 43 and n_{pop}(Upper Egypt/Nubia: Greek/Coptic) = 938 (z-test modified for finite population and denominator adjustment). A comparison of the smoothed data (three-month moving averages) reveals milder but still marked divergence: 44.1 per cent ($n = 37$) or 43.4 per cent ($n = 43$) of the Fayum data come from these months, against 31.6 per cent of the Greek and 29.2 per cent of the Greek and Coptic data from Upper Egypt and Nubia ($p < 0.0854$ and 0.0366). As a consequence, we are compelled to accept that most of the variance between the data from the Nile valley and the Fayum is not coincidental.

Various sources of reporting bias that might account for this difference are conceivable but none of them provides a persuasive explanation. Thus, potential inequalities in the age distribution or the social status of the deceased are impossible to determine but *a priori* unlikely to be particularly pronounced. There is no obvious reason why the testimonies from the Fayum should pertain to a significantly different cross-section of the general population than the corresponding texts from the adjacent Nile Valley. From a purely

---

Pauni: Lefebvre (1907) nos. 77, 111; Epeiph: Lefebvre (1907) nos. 105, 727 = *I.Fay.* I 41, *I.Fay.* III 198, 216; Mesore: *I.Fay.* I 59; Thoth: Lefebvre (1907) nos. 86, 102; Phaophi: Lefebvre (1907) 96, 787; Hathyr: Lefebvre (1907) nos. 792; Choiak: Lefebvre (1907) 94; *SB* 3949 = *I.Fay.* I 43. There are also six Coptic texts: *KSB* I 747 (?), Crum (1902) nos. 8423, 8441, 8584, 8698. None of the mummy labels discussed in the previous section is known to have come from the Fayum.

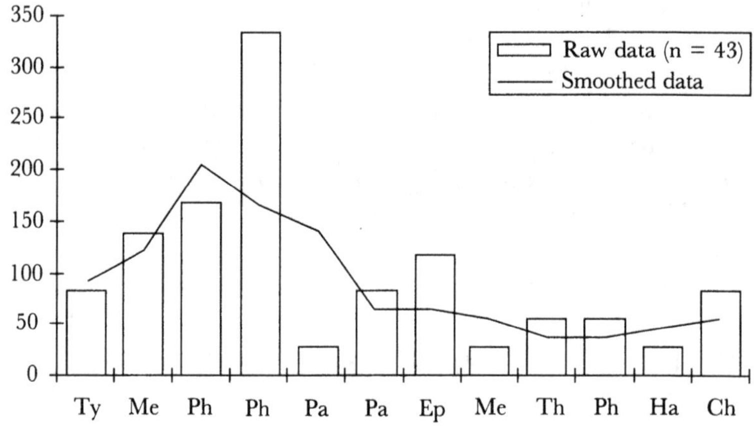

Figure 1.11 Seasonal mortality in the Fayum according to Greek and Coptic funerary inscriptions

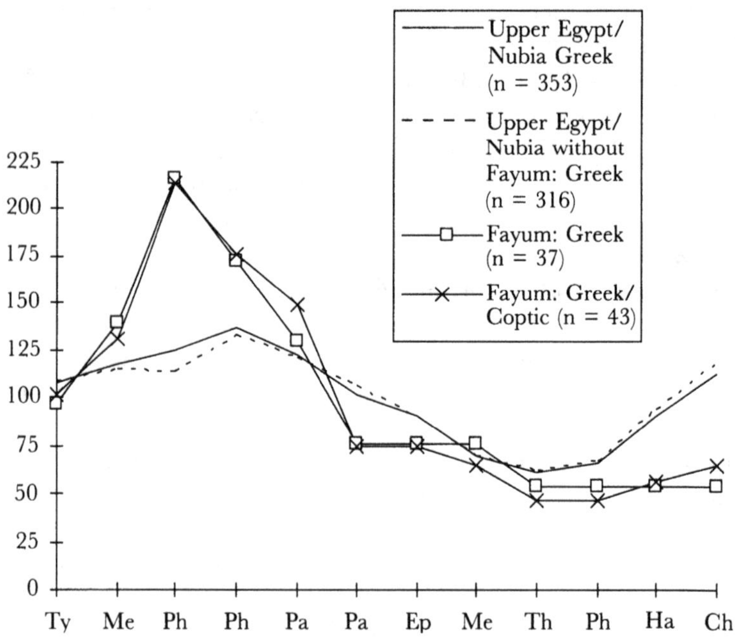

Figure 1.12 Seasonal mortality in the Nile Valley and in the Fayum according to Greek and Coptic funerary inscriptions (smoothed data)

statistical perspective, the odds strongly favour the conclusion that the observed discrepancy is a reflection of genuine differences rather than merely a function of insufficient or biassed evidence.[40]

2.4. *Lower Egypt: funerary inscriptions*

Several communities in Lower Egypt provide substantial sets of evidence of seasonal mortality. However, these data differ in important respects from the evidence from Upper Egypt and Nubia. First, hardly any published Coptic tombstone inscriptions can reliably be attributed to the Delta region. This lack of early medieval evidence seriously limits the scope of analysis. Second, Greek inscriptions do exist in sizeable numbers but are very unevenly distributed over the region. In fact, most of these 306 texts were found in only three settlements. Epitaphs from Terenouthis dominate the sample with 190 references, or 62.1 per cent of the total. Fifty-seven texts (or 18.6 per cent) come from the capital of Alexandria, and forty-three to forty-five (around fourteen per cent) from Leontopolis. A mere handful were uncovered in other findspots. By contrast, the texts from the Nile valley, albeit not randomly distributed, are more widely scattered across the region and thus more representative of the region as a whole.

To make matters worse, the two most prominent sources of data from Lower Egypt—Terenouthis and Alexandria—are hardly typical of the Nile Delta itself. Alexandria stands out for two reasons. It was the second largest city of the Roman empire and may well have generated a distinct metropolitan mortality regime. Perhaps even more important, it is situated on the northern coast at the northwestern corner of Lower Egypt right at the edge of the Delta, and was thus subject to different climatic conditions than the Delta proper. Terenouthis (El Tarrana), on the other hand, lies west of the westernmost tributary of the Nile, some forty-five miles northwest of modern Cairo, on the fringe of the cultivable land where it meets the Libyan desert. It is not strictly speaking part of the Nile Delta and likewise belongs to a somewhat different ecological zone.

[40] It is, however, true that most epitaphs from the Fayum come from Hawara, a village at the eastern fringe of the Fayum next to the Bahr Yussuf about halfway between the Lahun gap and Arsinoe. We cannot tell to what extent local conditions were typical of the Fayum in general.

Most of the remaining data come from Leontopolis (Tell el Yahoudijeh), a city in the South-East of Lower Egypt, east of the easternmost tributary of the Nile not far from Memphis. Thus, the interior of the Delta, home to at least half or perhaps up to two-thirds of the population of Roman Egypt,[41] remains hidden from our view.

Against this rather unpromising background, it seems best to approach the three main samples (Alexandria, Terenouthis, and Others, i.e., Leontopolis combined with sundry references) as discrete units in an attempt to elucidate and compare *local* conditions (Table 1.4).

As expected, the Alexandrian data diverge from the remainder. The jagged pattern of the raw data is largely a function of small sample size: converted into three-month moving averages, no consistent pattern emerges (Fig. 1.13). Although mortality appears mildly elevated during the first half of the year, this concentration might just as well be fortuitous ($p < 0.5092$). The largely aseasonal character of the mortality distribution distinguishes this sample from other local or regional data sets and thus requires explanation. It is possible that

Table 1.4 Monthly distribution of deaths in Lower Egypt according to Greek funerary inscriptions[42]

	Terenouthis	Alexandria	Others	Total
Tybi	25	4	6	35
Mecheir	18	7	7	32
Phamenoth	12	3	4	19
Pharmouthi	12	5	2	19
Pachon	7	7	1	15
Pauni	20	5	10	35
Epeiph	14	4	5	23
Mesore	9	3	3	15
Thoth	7	4	4	15
Phaophi	21	6	3	30
Hathyr	27	3	8	41
Choiak	18	6	6	30
Total	190	57	59	306

[41] Bagnall (1993) 19–20 speculates that in late antiquity, close to two-thirds of arable land in Egypt was located in the Delta region, perhaps up from a somewhat smaller share in previous periods. This implies a similar distribution of the population. The situation is similar today: Yates and Strzepek (1998) 263, 264 tab. 1.

[42] Sources: see Appendix 1.

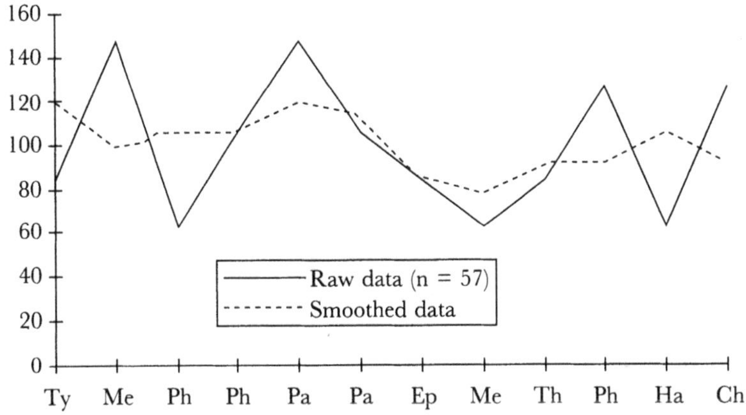

Figure 1.13 Seasonal mortality in Alexandria according to Greek funerary inscriptions

the sample is too small to reveal existing seasonal variation or that it is not representative of the urban population as such. For instance, we may be looking at wealthy suburbanites who had the means to evade seasonal mortality crises. Even so, when we compare the Alexandrian pattern with that attested for the next largest city in ancient North Africa, late Roman Carthage, a comparable lack of seasonal variation can be observed (Fig. 1.14).[43] The Carthaginian data are almost three times as numerous as the references from Alexandria and do not show any sign of extreme socio-economic bias. In the mid-eighteenth century, Naples, another large Mediterranean coastal city, experienced similarly low levels of seasonal mortality variation.[44] The causes of this apparent trend are obscure but doubtless merit further investigation. Comparative evidence of disease and seasonality in early modern Alexandria will be discussed below.

The bulk of the Lower Egyptian evidence comes from Kom Abu Bellou, the necropolis of the city of Terenouthis. This archaeological site has proven exceptionally fertile: some 6,000 tombs with perhaps 700 to 800 epitaphs have so far been discovered.[45] The dating of

---

[43] Based on Ennabli, ed. (1975, 1982, 1991), discussed by Scheidel (1996a) 157–63.

[44] Petraccone (1974) 158; see figs. 4.31–2 in Scheidel (1996a) 162.

[45] Hawwass (1979) 78 and Bingen (1987) 4 n. 3 (tombs); Wagner (1994) 179 n. 4 (epitaphs). The final report of the excavation at Kom Abu Bellou undertaken by the University of Michigan in 1935 is currently being prepared for publication by T. G. Wilfong.

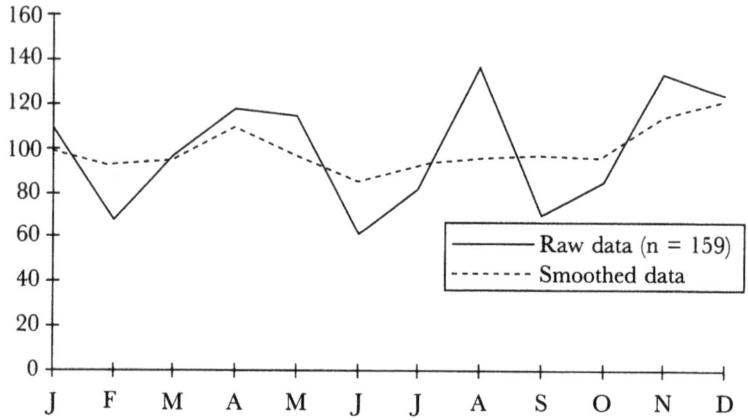

Figure 1.14 Seasonal mortality in Carthage according to Latin funerary inscriptions

many of these stelae remains controversial. Formerly mostly assigned to the second half of the third and the first half of the fourth centuries CE, some can be shown to originate from the reign of Augustus, and it now appears possible that the majority of the texts were set up in the period of the Principate.[46] This, if correct, would make them the earliest quantifiable evidence of seasonal mortality in world history. At any rate, all these epitaphs were produced for a single community over the course of no more than fifteen generations, and thus enable us to glimpse the local mortality pattern in much the same way as do the cemeteries of the Coptic monasteries in the Nile valley. The springtime mortality peak that is so characteristic of Upper Egypt is completely absent from this sample; that season registers the annual *minimum* of the death rate. Instead, we find a marked surge from October to January, preceded by a lesser increase in June (Fig. 1.15).

The peak in November would be much more extreme were we to include a group of forty-one or more cases of death recorded for

[46] Bingen (1987) 5–6 argues against the conventional 'late' dating propounded by Hooper (1961) 3–4. According to Parlasca (1970), the dates of the stelae range from the reign of Augustus to the fourth century. See most recently Cribiore (1997) 7. Demotic stelai from the same site also date from the first two centuries of Roman rule: D. Devauchelle in Abd el-Hafeez abd el-Al, Grenier and Wagner (1985) 87; Winnicki (1992) 357. The tombs of the Graeco-Roman cemetery range from the third century BCE to the fourth century CE; coins date back to the first Ptolemies: Hawwass (1979) 78.

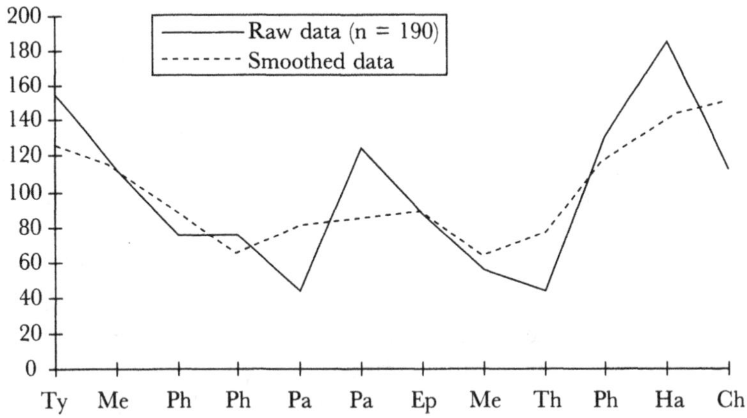

Figure 1.15 Seasonal mortality in Terenouthis according to Greek funerary inscriptions

a single day, the eleventh day of the month Hathyr in the twentieth year of an unnamed emperor, probably 7 November 154, 8 November 179, or 9 November 211.[47] This singular clustering must be evidence of some kind of disaster whose precise nature remains unknown. The fact that about ninety per cent of the victims were children, mothers and grandmothers suggests an accident such as the collapse of a large building, the sinking of a barge or a fire in a setting from which adult men had been excluded, rather than an epidemic or an attack by which the latter would have been affected in like manner.[48] The grown male survivors appear to have provided for the numerous and costly epitaphs, which were often adorned with elaborate reliefs. Other tombstones that refer to the month of Hathyr

[47] Discussed by Bingen (1987) (on thirty-three cases; briefly summarised in *SEG* XXXVII 1641) and updated by Bingen (1996) 333. In (1987) 14, he prefers 8 November 179; in (1996) 334, he considers 7 November 154 equally plausible. The data come from fifteen dated epitaphs listing forty-one individuals; several undated ones also appear to belong to the same group; all texts are listed by Bingen (1987) 6–10, (1996). Cf. also (1987) 13 n. 28.

[48] Thus Bingen (1987) 12–13 *contra* Casanova (1985), who regards this as evidence of an epidemic. That explanation does not account for the age and sex bias, nor is it readily consistent with the careful execution of the monuments. For comparative purposes, one might consider the case of the Spartan ephebes allegedly killed in a gymnasium which collapsed during an earthquake (Plutarch, *Cimon* 16.5). On 30 July 1999, the BBC reported that a fire in a tent at a wedding party in Saudi Arabia had killed thirty-seven women and children and wounded 132 others; the women and children had been segregated in keeping with tradition.

and can be dated come from different years and are therefore not related to this event. This case demonstrates how small samples can easily be distorted by isolated anomalies. All the same, such events must have been rare. While epidemic outbreaks could skew the regular mortality pattern, their victims were less likely to receive proper tombstones: the incidence of formal commemoration must have been inversely proportional to the severity of a mortality crisis.[49] Violent disruptions, such as war or raids by bandits, may also have left little room for epigraphic ritual.

The data from Leontopolis and other locations in the Delta point to a precipitous rise in June, much stronger than in Terenouthis, and further peaks during the cool season (Fig. 1.16). Except for the strong concentration of deaths in June, which may partly be a fluke caused by the small number of cases overall, this pattern quite closely resembles the seasonal distribution for Terenouthis (Fig. 1.17). This convergence may be taken to indicate that the local disease envi-

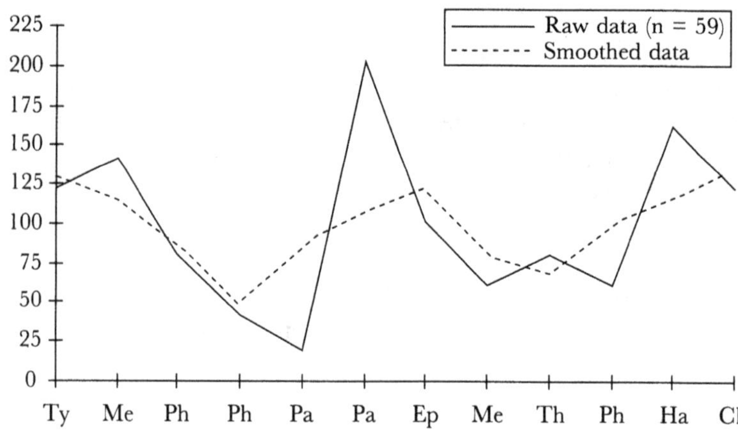

Figure 1.16 Seasonal mortality in Lower Egypt outside Alexandria and Terenouthis according to Greek funerary inscriptions

[49] This is not to say that victims of epidemics never received tombstone inscriptions: see, e.g., *CIL* III 5567 (Rosenheim/Noricum), set for parents, wife and daughter killed *per luem* in 182 CE. A recently discovered bronze inscription from Virunum (Noricum) refers to (epidemic) *mortalitas* among the members of a religious collegium in 183 CE; five out of thirty-four died. Both cases should presumably be associated with a late phase of the 'Antonine plague'; see Breitwieser (1995). However, during severe epidemics, victims would often be buried in less elaborately marked graves or even in mass graves, or would lack relatives willing to commemorate them. See below, n. 296.

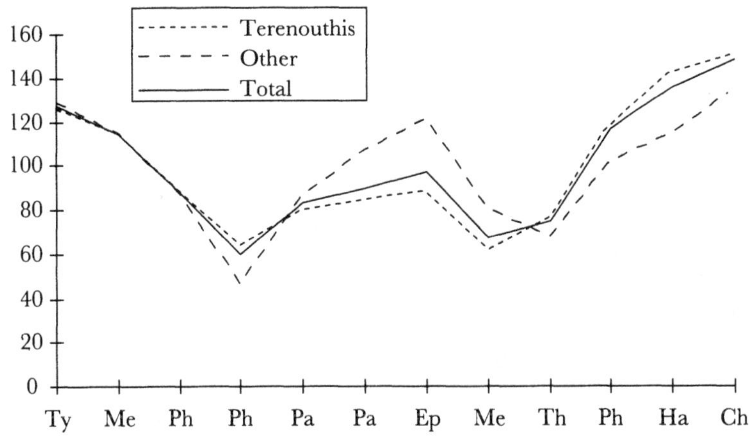

Figure 1.17 Seasonal mortality in Lower Egypt outside Alexandria according to Greek funerary inscriptions (smoothed data)

ronments of two communities at opposite margins of the Delta shared certain important characteristics. To what extent these peculiarities are representative of Lower Egypt in general remains an open question.

A comparison of the three main patterns attested in Upper Egypt and Nubia, Lower Egypt, and Alexandria highlights conspicuous regional differences (Fig. 1.18). The data from the Nile valley (including the adjusted dates on mummy labels) generate a smooth, wave-like unimodal distribution that in terms of shape and structure resembles other seasonality patterns derived from far superior evidence and that is readily consistent with intra-annual variation in environmental conditions. The sample from Lower Egypt, which is dominated by only two sites, exhibits a more complex bimodal distribution with a mortality peak at the end of the year which is of a similar magnitude as the spring peak in Upper Egypt, and a secondary increase in the middle of the year. The aseasonal pattern for Alexandria falls in between these two curves.

2.5. *Age-specific seasonal mortality*

Seasonal mortality varies with age. In historical Mediterranean populations, for instance, children would often die in the hot season and the elderly when the weather was cold and wet.[50] This raises two

[50] See, e.g., Ferrari and Livi Bacci (1985) 280 tab. 5 (Italy in 1869). For classical

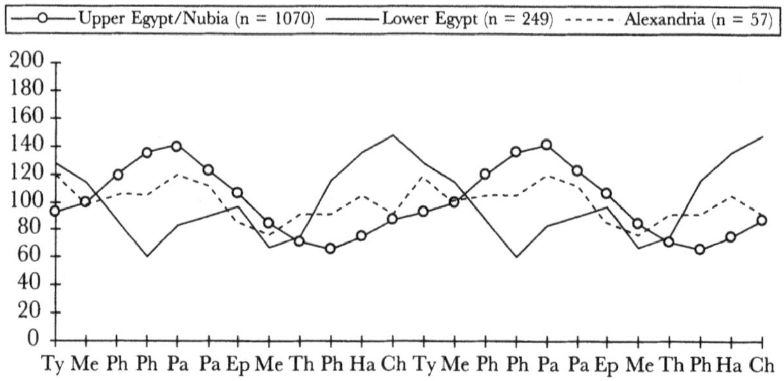

Figure 1.18 Seasonal mortality in Egypt and Nubia (smoothed data)

crucial issues, differential representation of age groups in the funerary record, and variation between age-specific patterns of seasonal mortality. The evidence from ancient and early medieval Egypt offers only very limited opportunities for an investigation of these problems. The largest regional samples, the Greek and Coptic inscriptions from Upper Egypt and Nubia, rarely contain references to ages at death. Only the mummy labels of Upper Egypt and the epitaphs of Terenouthis record both the age of the deceased and the date of death with sufficient frequency to permit some rudimentary quantitative evaluation.

The epitaphs from Terenouthis contain 111 dated references to age at death (Table 1.5). The small size of the sample makes it necessary to narrow the matrix by consolidating small units into more substantial subsamples of similar sizes (Table 1.6).

A comparison of the resultant age-brackets reveals a striking discrepancy between the seasonal patterns for children and teenagers on the one hand and for adults on the other. At the same time, there is no significant difference between the two adult age groups. During the first twenty years of life, 40.5 per cent of all deaths fall into a four-month period from May to August. By contrast, only 18.9 per cent of adult deaths occur during these months. In the complete sample of 190 dated cases of death (with and without ages), 25.9 per cent of all events can be placed in that period: the thirty-

antiquity, compare Shaw (1996) 119–21, on the late antique city of Rome, and Scheidel (1996a) 158 fig. 4.25, on Altava in Mauretania Caesariensis.

Table 1.5 Age-specific seasonal mortality according to the funerary inscriptions of Terenouthis (1)

	0–9	10–9	20–9	30–9	40–9	50–9	60–9	70+	Total
Tybi	1	3	2	2	1	2	1	1	13
Mecheir	–		1	–	3	2	3	–	110
Phamenoth	1	1		–	–	1	3	–	28
Pharmouthi	1	1	–	2	–	–	2	–	6
Pachon	2	1	–	–	–	–	–	–	3
Pauni	4	3	–	2	2	–	2	–	13
Epeiph	2	1	–	1	–	2	–	–	6
Mesore	2	–	2	1	–	–	1	1	7
Thoth	–	1	–	–	1	1	1	–	4
Phaophi	2	3	2	1	3	1	2	–	14
Hathyr	2	–	2	3	3	2	2	–	14
Choiak	4	1	1	1	1	3	1	1	13
Total	21	16	9	16	14	17	12	6	11

Table 1.6 Age-specific seasonal mortality according to the funerary inscriptions of Terenouthis (2)

	0–19	20–49	50+
Tybi	4	5	4
Mecheir	1	5	4
Phamenoth	2	1	5
Pharmouthi	2	2	2
Pachon	3	–	–
Pauni	7	4	2
Epeiph	3	1	2
Mesore	2	3	2
Thoth	1	1	2
Phaophi	3	6	3
Hathyr	2	8	4
Choiak	5	3	5
Total	37	39	35

seven pre-adult cases are unlikely to form a *random* subsample of that group ($p < 0.0244$). By necessity, the divergence between the young and adults is inverted for the cool season: 40.5 per cent of all deaths under age twenty took place from September to February, against 63.5 per cent of all adult deaths. The seasonal pattern for children and teenagers combines a principal peak centred on June with a lesser rise that mirrors the much stronger surge in mortality among adults at the beginning of the winter (Fig. 1.19). As will be clear from Figure 1.20, the weak rise in the middle of the year in the grand total for Terenouthis is caused in its entirety by pre-adult mortality. The adult death rate registers an annual minimum at that time of the year. This suggests that while the young were subject to the same seasonal health hazards as adults, they were more heavily affected by diseases of the hot season that seem to have spared older residents.

Among the mummy labels, only forty-five texts bear references to both the month of death and the age of the deceased. In this set of data, it appears that children and teenagers were disproportionately more likely to die early in the year than adults (Table 1.7 and Fig. 1.21). None of the sixteen deaths under age twenty falls into the last third of the year, compared to seven out of twenty-nine adults, or 24.1 per cent. Likewise, thirty out 132 of all dated deaths on mummy labels (with and without ages), or 22.7 per cent of the total, occur during that period. Despite the very small number of references, these discrepancies are statistically highly significant ($p < 0.0004$ if n(age 0–19) = 16 and n_{pop}(all ages) = 45, and $p < 0.00003$ if n(age 0–19) = 16 and n_{pop}(all dates) = 132).

Both the epitaphs from Terenouthis and the mummy labels of Upper Egypt indicate that the seasonal distribution of mortality varied with age. This phenomenon is much more safely attested by comparative evidence of far superior quality that will be considered in section 2.6. This observation leads to a crucial premise: the seasonal mortality pattern of undifferentiated samples of data is determined by the relative representation of different age classes. Thus, grand totals may conceal significant differences between distributions that are characteristic of specific age groups. More importantly, if certain age groups are heavily overrepresented or underrepresented in the record, the resulting overall pattern gives a misleading impression in that it does not reflect the mean seasonal mortality distribution for the population as a whole. For the purpose of determining the underlying causes of death, it is therefore essential to establish whether the

Table 1.7 Age-specific seasonal mortality according to mummy labels

	Ty	Me	Ph	Ph	Pa	Pa	Ep	Me	Th	Ph	Ha	Ch
0–19	1	2	4	1	3	1	1	3	–	–	–	–
20+	1	4	1	4	6	3	1	2	3	1	2	1

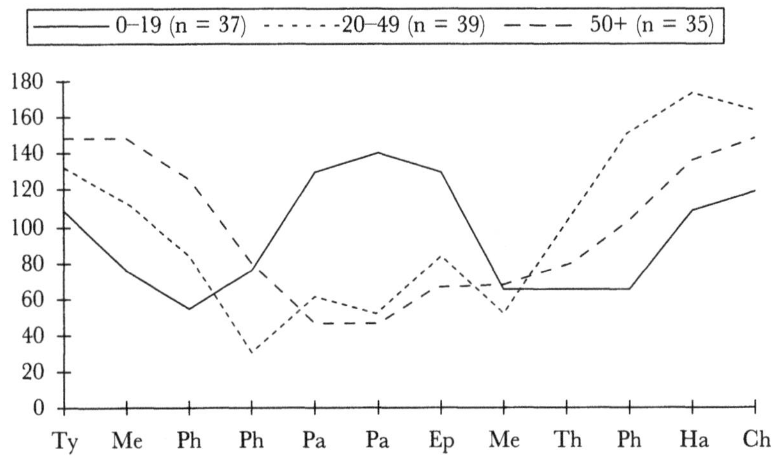

Figure 1.19 Seasonal mortality at specific ages in Terenouthis (1) (smoothed data)

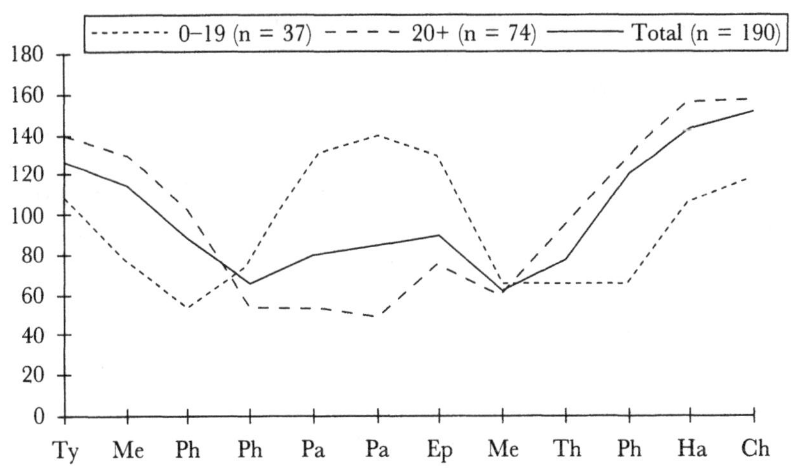

Figure 1.20 Seasonal mortality at specific ages in Terenouthis (2) (smoothed data)

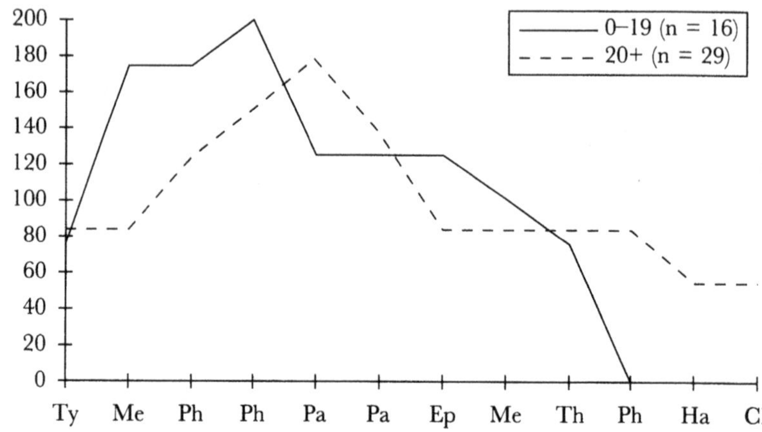

Figure 1.21 Seasonal mortality at specific ages according to mummy labels (smoothed data)

attested seasonal distributions evenly cover the entire population or give disproportionate weight to select age groups.

It has long been recognised that ancient tombstone inscriptions privilege particular segments of the population and tend to neglect or even conceal others. As a general rule, small children and especially infants are less frequently commemorated than their share in total mortality would require, whereas teenagers and young and middle-aged adults dominate the epigraphic record.[51] The same distortion is present in Egyptian epitaphs and mummy labels (Table 1.8).[52]

When we set the attested age-specific rates of commemoration against the predictions of a suitable Model Life Table (choosing Model West Mortality Level 3 Females [e_0 = 25] as a rough approximation of the actual age distribution), we find that in the ancient texts, deaths between ages ten and thirty-nine account for exactly one-half of all recorded cases, against one-fifth of all actual deaths. One in nine recorded deaths occur from age sixty onward, compared to one in six in real life. Deaths during the first decade of life amount to a mere fifth of the attested total, although almost half of all children would not survive beyond age ten. To some extent, this divergence is due to the almost complete suppression of infant

[51] See the references cited in n. 2. Only Sgarlata (1991) still maintains a pre-Hopkins vision of epigraphic age-data (but cf. also Suder (1990)).
[52] Cf. briefly Boyaval (1988) 68–70.

Table 1.8 Age-specific incidence of deaths according to funerary inscriptions and mummy labels (in per cent)[53]

Age	Upper Egypt Mummy labels (n = 557)	Upper Egypt Inscriptions (n = 207)	Lower Egypt Inscriptions (n = 499)	Expected (West 3 Females)
0/(1)–9	21.4 (20.1)	13.0 (12.6)	20.0 (18.9)	48.8 (26.2)
10–19	18.1 (18.4)	11.6 (11.7)	15.6 (15.6)	5.4 (7.8)
20–29	23.2 (23.5)	19.3 (19.4)	19.0 (19.3)	7.1 (10.2)
30–39	11.5 (11.7)	15.0 (15.0)	14.4 (14.6)	7.4 (10.7)
40–49	8.1 (8.2)	9.7 (9.7)	10.0 (10.2)	6.8 (9.8)
50–59	8.3 (8.4)	13.5 (13.6)	10.2 (10.4)	7.7 (11.1)
60–69	6.3 (6.4)	7.2 (7.3)	6.4 (6.5)	8.8 (12.7)
70+	3.2 (3.3)	10.6 (10.7)	4.2 (4.3)	7.9 (11.4)

mortality in our documents. However, even if we exclude death during the first year of life from our calculations, the predominance of cases from ages ten to thirty-nine changes little: they are still almost twice as numerous as expected. Only the underrepresentation of child mortality is less extreme than before, with an attested rate of 18.4 per cent against a prediction of 26.2 per cent. In general, teenagers and young adults are considerably overrepresented at the expense of both children and the elderly.

The most extreme features of this bias become apparent when we take a closer look at the documentation of death in early childhood. Recorded deaths in infancy correspond to a paltry 4.2 per cent of expected cases. Hence, infants were on average about forty times less likely to be commemorated than persons who died between ages ten and thirty-nine. As between one-quarter and one-third of all deaths must have occurred during the first year of life, this discrepancy necessarily results in a massive distortion of the pattern. Had infants more frequently died at different times of the year as adults, this would be impossible to discover from the epigraphic evidence. Hence, a consolidated seasonal pattern that took proper account of all age groups might well differ from the skewed attested distribution.

[53] Sources for Table 1.8: Boyaval (1975) 63–6 (mummy labels); (1976b) 221, 240 (epitaphs/Upper Egypt); ibid., 219, 238–9, Wagner (1972), El-Nassery and Wagner (1978); El-Sawy, Bouzek and Vidman (1980); Abd-el Hafeez abd el-Al, Grenier and Wagner (1985); Wagner (1994a, b); Cribiore (1997) (epitaphs/Lower Egypt). Expected distribution: Coale and Demeny (1983) 43. For doubts about the suitability of standard model life tables, see below, Chapter 2.

Conversely, had infant mortality peaked at the same time of the year as the adult death rate but to an even larger extent, the actual seasonal concentration would have been more pronounced than our texts suggest (cf. below, Fig. 1.28).

Strictly speaking, we cannot be sure whether those texts which name the month of death but do not include the person's age suffer from the same bias as the two samples under review. Indirect means of investigation, however, strongly suggest that this is indeed the case. If we compare the age distribution of the data from Terenouthis that give both ages and dates with those that do not date deaths, no significant differences emerge (Table 1.9). Moreover, the seasonal distribution of the former is virtually identical with that of the grand total of dated epitaphs from that site (Fig. 1.22).

The same is true for mummy labels. There is hardly any difference between the age distribution of dated mummy labels and all mummy labels (Table 1.10). Again, the seasonal patterns for texts with dates and ages and for those with dates only closely resemble each other (Fig. 1.23).

Table 1.9 The age-specific incidence of deaths according to the funerary inscriptions of Terenouthis (in per cent)

Age	Texts with dates and ages (n = 111)	All texts (n = 385)
0–19	33.3	36.1
20–39	22.5	29.1
40–59	27.9	23.1
60+	16.2	11.7

Table 1.10 Age-specific incidence of deaths according to mummy labels

Age	Dated texts (n = 55)	All texts (n = 557)
0–19	36.4	38.5
20–39	36.4	35.2
40–59	20.0	16.6
60+	7.3	9.7

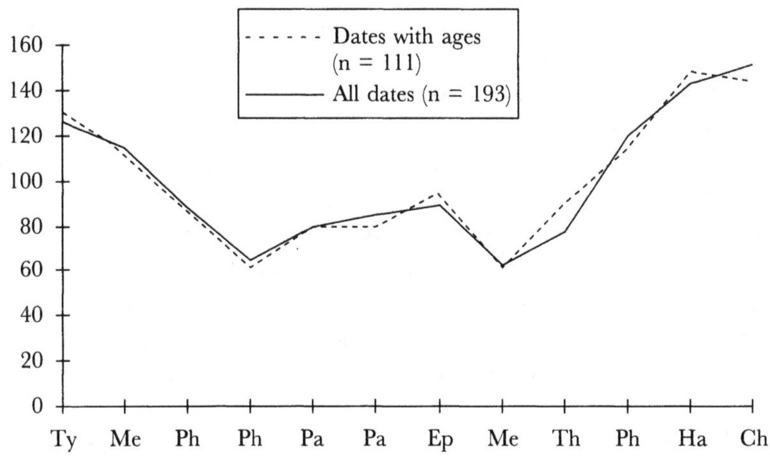

Figure 1.22 Seasonal mortality according to specific samples of the funerary inscriptions of Terenouthis (smoothed data)

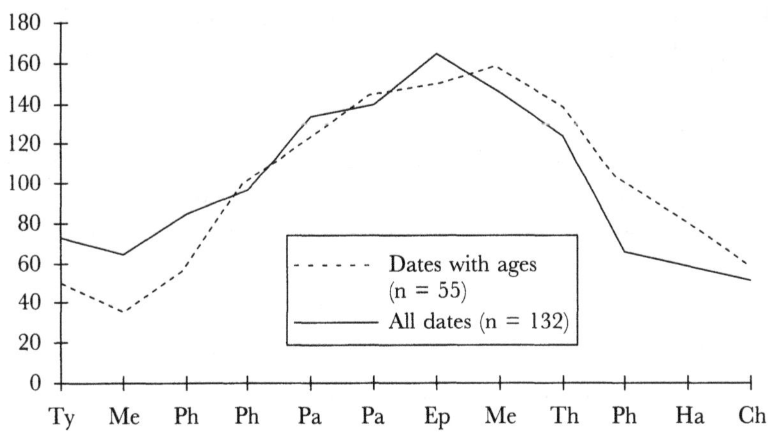

Figure 1.23 Monthly incidence of unadjusted dates in specific samples of mummy labels (smoothed data)

By analogy, we may assume that the Greek funerary inscriptions from Upper Egypt show a comparable age bias. The position of the Coptic evidence, most of which derives from three large monasteries, is perhaps somewhat more ambiguous. The age structure of a monastic community would not have been the same as that of the general population. These epitaphs probably give even greater prominence to adults than other sets of data but, unlike the evidence set out in Table 1.8, may also emphasise death in old age.[54] A number of Nubian inscriptions for aged bishops and other dignitaries seem to confirm that suspicion.[55] Even so, the relatively large number of surviving documents suggests that ordinary monks also frequently received tombstones, and that these texts cover the whole adult life phase. Thus, with regard to age bias, our various samples may be put on roughly the same footing. As far as we can tell, all of them are largely silent about infants, conceal much of child mortality, and accord undue weight to teenagers and adults in the prime of life.

In short, the ancient and Coptic evidence of seasonal mortality in Egypt does not provide us with a balanced picture. The attested patterns predominantly reflect mortality in what is usually considered to be the most vigorous and disease-resistant segment of the population. We must also bear in mind that in a country where most people lived at or near subsistence level and stone was scarce, only a small minority could afford any tombstone inscriptions at all.[56] In general, with the possible exception of certain categories of slaves, everyone whose death and burial left a mark in the written record will have come from a relatively privileged segment of the population.[57] Coptic monks who were commemorated with tombstones must perforce be included in this category. Thus, the attested patterns of

---

[54] Cf. Boyaval (1992) 178–9, for the high mean age of persons in Greek ecclesiastical commemorations compared to all other Greek inscriptions: twenty-two references, mean age 48.7, vs. 105 other references, mean age 37.2.

[55] See Kubinska (1974), for bishops aged seventy-eight (no. 4), eighty-two (no. 7), sixty-nine (no. 8), eighty-eight (no. 9), seventy (no. 10), seventy-five (no. III), sixty-one, ninety-three, sixty-seven and ninety-five (pp. 54–9).

[56] As Bowman (1990) 186, puts it, 'the poor would end up simply as plainly bandaged mummies, soaked in pitch and consigned, with a label bearing the name of the deceased, to a communal pit or graveyard'.

[57] See Scheidel (1996a) 90–1. Egyptian tombstone inscriptions show lower levels of digit preference than mummy labels; this could be taken to indicate that they come from a superior socio-economic background (ibid., 84–5, 91).

mortality were not affected by factors such as periodic malnutrition or seasonal income fluctuations in peasant households.[58] For the most part, we are looking at the deaths of reasonably affluent people in the prime of life. This double bias makes the observed high levels of seasonal variation all the more intriguing.

The surviving material is also skewed in favour of urban and monastic contexts. Although Terenouthis and Leontopolis had not been elevated to the status of nome capitals and technically counted as mere 'villages', both appear to have been substantial communities, quite possibly with thousands of residents. Even in the case of Terenouthis, however, it is impossible to tell how many of the deceased had resided in the settlement itself. We can only assume that the levels of material well-being and acculturation that underpinned the habit of epigraphic commemoration were most frequently found in an urban setting. Large monasteries were also local foci of high population density.[59] As a consequence, the mortality patterns of village communities may well remain largely undocumented.[60] It is unclear to what extent this might affect our study. On the one hand, population density was very high by any pre-modern standard throughout the country, some Egyptian villages were large and would not greatly differ from small towns, and settlements of different sizes would share crucial climatic, hygienic and social conditions. On the other hand, urban centres could very well have created their own demographic 'micro-climate' (cf. below, Chapter 2).

[58] Among the poor, these factors could have influenced both the actual distribution of deaths and the incidence of commemoration. Although the trough in the incidence of commemoration in August and September in both Upper and Lower Egypt coincides with the peak of the inundation, when much of the land was flooded, we have no reason to assume that the observed distribution arose because funerals were deferred or burial sites were inaccessible, or that it was otherwise linked to this event: the dates refer to the time of death, not of interment; individuals who could afford tombstones must have been able to store corpses for some time; it may have taken stone-cutters some time to finish and deliver tombstones; there was no sharp upturn in commemorations when the waters receded; and, most important, the mummy labels also show the same pattern.

[59] See Guillaumont (1991) 1662–3 for evidence of the substantial size of Coptic monasteries in Egypt.

[60] Wagner (1993) discusses the underrepresentation of villages in Egyptian epigraphy of the Graeco-Roman period.

2.6. *Comparative evidence*

The evidence from ancient and early medieval Egypt needs to be evaluated within the context of comparative data on seasonal mortality. Patterns of seasonality in populations that share climatic conditions often resemble one another. For the nineteenth century, for example, we can find a pattern with a spring peak of deaths in northern and northwestern European countries such as England, Scotland, and the Netherlands that contrasts with an autumnal peak in the Mediterranean, as in Spain and Italy. France and Germany occupy an intermediate position with both the northern spring peak and an additional summer peak.[61] Moving farther south, we can see that the autumn surge of the northern Mediterranean changes to a spring peak precipitated by an earlier onset of high temperatures. The principal difference, it seems, lies between a 'northern' and a 'southern' seasonality pattern created by different types of disease environments, with a high incidence of respiratory illnesses in the former and of intestinal infections in the latter.

Here, we will focus on two different categories of comparative material: contemporaneous, i.e., ancient, sources from outside Egypt, and more recent data from Egypt itself. Other epigraphic samples from the ancient world tend to share the social and age-specific biases of the Egyptian texts in privileging adults and the well-to-do, thereby facilitating direct comparison. Egypt's eastern neighbour Palestine provides funerary records from the same period and a similar ecological setting. Patlagean gathered two samples of pertinent inscriptions dating from the fourth to seventh centuries CE comprised of 105 references from Palaestina Tertia (southern Palestine) and sixty-five items from Moab (the Transjordanian steppe). The larger of the two generates a seasonal pattern similar to that for Upper Egypt and Nubia (tombstones and mummy labels combined), although it peaks one month later and shows a somewhat higher amplitude of variation. The data from Moab, by contrast, are heavily concentrated in the month of June (Fig. 1.24).[62]

The smoothed data clarify the unimodal distribution of the Palestinian data. Employing three-month moving averages, the relatively late peak in Moab can be shown to coincide with the surge

---

[61] Wrigley and Schofield (1981) 296–8.

[62] Based on Patlagean (1977) 92–4.

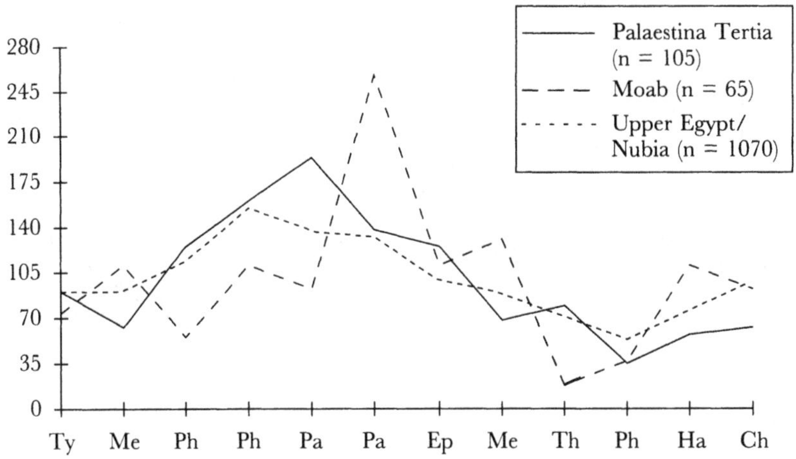

Figure 1.24 Seasonal mortality in Palestine according to Greek funerary inscriptions

in mortality in the Coptic monastery of Sakinya in Nubia. On the face of it, conditions in the Nile valley and in the most arid parts of Palestine were broadly similar. This, in turn, serves to emphasise the distinctness of the local evidence from Lower Egypt.

The largest body of ancient evidence of seasonal mortality comes from the city of Rome. Drawing on early Christian epitaphs from the catacombs that encircled the former capital of the empire, Brent Shaw gathered a total of almost 4,000 references to the month of death.[63] Ranging mostly from the fourth to the sixth centuries CE, the bulk of these texts were set up during the fifty-odd years before the first sack of Rome in 410 CE.[64] Shaw also established a much smaller sample of 244 references from various locations in late Roman southern Italy that show the same characteristics as the metropolitan data.[65] In Figure 1.25, these Italian data sets are compared to two different samples of the Egyptian evidence, namely, the grand total of 1,070 references from stelae and mummy labels from Upper Egypt and Nubia, and a narrower selection of 674 data from the Nile valley from the Thebaid to Memphis. The Italian and Egyptian data generate two

[63] Shaw (1996) 115 fig. 5. As noted above, his sample supersedes the previous collection by Nordberg (1963). For discussions of seasonal mortality in ancient Rome, see above, nn. 6–7.

[64] Shaw (1996) 106 figs. 1–2.

[65] Ibid., 115 fig. 5 (Rome), 127 fig. 19 (southern Italy, *regiones* I–V).

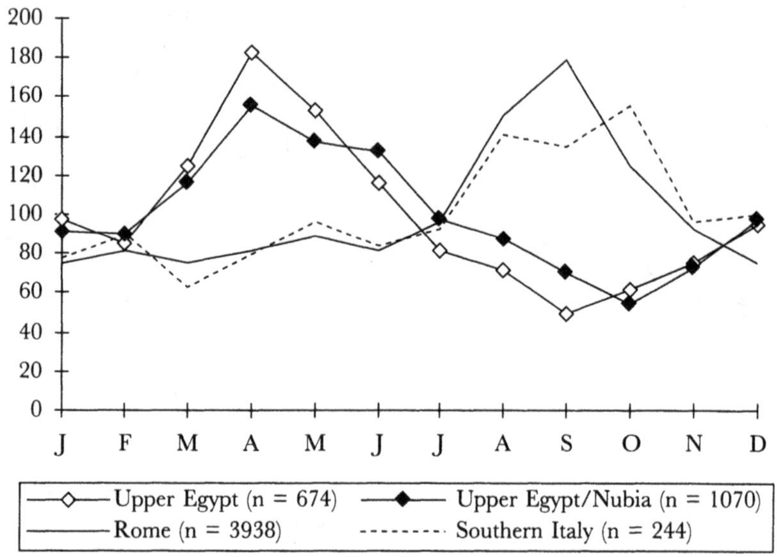

Figure 1.25 Seasonal mortality in ancient Upper Egypt and Italy

unimodal distributions of similar shape: the Egyptian peak in April corresponds to an Italian peak in September. The extent of seasonal variation (between the highest and the lowest monthly incidence of deaths) is the same in Rome (104 index points) as in Upper Egypt and Nubia (101 index points). The seasonality index for the more homogeneous Upper Egyptian material varies by 133 points.

Individual locations score even higher, above all Saqqara (a shift by 208 index points from May to September). The smoothed figures control for the small size of local samples but still produce high levels of intra-annual variation: 114 index points for Saqqara, 110 for Sakinya and ninety for Terenouthis, compared to eighty-four for Rome in general and ninety-two for Roman adults aged twenty to forty-nine.

In the Rome sample, the pattern for the age group from twenty to forty-nine years barely differs from the overall distribution; again, albeit to a somewhat lesser degree than in Egypt, these data are dominated by individuals who died as young and middle-aged adults.[66]

[66] 857 references from Rome pertain to persons aged twenty to forty-nine, compared to 706 for children under the age of ten and 313 for persons upwards from age fifty: Shaw (1996) 118 fig. 9, 120 figs. 11–12. Thus, the first group is about three times as numerous relative to children and the elderly as expected. In the

By and large, the best attested sites in Egypt and Nubia experienced similar levels of seasonal mortality variation as the city of Rome. The same is true for the Palestinian data presented above. It is therefore safe to say that strong seasonal fluctuations in the death rate of adults were not unique to a single part of the ancient Mediterranean. However, the epigraphic record merely sheds tiny spots of light on what must have been a whole range of mortality regimes. The lack of properly quantifiable evidence from most provinces of the Roman empire makes it impossible to assess the representative nature of the extant documentation.[67]

Pertinent evidence from more recent periods partly alleviates this dilemma by enabling us to interpret ancient conditions within a broader context. In Egypt, relevant national statistics have been published since the 1920s. Figure 1.26 shows the seasonal distributions

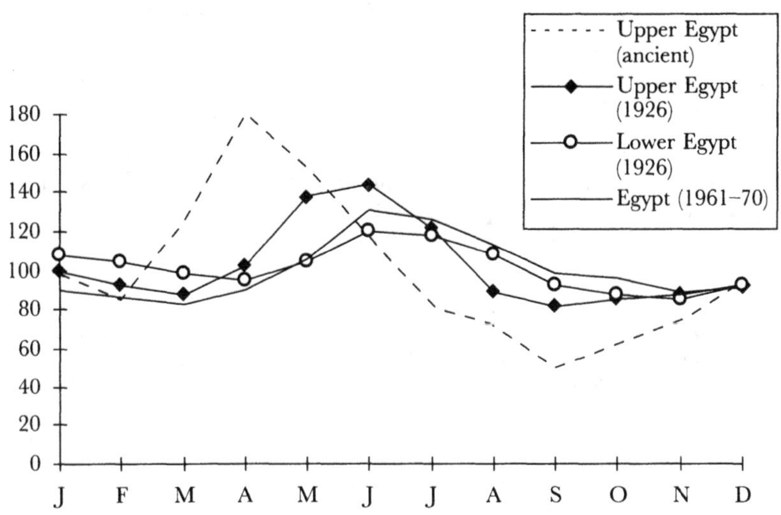

Figure 1.26 Seasonal mortality in ancient and modern Egypt

Egyptian data (see above, Table 1.8), adults aged twenty to forty-nine are more heavily overrepresented relative to children under ten (5.5 times) but less so relative to people over fifty (more than twice).

[67] In Altava in Mauretania Caesariensis, mortality under age fifty soared from September to January: Scheidel (1996a) 158 fig. 4.25. Other samples of evidence of seasonal mortality in the Roman world fail to produce similarly clear-cut patterns: cf. Shaw (1996) 127 fig. 18 (North Italy) 129, fig. 23 (Gaul/Germany), 130 fig. 24 (North Africa). See also the evidence from Carthage, above, Fig. 1.14. The data from late antique Spain are probably unreliable (Shaw, 129).

of deaths in Upper Egypt and Lower Egypt as reported for 1926, the average pattern for the whole country during the 1960s, and the curve for the ancient Nile valley north of Aswan.[68] By the early twentieth century, seasonal variation had dropped to lower levels: thirty-five index points in Lower Egypt and sixty-two in Upper Egypt for 1926, and forty-eight in the 1960s, compared to 101 or 133 points in the ancient and medieval data, depending on the scope of the samples. As the scale of seasonal mortality variation is negatively correlated with the level of development (see below, section 3.1), the higher rate for Upper Egypt may reflect the fact that from the nineteenth century onward, living conditions in the Delta had improved faster than in the south.[69] Considering that Lower Egypt accounted for a larger share of the total population than Upper Egypt, it appears that the overall level of variation had not changed much between the 1920s and the 1960s.

In Upper Egypt in the 1920s, mortality peaked in the late spring and early summer from May to July, followed by a more moderate rise in Lower Egypt during the summer months.[70] While the former pattern differs significantly from its ancient counterpart, the ancient and modern distributions for Lower Egypt seem all but incompatible. The data from the Fayum show a similar 'time shift' as the evidence for Upper Egypt (Fig. 1.27).

---

[68] Data for 1926: *Annuaire statistique 1926–1927* (Cairo 1928), 60–1, tab. IV. This is also one of the two years chosen by Shaw (1996) 124 as being typical of the general pattern (i.e., free of unusual epidemics). The annual statistical yearbook for Egypt was first published in 1909 by the Statistical Department of the Ministry of Finance under the title *Statistical Yearbook of Egypt for 1909, vol. 1* (Cairo 1909), and continued as *Annuaire statistique de l'Egypte*. The earlier issues that are available to me (vols. 1–7 for 1909–15) do not contain data on seasonal mortality; neither do the *Statistical returns 1880–1899* (Cairo 1900) published by the Egyptian Government. Data for the 1960s: Salem, Soliman and El Sayed (1973) 41 (mean for 1961–70).

[69] E.g., Baer (1982) 243–5.

[70] For some inexplicable reason, the official or officials who produced the official handbook of infectious diseases in Egypt that was issued in 1922 by the Ministry of the Interior contrived to remain unaware of the seasonal pattern revealed by the data gathered by the same government agency: 'The deaths below one year of age are usually more numerous in the autumn, and those above fifty years of age more numerous in winter, but those between 1 to 10 and 10 to 50 years of age remain fairly constant in the absence of epidemic disease' (*Infectious diseases handbook* (1922) 4). This assertion is clearly incompatible with the attested peak in the late spring and throughout the summer, and with the autumnal drop in mortality. Incidentally, the supposedly regular age-specific distribution of deaths reported on the same page is equally spurious (twenty per cent of all deaths are said to have occurred from birth to age one, against thirty per cent from ages one to ten, etc.).

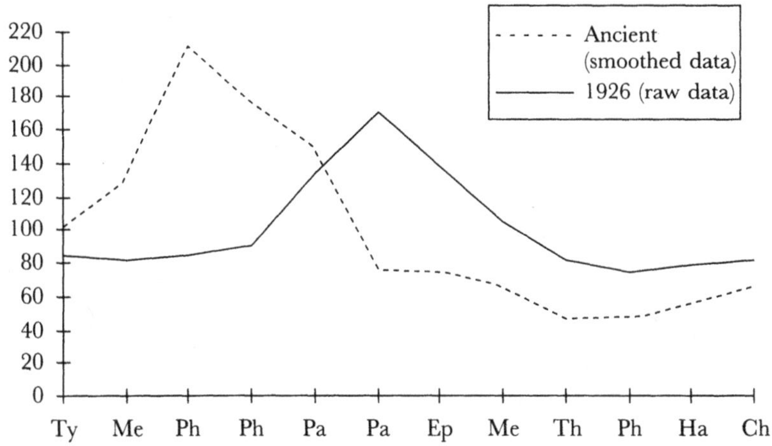

Figure 1.27 Seasonal mortality in the ancient and modern Fayum

However, it would be inappropriate to put ancient and modern data on the same footing. While the ancient and medieval data exclude, or reduce the importance of, certain age groups, the figures for the twentieth century are based on annual counts and aim to cover the entire population. Of course the latter are far from perfect. In the 1920s, official registration still suffered from serious problems: in the countryside, where most Egyptians lived, perhaps one-third of all deaths seem to have gone unrecorded.[71] It is a fair guess that many of these deaths occurred in infancy and early childhood. By the late 1960s, the bureaucracy had tightened its grip and it had become possible to demonstrate that seasonal mortality variation was significantly stronger among infants than later in life (Fig. 1.28).[72]

A similar difference between children and adults was first established for Cairo in the years from 1798 to 1801. These data, gathered by the French expeditionary forces that invaded Egypt in 1798, provide the earliest published modern evidence of seasonal mortality in that country. In this count, the precise meaning of the term 'enfants' remains unclear but may well include all cases up to puberty; these children account for 56.4 per cent of all recorded deaths. It catches the eye that adult mortality was subject to far less variation than the

[71] The attested Crude Death Rates for Lower Egypt and Upper Egypt outside the largest cities were 25.5 and 25.1 per 1,000, respectively. The actual rate must have been 40 per 1,000 or over: see below, Chapter 3, p. 214.

[72] Salem, Soliman and El Sayed (1973) 41.

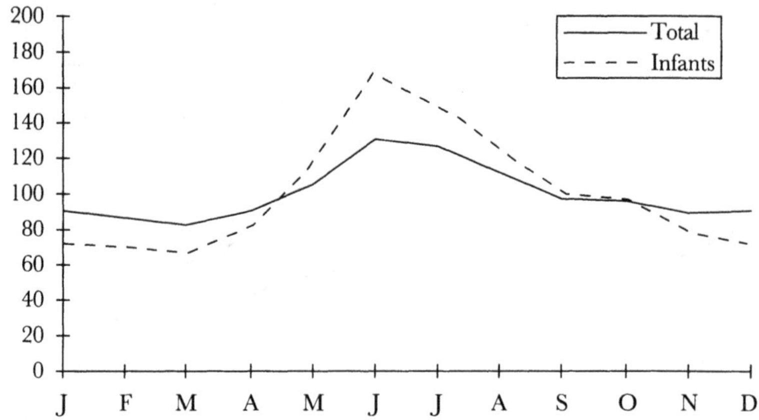

Figure 1.28 Seasonal mortality in specific age groups in modern Egypt, 1961 to 1970

ancient data suggest (Figs. 1.29–30).[73] Elevated adult mortality in the spring of 1799 is vaguely reminiscent of the (much stronger) peak in April documented by the Greek and Coptic epitaphs of Upper Egypt, while the winter peaks are rather more consistent with the ancient data from Lower Egypt. What matters here is that by and large (especially during the second period), juvenile and adult death rates of children and adults moved in tandem, and that the seasonal amplitudes are more pronounced for children than at mature ages.

The nineteenth-century physician Schnepp reproduced monthly counts of deaths in Cairo and Alexandria over a twelve-month period from August 1859 to July 1860 (Figs. 1.31–32).[74] The representative value of these distributions must not be overrated: Schnepp himself warns against regarding this isolated series as typical, and, more importantly, the underlying process of registration may itself have been defective.[75] At any rate, these data give us a rough idea of the seasonal patterns. In Cairo, the picture is less erratic than sixty years earlier, with a peak in child mortality during the summer and com-

[73] Desgenettes (1813) 311–19 (cf. also (1800)). The count for 1800 was interrupted by the Cairo uprising; the seasonal mortality pattern for the spring of 1801 was massively distorted by an outbreak of plague, and is therefore excluded: see below, Fig. 1.42.

[74] Based on Schnepp (1862b) 544–5.

[75] Schnepp (1862b) 546. For a discussion of the poor quality of Egyptian demographic data from that period, see below, p. 49. However, the administration was far better informed about these two major cities than about the villages, and in this case, the recorded totals cannot be wide of the mark: see below, n. 327.

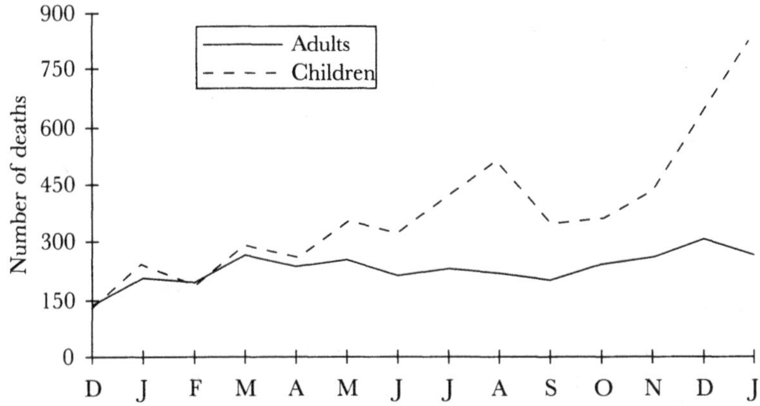

Figure 1.29 Seasonal mortality in Cairo, December 1798 to January 1800

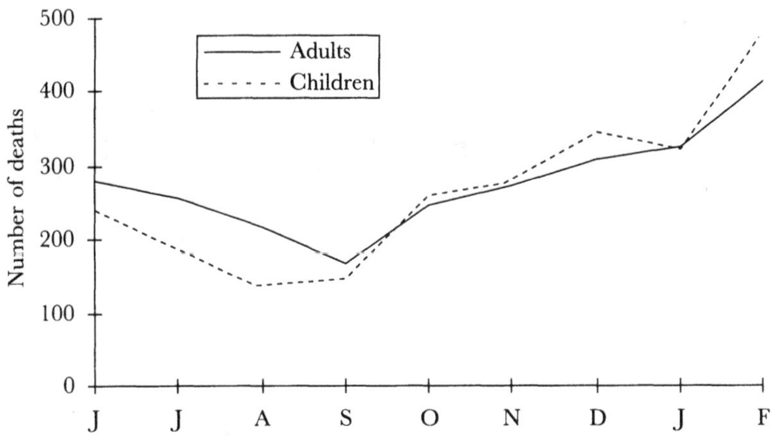

Figure 1.30 Seasonal mortality in Cairo, June 1800 to February 1801

paratively little variation for adults. The mortality plateau for adults in March and April has disappeared. Alexandria experienced broadly similar conditions.

By contrast, the data for 1798/1801 and 1859/60 differ conspicuously from those for 1926 (Fig. 1.33). By that time, the mortality peak in Cairo had shifted from mid-summer to the late spring. This new curve is consistent with the pattern for the Nile valley in general. However, in 1847 Pruner already reported that mortality in Cairo

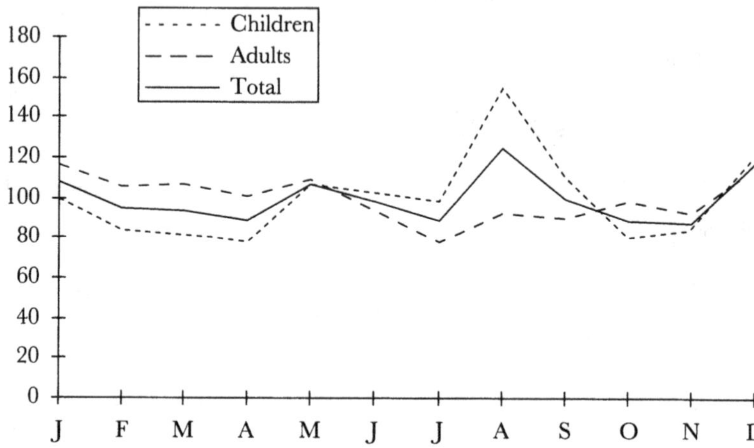

Figure 1.31 Seasonal mortality in Cairo, August 1859 to July 1860

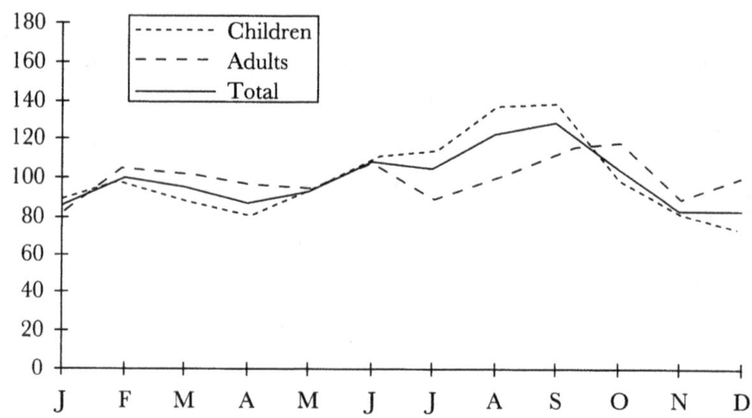

Figure 1.32 Seasonal mortality in Alexandria, August 1859 to July 1860

peaked from May to August.[76] Thus, it seems that the evidence from the 1920s can be reconciled with some data from the nineteenth century but not with others. The evidence from Alexandria is (even) more difficult to interpret and cannot support any generalisation.

Those samples from the nineteenth and twentieth centuries that differentiate the frequency of deaths according to age all make it

[76] Pruner (1847) 86 (with reference to years that were free of plague). He also stated that in Alexandria, the month of October registered the largest number of deaths.

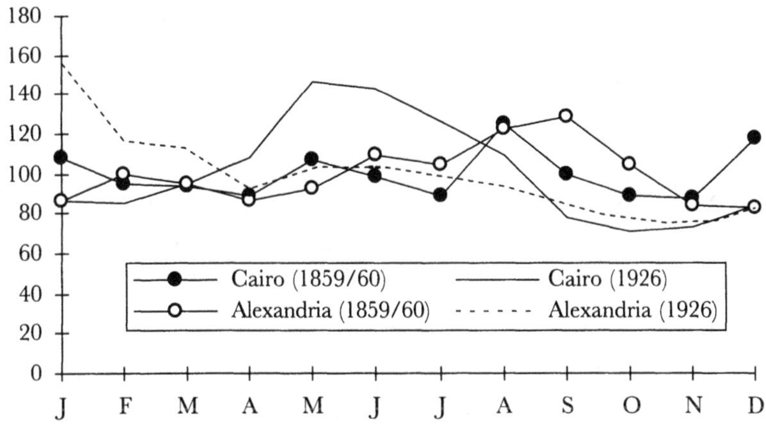

Figure 1.33 Seasonal mortality in Cairo and Alexandria, 1859/60 and 1926

clear that deaths in infancy and childhood were responsible for most of the observed seasonal variation and especially for distinct mortality peaks. In 'normal', non-crisis years, at least, adult mortality fluctuated only moderately across the seasons. A close parallel to nineteenth-century Cairo and Alexandria is provided by the national statistics for Italy in 1869 (Fig. 1.34).[77]

In both the Egyptian cities and in Italy after the middle of the nineteenth century, the very young succumbed to seasonal infections in numbers that were unheard of among adults who had successfully negotiated the hazards of childhood. In both cases, the conditions of that period stand in marked contrast to the mortality regime of the first millennium. The massive seasonal fluctuations in mortality attested by Egyptian and Nubian tombstone inscriptions and mummy tags that were heavily dominated by teenagers and adults are without parallel in the extant evidence for adult deaths from nineteenth century Egypt when average levels of life expectancy and quality of life had barely, if at all, improved on the standards of the Roman period. The same discrepancy emerges for Italy. It is seriously misleading to compare seasonality patterns from late Roman and modern Italy as if they had been derived from the same *type* of

[77] Based on Ferrari and Bacci (1985) 280 tab. 5. Comparable indices can be found in Bellettini (1987) 187–92 figs. 1–3; Petraccone (1974) 155–9, 171–3.

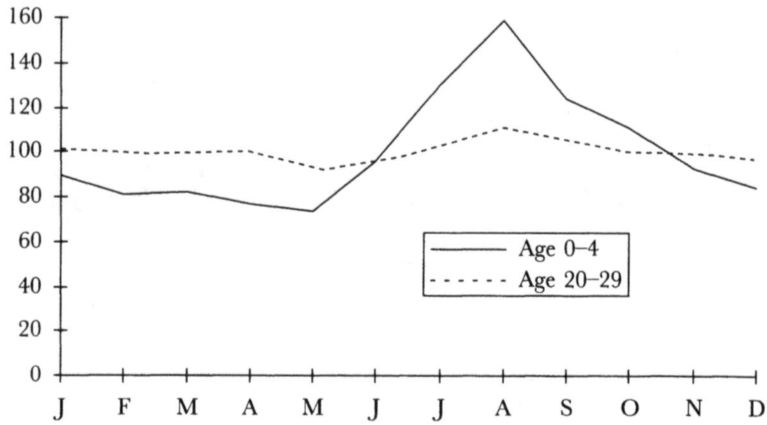

Figure 1.34 Seasonal mortality at specific ages in Italy, 1869

base populations.[78] The crucial difference lies in the relationship between infant and adult mortality: in ancient Rome, adult deaths were subject to the same swings as deaths in early childhood (Fig. 1.35),[79] whereas in the nineteenth century, as shown in Figure 1.34, the mortality distribution for young adults did not in the least replicate the pattern for small children. Somewhat paradoxically, the very fact that samples that tend to conceal early mortality bear some semblance to the results of more representative counts demonstrates that they reflect different mortality regimes.

Just how unusual were the seasonality patterns of ancient Egypt and Rome? For one thing, it is remarkable that the Egyptian samples register amplitudes of variation that equal those found in the city of Rome. As a rule of thumb, steep amplitudes are associated with high mortality levels as such. While it is impossible to infer vital demographic parameters such as the Crude Death Rate or life expectancy from seasonality patterns, there can be little doubt that in this respect, more is worse: an average intra-annual variation in excess of a hundred index points even among adults suggests extremely high levels of exposure to lethal infectious diseases.[80] This was surely

[78] Shaw (1996) 115–16 argues that the seasonal patterns for Italy from 1863–69 and for Central Italy in 1869 that produce summer peaks are therefore 'consistent' with the distribution for ancient Rome. In fact, however, this apparent match does not extend to include adult mortality.

[79] Source: Shaw (1996) 115 fig. 5, 118 fig. 9, 120 fig. 11.

[80] The same point has been made by Shaw (1996) 132–4, with respect to ancient Rome.

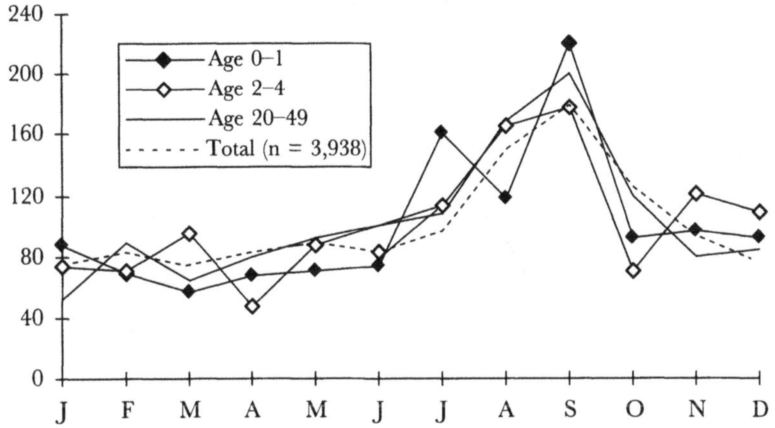

Figure 1.35 Seasonal mortality at specific ages in late antique Rome

true for the city of Rome, which is commonly regarded as a vast population sink—an idea receives ample confirmation in Sallares' new study of Roman malaria.[81] It is therefore interesting to find seasonal mortality fluctuation on a similar scale in both Egypt and Palestine, well outside a metropolitan setting.[82]

As we have seen above (Fig. 1.26), the Greek and Coptic documents from Upper Egypt, even though they largely conceal ancient child mortality, generate far higher seasonal amplitudes than the data from the early twentieth century. This observation is put into perspective by the fact that Egyptian seasonality in the 1920s was very substantial even by the standards of the Mediterranean of the *preceding* century. Thus, the former may be put on a par with conditions in the malarial and destitute southern parts of nineteenth-century Italy (Fig. 1.36).[83]

This means that the ancient Egyptian data, which are dominated by adults, document seasonal variation on a considerably larger scale than the more balanced evidence from the 1920s, which is itself consistent with high-mortality populations of the nineteenth century. We

[81] Sallares (forthcoming). See also Scheidel (forthcoming a).

[82] This problem was first noted by Scheidel (1996a) 163. To complicate matters further, the only other large ancient cities that provide evidence of seasonal mortality, Alexandria and Carthage, show little sign of massive variation: see above, Figs. 1.13–14.

[83] Spain: Wrigley and Schofield (1981) 297 tab. 8.4; Sicily and Foggia: Shaw (1996) 128 figs. 20, 21.

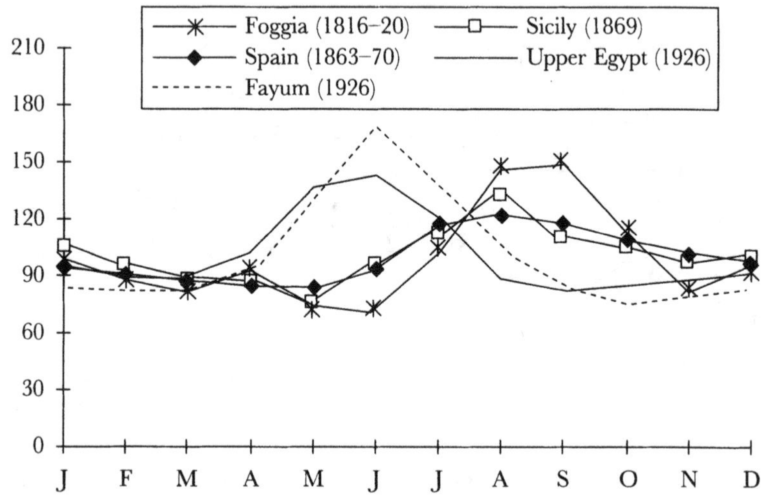

Figure 1.36 Seasonal mortality in the Mediterranean in the nineteenth and early twentieth centuries

may conclude that in Egypt in the first millennium CE, in much the same way as in late antique Rome, endemic seasonal infectious diseases must have taken a higher toll on adults than in other, more recent pre-modern populations.

The seasonal patterns for Terenouthis and Leontopolis deviate significantly from the Lower Egyptian distribution of the 1920s. In both periods, mortality peaked in June and July. In Terenouthis, this rise appears to have been caused by the deaths of individuals under the age of twenty (see above, section 2.5); the same was true for modern Egypt. However, the modern data show only a mild increase in mortality in the early winter that falls far short of the extreme peak in the fall and the early winter derived from the epitaphs of the Roman period. As I have observed above, conditions in Terenouthis and Leontopolis may not have been typical of the Delta as such, and it is tempting to dismiss the peculiarities of the ancient data as local anomalies. Alternatively, it is certainly not inconceivable that the disease environment of Lower Egypt had undergone significant changes during the intervening 1,500 years or so. In principle, the available evidence is simply insufficient to substantiate either interpretation.

This caveat notwithstanding, a seriously deficient national count from the late 1850s might be taken to corroborate some crucial features of the ancient data. According to government statistics reproduced by Schnepp, the mean annual number of deaths in Egypt over a thirty-six month period from 1857 to 1860 amounted to 102,500 cases. This figure is surely too low: since these statistics (quite plausibly) register some 21,300 deaths in Cairo and Alexandria for 1859/60, only about 81,200 deaths are supposed to have occurred in the remainder of the country.[84] Given a non-metropolitan population of around six million,[85] this implies a Crude Death Rate of 13 per 1,000, an impossibly low value that is characteristic of present western societies. The actual death rate must have been at least three times as high; thus, at least two-thirds of all deaths in the small towns and villages of Egypt went unrecorded. It is a fair guess that the inhabitants of towns are better represented than villagers, that cases from Lower Egypt dominate the record (both because a larger share of the population resided in the Delta and because of the relative backwardness of Upper Egypt that would have hampered registration), and that deaths in infancy and early childhood were less likely to be reported than fatalities among adults. We may also suspect some bias against the poor, and in favour of men. These deficiencies not only help to explain the differences between the distributions for the 1850s and the 1920s. They also tend to render this particular sample more similar to our biased ancient sources than any other modern count. A comparison with the ancient data yields some contradictory results (Fig. 1.37). The summer peak of the Roman period and the 1920s was entirely missing in the late 1850s. We can only speculate that this might be a function of severe underregistration of children in the latter sample. Instead, we find a moderate rise in the spring, centred on April, that overlaps with the much stronger surge in ancient Upper Egypt, and a more pronounced increase during the fall, which seems to echo the corresponding pattern in Terenouthis and Leontopolis. The closest parallel to the latter is provided by the 1926 data from the 'frontier districts' of Egypt, i.e., the Western Oases in the arid lands west of the Nile. Like the ancient texts, they point to a strong surge in mortality from November to January. Again, owing to discrepancies in the representation of different age groups, these two samples cannot be put on the same footing. Even so, this apparent match raises the possibility that the underlying disease environments may have shared important characteristics.

[84] Schnepp (1862b) 543 (mean for 1857–60), 543–5 (data for 1859/60).

[85] See below, Chapter 3, p. 212.

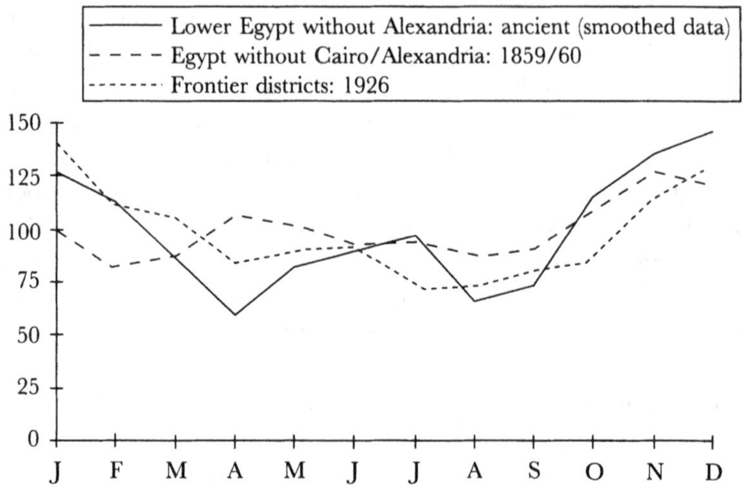

Figure 1.37 Regional seasonal mortality in ancient and modern Egypt

2.7. *Conclusions*

Quantifiable evidence of seasonal mortality from ancient and early medieval Egypt and Nubia is spread out over a thousand years and fourteen degrees of geographical latitude from Meroe to Alexandria. A little under 1,400 references are unevenly distributed over this very considerable time and space, many of them clustering at a few Coptic monasteries in the Nile valley and a couple of sites on the fringes of the Delta. Moreover, for all we can tell, funerary commemoration was skewed in favour of the productive members of society, neglecting children and perhaps also the elderly. To an historical demographer accustomed to the riches of more recent sources, analysis of such scanty bits of biased evidence may hardly seem worthwhile. For the student of antiquity, however, these data rank among the best that have survived from the period under review, and call for close scrutiny. From what we have seen so far, this undertaking need not be entirely hopeless. Scattered as they may be, the testimonies from the Nile valley, with only a single minor exception, readily fall into a smooth and intrinsically plausible pattern: a unimodal distribution of deaths that gradually rises in the winter, markedly peaks in the spring, and bottoms out in the early autumn. More modest in volume and more constricted in geographical (and chronological) provenance, the data from Lower Egypt hint at a different pattern, with a summer peak for the young and a strong surge in adult mortality during the cool months of the year. True to their ecological distinctness, the city of Alexandria and, to a lesser extent, the Fayum region appear to exhibit different characteristics; in both cases, however, the available data sets are exiguous. Comparisons with modern evidence show above all that in the first millennium of the Christian era, mortality varied more heavily over the course of the year than in the recent past. This is true in particular for teenagers and adults who appear to have succumbed to seasonal infections as readily as children did. In this, the conditions in early Egypt bore a close resemblance to the mortality regimes of neighbouring Palestine and the city of Rome in late antiquity. It is thus above all the *difference* between ancient and modern Egypt that catches the eye. In this section, I have tried to show that even allowing for all the various shortcomings of the evidence, ancient and modern, much of this difference ought to be considered genuine. This finding inevitably raises the question of the underlying causes: what made ancient Egypt different?

3. *Causes of seasonal mortality*

3.1. *The shifting ecology of disease*

There is no denying that 'the logical and empirical difficulties in (. . .) moving from observed patterns of seasonality to imputed patterns of disease are considerable'.[86] When analysed with due caution, however, evidence of seasonal mortality may point to underlying causes of death that would otherwise be impossible to identify, and enables us to weigh conflicting reconstructions against each other. The observed discrepancy between the ancient and modern Egyptian data is consistent with the premise that seasonal mortality patterns are inherently unstable and may change over time following shifts in the prevalence of particular clinical and contributing causes of death. Such changes may arise from the introduction or disappearance of certain diseases, an increase or reduction of their impact or frequency owing to variation in environmental conditions, including

[86] Landers and Mouzas (1988) 62–3.

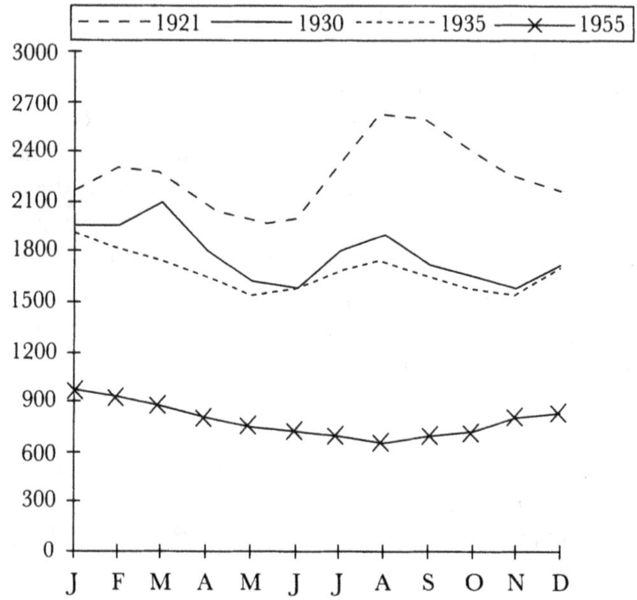

Figure 1.38 Seasonal mortality in Japan, 1921 to 1955 (monthly number of deaths per 1,000,000 population)

human intervention, the mutation of the pathogen concerned, and interaction with other diseases with which they are associated.[87] Human intervention in the form of improvements in hygiene, sanitation and water supply has been of pivotal importance in the massive reduction of death rates in recent history. This reduction usually went hand in hand with a contraction of seasonal mortality fluctuations. These parallel developments, exemplified in Figure 1.38, highlight the link between high mortality and high seasonal amplitudes.[88]

In the case of pre-modern Egypt, however, human intervention was not an issue. Living conditions, especially outside the large cities, did not significantly improve from ancient times to the late nineteenth century. Progress in hygienic measures was slow, and the departure of bubonic plague and the gradual eradication of smallpox in the nineteenth century may merely have restored the conditions of the

[87] Cf., e.g., Risse (1997) 175–6, drawing attention to what he calls the 'shifting ecology of disease'.

[88] Based on Sakamoto-Momiyama (1977) 67 fig. 4.8.

early Roman period.[89] Thus, at any rate well into the nineteenth century and to a large extent up to the late 1940s (when life expectancy finally began to increase steadily), there are no grounds for relating changes in seasonality to social, economic and medical developments.

Before the rise of modern science, mortality patterns would change independently of human behaviour.[90] We may assume, for instance, that the summer peak of deaths, strongly centred on August, in London and other parts of England in the sixteenth and seventeenth centuries disappeared around 1700, only to be replaced by a much broader 'cold winter plateau' from November to April, because of the weakening of dysentery and gastro-enteritis—yet we cannot tell for sure how the latter was brought about. In the absence of clear evidence of human intervention, climatic change and/or a change of pathogen have been regarded as the most promising explanations.[91] Other populations experienced comparable changes, the causes of which remain obscure.[92]

Pathogens constantly change due to mutation and the introduction of new strains from abroad. Recent western examples include fluctuations in smallpox mortality before the 1780s, some kind of streptococcal infection known as 'putrid sore throat' in the eighteenth century, and short-lived periods of scarlet fever in the early nineteenth century.[93] New fatal infections repeatedly became endemic for limited periods of time, thereby subjecting regional mortality patterns to sometimes significant changes. Plague is only the most notorious of these diseases; smallpox, the spread of louse-borne typhus in eighteenth-century Europe, the cholera epidemics emanating from India from the late eighteenth century onward, and diphtheria also come to mind. Egypt, at the crossroads of two continents and linked by the Nile to central Africa, the cradle of major infections, was continually exposed to novel pathogens. A high population density,

[89] For a comparative assessment of Roman and nineteenth-century Egypt, see below, Chapter 3.

[90] In some cases, of course, human action would indirectly affect the mortality regime. The proliferation of density-dependent infections facilitated by the spread of agriculture and then urbanisation is the most conspicuous example.

[91] Landers and Mouzas (1988) 76–7; Landers (1993) 205, 226–7, 239–40.

[92] For a similar shift from a summer peak to a winter peak in seventeenth- and eighteenth-century Geneva, caused by the decline of smallpox, see Perrenoud (1979) 429–30. In the first half of the seventeenth century, an early autumnal mortality peak that is missing in later evidence is documented for Podesteria di Lorea in the Venetian Dogate: Scheidel (1996a) 146 fig. 4.11 (malaria is a possible cause).

[93] Landers (1993) 240.

the result of the unusual fertility of the soil, must have helped new arrivals gain a foothold.

Long-term shifts in disease patterns create a major obstacle to any study of causes of death in populations that existed one or two thousand years ago and failed to produce pertinent statistics or even impressionist assessments. Moreover, climatic conditions, which influence the force and seasonal incidence of diseases, are also subject to long-term change.[94] Today, Egypt is an arid country with only trace rainfall from the southern border to just south of Cairo, limited rainfall in the Delta, and up to 200 mm in a narrow strip along the Mediterranean coast. It seems reasonable to expect similar conditions to have prevailed in antiquity.[95] This assumption, however, conflicts with meteorological data for Alexandria (or Lower Egypt) recorded in the second book of *Phaseis*, a compilation attributed to Claudius Ptolemaeus which thus apparently dates from the first half of the second century CE. According to this work, the winds mostly blew from the south, west and north-west. A comparable distribution is suggested by al-Biruni's survey (*c.* 1000 CE) of ancient sources for the Egyptian climate. This evidence is strongly at variance with data for modern Alexandria which document a prevalence of winds from the north, north-west and north-east. The seasonal incidence of winds reported by Ptolemy and al-Biruni is similarly erratic, with

[94] See especially Lamb (1977). Lamb (1995) provides a more recent synthesis. Cf. also Brown (1995). Sallares (1995) *inter alia* discusses climatic change in antiquity. A comprehensive assessment of the climate of ancient Egypt remains a desideratum. Modern research has focused on the climate of Egypt and the desert west of the country in the predynastic period. Hassan (1986b) traces climatic fluctuations in the Western Desert of Egypt since 8,300 BCE; see also Hassan (1988); Brewer (1991). For the Sahara, see Shaw (1981); Muzzolini (1985), esp. 13 fig. 1 (humidity fluctuations since 20,000 BCE); Casini (1990/91). Fayum: Ginter and Kozlowski (1986). For a brief survey of the ecology of the Nile valley during the past 10,000 years, see Raikes and Palmieri (1972). Prusakov (1997) discusses sand-drift in dynastic Egypt.

[95] In historical times, Egypt has always been arid; episodes of slightly greater rainfall than at present (such as under the Roman empire: Hassan (1986a) 65 tab. 1; see also Muzzolini (1985) 23) did little to alter this structural condition: Hassan (1988) 146. Mean temperatures in Roman Egypt were probably at least as high as today: low air temperatures appear to be correlated with low Nile floods and low rainfall in the Western Desert (Brewer (1991) 299), and during much of the Roman period, humidity and flood levels seem to have been *relatively* high (for humidity, see the preceding references; for floods, see below, n. 103). According to Burns and Denness (1985) 220 fig. 13.11, 222 (followed by Laronde (1989) 129), temperatures in Tripolitania increased from around 200 BCE and peaked from the first to the mid-third centuries CE at 1–1.5°C above current levels. In the Near East, a cool phase preceded the Roman period: Neumann and Parpola (1987) 162.

frequent west winds during the summer months which now very rarely occur in that season.[96] Their references to precipitation are even more problematic (Table 1.11).

Table 1.11 Monthly distribution of reported raindays at Alexandria according to Ptolemy and al-Biruni, and at present (in per cent)[97]

	J	F	M	A	M	J	J	A	S	O	N	D
Ptolemy	13	10	–	17	10	3	7	–	10	13	10	7
al-Biruni	9	6	3	22	19	6	–	–	6	3	13	13
Present	26	14	12	2	2	–	–	–	–	2	17	24

If we were to believe the ancient reports, between one-third and one-half of the annual raindays would have fallen into the period from April to July, which is currently characterised by negligible levels of precipitation. These rainfalls would have coincided with winds from the west, south-west and south. This scenario is implausible for several reasons. Most of the annual precipitation in the eastern Mediterranean, including Alexandria, is caused by a relatively small number of winter cyclones. Recent computer simulations have shown that even significant shifts in the mean temperature would merely result in a limited amount of redistribution of regional rainfall.[98] The alleged frequent presence of rain-bearing winds at a different time

[96] Hellmann (1916) remains the fundamental discussion of the Egyptian weather records in *Phaseis*. Ancient and modern winds: ibid., 335–6. The ancient 'Egyptian' references in al-Biruni's *Chronology* are broadly similar to the evidence of *Phaseis* but frequently differ in points of detail (see Oliver (1991) 441–2). Oliver (1991) 449 fig. 6 compares the percentages of winds from cardinal directions in Alexandria as reported by Ptolemy, al-Biruni and at present (north: 16/14/67, east: 3/6/13, south: 44/35/10, west: 37/45/10). By contrast, Ptolemy's account of storms tends to fit the modern pattern: Hellmann, 336–7.

[97] Based on Oliver (1991) 448 tab. III. Because *Phaseis* records specifics for only 171 days and al-Biruni for 155 days of the year, the monthly incidence has been expressed as a percentage of the total annual number of raindays.

[98] Segal *et al.* (1994) model the effects of a doubling of current levels of CO_2 in the atmosphere (and the concurrent rise of the temperature) on precipitation in the eastern Mediterranean: in two of three scenarios, Alexandria receives somewhat less rain than today, and a bit more in the third. The properties of these cyclones appear to have varied in historical time: their temporary failure to penetrate Greater Syria may have affected the climate in eleventh-century BCE Mesopotamia (Neumann and Parpola (1987)). According to an earlier more general model, global warming might lead to an increase in precipitation in certain parts of the world, including Egypt: Wigley, Jones and Kelly (1980) 20 fig. 2; this, however, is of little relevance for the country south of the Delta.

of the year could only be explained with reference to considerable differences between the ancient and modern climates of the entire Mediterranean.[99] No compelling independent evidence of such discrepancies has so far come to light; instead, recent studies tend to emphasise broad climatic similarities between the ancient and the contemporary Near East.[100] What is more, a comparison of the detailed descriptions of Mediterranean winds given by Aristotle and Theophrastus in the second half of the fourth century BCE with modern conditions supports the conclusion that 'the winds of classical antiquity were essentially the same as they are today'.[101] It therefore seems unwise to put too much faith in the reliability of *Phaseis* and similar compilations from antiquity.[102] There is no good reason to believe that the climate of ancient Egypt south of the littoral, and

---

[99] For clouds from the south to bring rain to Alexandria, they would need to travel from Ethiopia all across Sudan and Egypt: this is most unlikely, despite the fact that up to 3000 BCE, the monsoon rains appear to have extended farther north than at present; the last great northward penetration of the monsoon which produced a rainy season in Nubia is recorded for 683 BCE (Lamb (1977) 619). Alexandria is well outside the possible remit of any such phenomenon. Rain from the south-west, i.e., the Libyan desert, is equally improbable. Oliver (1991) 451 notes that a more southerly extension of upper air westerlies would indicate a cooler climate in Europe: this is incompatible with the view that its climate was *at least* as warm in Roman times as at present (see Sallares (forthcoming), and in the next footnote).

[100] Wagstaff (1985) 220–1 doubts any progressive desiccation of the region after late antiquity, and thinks that the period from 400 to 700/800 CE may have been drier than before. Rubin (1989) 76–7 also favours the view that in the late antique Negev, rainfall was not necessarily higher than it is now. However, Issar and Yakir (1997) now maintain that Roman Palestine was cooler and more humid than at present. See Neumann (1991) 461 for the view that under the early Roman empire, the Black Sea region was slightly warmer than today, and in general Lamb (1995) 157.

[101] Murray (1987), based on Aristoteles, *Meteorologica* 2 and Theophrastus, *De Ventis*. He finds a 'good' fit between ancient and modern data for the south-western corner of the Mediterranean Sea north of Egypt (30–35°N, 30–35°E): 152–3. In general, the goodness of fit improves as one moves from Gibraltar to the eastern Mediterranean, and peaks for mainland Greece, which suggests that apparent local differences are a function of deficient information rather than pointers to intervening change (156). It is interesting to note, however, that the ancient observers commonly reckon with a higher incidence of southerly winds than documented today (158). This finding is consistent with the ancient Egyptian data (which are not considered by Murray, who speculates that either the climate did change or the ancient philosophers felt a need to balance the existing north winds with spurious south winds).

[102] Hellmann (1916) 333, 339–40 comments on the various shortcomings of these sources. The Egyptian calendar of Antiochos (*c.* 200 CE), for instance, reckons with no fewer than nineteen unspecified changes in the weather from May to September, whereas today, almost continuous heat and dryness are typical of these months (ibid., 340–1). Computer simulations may show whether the ancient data can be related to any meaningful climatic pattern.

in particular that of the Nile valley, the main source of our demographic evidence, was substantially different from today's.

The mean flood levels of the Nile could vary considerably within a span of not more than a few centuries.[103] For the purposes of our study, it is, however, reassuring that the overall timing of the inundation appears to have been constant for millennia. Starting at the time of the summer solstice, the rise continued until the river began to overflow in mid-August in Upper Egypt and a few weeks later in the North, and peaked in September. The floods receded during the autumn, although some fields were not free from water until December.[104] The modern dam projects at Aswan were the first to interfere with this pattern.

Climatic variation is instrumental in creating seasonal patterns of disease and death. The main factors determining the transmission of infections are precipitation and temperature. They affect disease by way of the breeding of vectors and the survival and proliferation rate of pathogenic organisms in the environment.[105] Other agents that are involved in the shaping of the seasonal death rate are immaterial in the specific context of the Egyptian evidence. Seasonal malnutrition, which may affect mortality by increasing susceptibility to infections, cannot have played a significant role in the lives of individuals who were able to afford tombstones or embalmment.[106] The impact of seasonal variation in the birth rate on the incidence of deaths is invisible in samples that conceal neonatal mortality.[107] As

---

[103] The history of flood levels has been studied by Popper (1951) and Said (1993) 127–69. Cf. also Hassan (1988) 143 for the sixth millennium BCE, and in general (1981b). These fluctuations are caused by long-term variation in the monsoon rains in East Africa, which are not unusual and can still be observed today: e.g., Nicholson (1981); Conway and Hulme (1993). Flood levels in the (early) Roman period seem to have been relatively high (thus Said (1993) 152–5), although owing to the lack of serial quantitative data some uncertainty remains (Lamb (1977) 140). The eighth to eleventh centuries registered a low, especially during the first half of that period: Popper (1951) 182 graph 5; cf. Said (1993) 162. Lamb (1977) 425–6 and 426 fig. 17.1 reckons with low levels beginning with the fourth century, and observes correlations between flood levels of the Nile and water levels in Central African lakes (also 470).

[104] See, e.g., Palanque (1903) 20 (onset of inundation in antiquity); Bagnall (1993) 21; Khattab (1982) 60, 63, 65 (late Middle Ages); Antes (1801) 62–109, esp. 78, 81.

[105] For a survey of the seasonal ecology of disease, see Chambers, Longhurst and Pacey, eds. (1981) 102–34.

[106] Various contributions to Chambers, Longhurst and Pacey, eds. (1981) deal with the seasonality of rural poverty in the developing world. See above, pp. 34–5.

[107] Seasonal birthing patterns in ancient populations are discussed by Shaw (2001).

we have seen, seasonal mortality variation is also an age-specific phenomenon. Under conditions of low life expectancy, the probability of dying of infectious diseases is highest at the youngest ages; hence, variation in the monthly distribution of deaths is most pronounced very early in life. A strong seasonal prevalence of a different set of causes of death at higher ages may result in a bimodal distribution, as for instance in early modern London where a 'child peak' caused by water- and food-borne infections went together with a 'winter peak' of respiratory diseases.[108] As a general rule, it is for the most part in childhood that (endemic) infectious agents are first encountered, and hence it is children who bear the heaviest burden of infectious disease. That some diseases are more likely than others to affect the seasonal pattern of mortality is well brought out by the comparison of all deaths to deaths of 'fevers' in Tendernden in Kent from 1712 to 1742 undertaken by Mary Dobson. In this case, seasonal variation for all 'fevers' (110 index points) is twice as high as for all causes combined (fifty-five points). About thirty per cent of identified causes of death were listed as 'fevers'.[109] In the absence of these 'fevers', seasonal variation overall would have been much weaker. These two examples help define the focus of the present study. Thus, with regard to ancient Egypt, we need to identify diseases which—or the lethal effects of which—were largely confined to a particular part of the year and which struck down adults as regularly as other afflictions (or the same ones?) would dispose of small children. A sophisticated analysis of the link between seasonal mortality and causes of death in the mould of Landers' study of early modern London, for instance, is obviously well beyond our reach.[110] Instead, I will attempt to interpret the attested seasonality patterns in the multiple context of written and material evidence from antiquity, medical descriptions and statistical data from early modern Egypt, and comparative material from other populations.

3.2. *Disease and climate in Egypt: the pre-modern tradition*

In the fifth century BCE, Herodotus, who may or may not have visited the country, declared that

[108] Landers (1993) 229 fig. 6.8.
[109] Dobson (1997) 251, 253 fig. 5.4, 255.
[110] Landers (1993) ch. 6 (202–41). See also Wrigley *et al.* (1997) 322–47.

> the Egyptians are the healthiest of men, next to the Libyans; the reason of which to my thinking is that the climate in all seasons is the same; for change is the great cause of men's falling sick, more especially changes of seasons (2.77).

Even by Herodotean standards, this would seem an extraordinary claim.[111] Of thirty-four adult skeletons excavated in Abydos in Upper Egypt, ranging from the twenty-first to the fourth centuries BCE, all but one exhibit evidence of disease, including degenerative, traumatic and infectious lesions, and all remains of children display extensive pathology.[112] Hyksos skeletons from the Delta provide ample documentation of extreme ill-health.[113] Papyrus letters from late antiquity betray great concern over various illnesses.[114] In 1599, Mustafa Ali observed that 'most of the people of Egypt are affected by some disease or ailing'.[115] A few years earlier, an Italian visitor to the country had elaborated on that theme: according to Prosper Alpinus, Egypt was rife with ocular inflammations, leprosy, elephantiasis, 'extremely frenzied deliriums' that killed within hours, smallpox among children, and many other afflictions including fevers and stomach disorders. What is more, he went out of his way to stress that while such diseases were also known to other peoples, they were nowhere as continually present as in Egypt: every year children would succumb to smallpox; 'numerous pestilential fevers' raged on an annual basis, and 'innumerable people were afflicted and tormented by stomach disorders'. All these diseases also occurred in epidemic form.[116] Throughout the following centuries, western observers concurred.[117] Looking back in 1799, Sonnini acknowledged that 'the climate of Egypt has long been deemed the focus of the most dreadful maladies'.[118]

---

[111] As Lloyd (1976) 332 puts it in his extensive commentary of Herodotus' description of Egypt, 'the appalling condition of native health in Egypt today excites considerable astonishment at this statement'.

[112] Baker, Kealhofer and Richards (1989) (seven children, twenty-seven adults).

[113] Winkler and Wilfing (1991) found an extremely high degree of deficiency diseases and anemic states caused by periodical malnutrition, attacks by parasites and infectious diseases. The osteological sample suggests a mean life expectancy at birth of 18.6 years (n = 247).

[114] Barrett-Lennard (1987) 247–50, with Bagnall (1993) 185–6. See also *O.Claud.* 174, 222–3.

[115] Tietze (1975) 42.

[116] Alpin (1980) 87–9 (bk. I, p. 50). Alpinus' work on the medicine of the Egyptians, based on his stay in the country from 1581 to 1584, provides an invaluable survey of health conditions in pre-modern Egypt.

[117] E.g., Volney (1788) 240–58 (ch. 17: 'On the diseases of Egypt').

[118] Sonnini (1799) 15. His own disagreement with this view flies in the face of

After their invasion of Egypt, the French founded a journal called *La décade égyptienne*. While the first issue of this 'journal littéraire et d'économie politique', published in 1799, was given over to the study of antiquities and literature, the next year's articles reveal a telling preoccupation with a host of local diseases, among which diarrhoeal conditions loom large. Reality had swiftly caught up with an idealised vision of the country. Following in Napoleon's footsteps, the British army inevitably made the same discovery: 'In no country are the inhabitants afflicted with more dreadful disorders, many of which must be attributed to the vices of the people, yet the most fatal unhappily proceed from causes which civilization and art cannot altogether controul [*sic*].'[119]

The Hippocratic writers prove a more trustworthy guide than Herodotus: the treatise on *Airs, Waters and Places* correctly maintains that the inhabitants of hot regions commonly suffer from diarrhoeas, dysentery, convulsions and eye infections. Egypt is a classic case. The allegedly aseasonal character of its climate was not quite as obvious to other ancient observers: Marcus Diaconus, in his biography of Porphyry, contrasts conditions in Egypt with those in Palestine where the temperature differed more between day and night than between seasons.[120] In fact, temperatures in Egypt today vary greatly between the winter and summer: from 11–20°C (January) to 23–30°C (July) in Alexandria, from 8–16°C degrees (January) to 21–36°C (July) in Cairo, and from 10–23°C (January) to 26–41°C (July) in Aswan. Paradoxically, Egypt was well suited to confirm Herodotus' belief that climatic change was associated with health hazards. The epigraphic evidence of seasonal mortality variation can be supplemented by the accounts of travellers to Egypt who for centuries have drawn attention to the characteristic patterns. In the 1580s, Prosper Alpinus noticed that the dry hot season from March to May caused a great

---

overwhelming evidence to the contrary: his claim that violent fevers and malaria were unknown in Egypt (19) verges on the bizarre, but needs to be seen as a propagandistic effort to justify France's involvement in that country. Wilson (1803) 252 noted that Sonnini was partial. Echoes of this debate can still be found in Frank (1820), who called Egypt one of the healthiest regions in the world (4 [—incidentally the very page where he averred that Egyptian smallpox spared hardly one in ten thousand!]), and contrasted it with the malarial desolation of the Pontine Marshes and Latium (37).

[119] Wilson (1803) 252.

[120] *Vita Porphyrii* 4. Ancient Egyptian medical texts show some awareness of the seasonal prevalence of certain diseases: Lloyd (1976) 333.

expansion of 'many epidemics and deadly diseases'. In that season, 'infernal winds' blew many into the arms of Charon; this was also the time of pestilential fevers and deliriums. The body was so weakened by the heat that it rejected nourishment and fought dehydration. By contrast, despite continuing heat, the summer months were said to be healthy and free of disease, as were the months of September and October.[121] Jean Coppin, in the mid-seventeenth century, declared the *khamseen* season to be the worst time of the year, when large numbers of people were known to die.[122] Around 1800, according to French sources, various fevers and dysenteries abounded in hot weather. 'The spring, which in Egypt is the summer of our climates, brings with it malignant fevers, which soon arrive at a crisis.'[123] These accounts mainly focused on the northern confines of Upper Egypt in the Cairo area. The inhabitants of the Nile valley were said to suffer more under the *khamseen* than the people of the Delta: 'a son apparition, (. . .) on éprouve un malaise general, une prostration complete, souvent suivie d'ophthalmie, ce cephalalgie, d'apoplexie, de dysenterie aigue; sous l'influence de ces vent funeste, l'état des malades s'aggrave, et, s'il régne une épidémie, la mortalité s'accroît dans des proportions sensibles.'[124] Yates called this 'the sickly season in Egypt', when the hots winds were 'exciting the most malignant diseases, and generating swarms of insects'.[125] Conversely, Richard Pococke, presumably with reference to Lower Egypt, stated in 1740 that 'the most unhealthy time is when the perspiration is stopped by the cold'.[126]

References such as these to the hazards of the spring in the Nile valley and the effect of the cold farther north appear to tally well with the seasonal mortality patterns of ancient sites. For our present

[121] Alpin (1980) 41–2, 44 (bk. I, pp. 22–4).

[122] *Voyages* (1971) 295: 'C'est alors qu'ils sont attaquez de beaucoup de maladies & souvent de la peste, & principalement quand leur Romadan vient à tomber dans cette saison, c'est une chose immanquable qu'il meurt une grande quantité de monde.'

[123] Barbès (1800) 203; Volney (1788) 251 (quote).

[124] Clot-Bey (1840) I 17. Frank (1820) 33 considered the months from March to May and from June to September the least healthy and the healthiest parts of the year, respectively.

[125] Yates (1843) 51 and 384. 'During this period, the whole atmosphere looks wild and lurid; the skin is hot, the tongue perched, the eyes suffused and bloodshot, the temples burn and throb, and the most distressing thirst is experienced—symptoms which are often the fore-runners of purulent ophthalmia, and of the most loathsome diseases' (51).

[126] Pococke (1743) 196.

purposes, medical information that predates the gradual opening of the country to European influences in the nineteenth century *a priori* deserves special attention. At the same time, the vague and prescientific nature of these early descriptions easily frustrates attempts to locate the underlying conditions within the framework of modern medical taxonomy. Moreover, the disease environment of ancient Egypt itself still awaits comprehensive examination.[127] Against this less than promising background, I will review evidence for each of the major diseases of Egypt in order to narrow the range of possible interpretations and specify the most likely causes behind the attested mortality profiles from antiquity.

3.3. *Diarrhoeal diseases*

'Diarrhoeal diseases' are an umbrella term for a variety of conditions.[128] They can be grouped with enteric fevers, i.e., typhoid and paratyphoid, which will be considered separately in the following section. Acute diarrhoeas include watery diarrhoeas caused by bacteria and bloody diarrhoeas, such as bacillary and amoebic dysentery. The symptoms caused by other agents, such as salmonella, are usually grouped under the general heading of food poisoning. Still other kinds of diarrhoeal diseases are caused by rotaviruses or arise from unknown causes. Diarrhoea developed with the growth of large sedentary societies, and is ultimately a socially induced disease whose origin is civilisation itself.

Although diarrhoeas can occur in all seasons, hot season epidemics are very common. While deaths are possible at all ages, fatal outcomes are most common among infants and young children. Deaths among adults are rare, but more frequent among the elderly. In past centuries, summer diarrhoea of infants was common in Britain as well as other countries.[129] To give but two examples, in Chicago in

---

[127] Pertinent studies include Sandison (1980); Harer (1993); Buikstra, Baker and Cook (1993). See also Andorlini Marcone (1993); Bagnall (1993) 184–8; Marganne-Mélard (1996); and cf. briefly Adamson (1982). Nunn (1996) 64–95, provides the most recent summary of modern research. Ostraca found on the Mons Claudianus site in the desert between the Nile and the Red Sea are the most recent addition to our knowledge of disease in Roman Egypt: see *O.Claud.* 83–118 and esp. 191–223, discussed by Cuvigny (1992, 1997). On diseases in the classical world in general, see Jackson (1988) 170–86; Grmek (1989); Sallares (1991) 221–93.

[128] For a brief survey, see Mata, Kromal and Villegas (1980).

[129] For Britain, see esp. Landers (1993) 208 tab. 6.2: from 1670 to 1679, death

the years from 1867 to 1895, between seventy-eight and ninety per cent of all deaths from diarrhoea were recorded from June to September, and in Japan in the 1890s and 1900s, the monthly incidence of mortality from gastro-enteric diseases varied strongly by 150 index points between January and August/September.[130] Summer diarrhoea of this kind is still common in developing countries. Studies in India have shown that diarrhoeas among adults follow a similar seasonal distribution to that among infants, and epidemics of infantile diarrhoea may be accompanied by infections among adults. This points to infections of adults who failed to acquire (lasting) immunity through exposure during childhood.[131] Food poisoning is primarily a disease of older children and adults, resulting from the contamination of foods with bacteria. This usually occurs during warm months, and we must assume that diarrhoea caused by the ingestion of contaminated food is very common in developing countries.

Dysentery is an inflammation of the large bowel with consequent passage of blood and mucus in the stools. Bacillary dysentery is caused by *Shigella* spp., the amoebic variety by *Entamoeba histolytica.* Modern treatment has greatly reduced the impact of dysenteries. For earlier times, a reference work of 1913 quotes a minimum fatality rate of twenty per cent. In the nineteenth century, mortality for bacillary dysentery may have been around thirty per cent, though figures from forty to sixty-five per cent are also reported. The most severe attacks of bacillary dysentery were due to *Shigella dysenteriae*, with fatality rates of up to fifty per cent.[132]

Diarrhoeal diseases must continually have been present in Egypt, and explicit references range over several centuries. In the late sixteenth century, Prosper Alpinus claimed that every year, 'innumerable people were afflicted and tormented by stomach disorders', which, in conjunction with his reference to 'numerous lethal pestilential fevers', points to a wide range of diarrhoeal diseases including enteric fevers. Back then, dysentery and 'bilious diarrhoea' were treated by bloodletting, as, incidentally, were many other diseases

---

from what contemporaries called 'griping in the guts' (probably bacillary dysentery) up to age two was heavily concentrated from July to September.

[130] Chicago: Sakamoto-Momiyama (1977) 66 fig. 4.7, 67; Japan: ibid., 21, 33 fig. 2.3. Cf. above, Fig. 1.38.

[131] Drasar, Tomkins and Feachem in Chambers, Longhurst and Pacey, eds. (1981) 105.

[132] Rogers (1913) 114–115, 284–5; Lancaster (1990) 74.

from smallpox to plague.[133] Father Gonzales, in the 1660s, listed local remedies for dysentery.[134] According to a member of the French forces, the months preceding and including August and September were characterised by diarrhoea and dysentery. The latter took the form of what was called gastritic fever and 'bilious fever', and could be worsened by concomitant malaria infections.[135] 'Bilious fevers' were also evoked by John Antes, who stated that 'putrid and bilious fevers were common in spring among some classes of people, particularly in May and June'.[136] Even the sanguine Sonnini referred to dysentery. References to the age-specific incidence of such diseases are usually missing. Only one French source reported that in Damietta in the Nile Delta, old people had died of dysentery. In 1820, Frank devoted considerable attention to Egyptian dysentery, a disease 'dangerous, difficult to cure and often lethal' which he considered second only to the plague.[137] Twenty years later, Clot-Bey likewise regarded dysentery as very common, more so in Lower than in Upper Egypt, and Hirsch later called the Nile valley from the Sudan up to the sea one of the most lethal areas of dysentery in Africa. It killed mostly in the months that followed outbreaks of plague, i.e., during the summer, and sometimes occurred as an epidemic. During a trip to the Thebaid, Yates encountered fevers and dysentery that killed thousands when hot winds raised the temperature above 30°C.[138] Pruner located annual the peaks of dysentery in the spring and the early autumn. In Alexandria in the 1860s, dysentery, gastritic fever and diarrhoea flourished from June to August. It was also endemic at the end of the summer, lasted throughout the fall, but never extended into the winter. At that time, dysentery was said greatly to ravage the whole country.[139] Three quarters of identified cases were bacillary, one-eighth amoebic. Amoebas were rare in small chil-

---

[133] Alpin (1980) 89 (bk. I, p. 50). Bloodletting: ibid., 185 (bk. III, p. 113) (dysentery and diarrhoea), 165 (bk. III, p. 95) (other diseases).

[134] *Voyage* (1977) (= 1673) 448, 457, 514, 533 (= bk. VI pp. 369, 374, 405, 416).

[135] Bruant (1800) 52–3.

[136] Antes (1801) 130. His peculiar claim that this season was nevertheless very healthy is clearly incompatible with the accounts given by other observers of his day.

[137] Sonnini (1799) 23; Savaresi (1800a) 89 (Damietta); Frank (1820) 179–223, at 192 and 181 ('morbus, post pestem maxime in Aegypto timendus, est dysenteria').

[138] Clot-Bey (1840) I 350; Hirsch (1886) 199; Yates (1843) 525–6. According to Pruner (1847) 212, dysentery was not particularly common on the coast but malignant and widespread from the upper Delta southwards.

[139] Pruner (1847) 214; Dikaios (1862) 501–02 (Alexandria); Schnepp (1862b) 562.

dren, who were heavily affected by bacilli.[140] At the beginning of the twentieth century, Craig studied the correlation between the death rate, humidity and temperature in Cairo and Alexandria. Mortality from dysentery in particular was found to peak a few weeks before the temperature maximum.[141] In the 1950s, a study of diarrhoea in a group of children in Egypt showed that more than ninety per cent had a *Shigella* infection during the year. Three seasonal peaks were observed, in the spring, late summer, and winter. According to a public health guide published in 1970, gastro-intestinal diseases were then still the most serious health hazard in Egypt. In rural areas, infantile diarrhoea accounted for more than half of infant deaths.[142]

Evidence from antiquity is meagre by comparison. Ancient Egyptian medical texts sometimes refer to diarrhoea, swollen belly, and pain in the anus.[143] A desire to 'cool the anus' may also be suggestive of violent diarrhoea.[144] Haematuria was 'probably' common in ancient Egypt.[145] Even so, diarrhoeal complications do not nearly play as important a role in the sources as one might expect. On the contrary, these writings reveal a much stronger interest in constipation.[146] This bias tells us more about the medical profession than about the actual prevalence of certain diseases in antiquity. There can be no doubt that in the ancient world, very much as in better documented underdeveloped societies of the past and present, diarrhoeal diseases were a leading cause of mortality in infancy and early childhood.[147] Even so, the extant medical treatises of the Greek and Roman periods paid scant attention to this problem; their Egyptian counterparts merely conformed to a general trend.[148]

---

[140] Jagailloux (1986) 260.

[141] Craig (1908), (1912), esp. 247.

[142] Higgins and Floyd (1955); *Area Handbook* (1970) 125.

[143] Manniche (1989) 73, 80–2, 86, 97, 103–4.

[144] It is conceivable, however, that the need to 'cool the anus' arose from painful schistosomiasis of the rectum: Nunn (1996) 69, 90–1. Haemorrhoids are another possibility: Kolta (1984) 163.

[145] Sandison (1980) 30.

[146] Leca (1971) 188–90; Nunn (1996) 90. The same is true for Coptic medicine: Worrell (1935) 36, 191; Till (1951) 24.

[147] Cf. Scheper-Hughes (1992) 314–15, 321–2, 366–8.

[148] Bertier (1996) and Hummel (1999) provide recent surveys. Aretaios showed some passing interest in infantile diarrhoeas (Hummel 224); Galen vol. 13, pp. 288–9 ed. Kühn refers to dysentery of children. Cf. also Plinius, *Naturalis Historia* 28.258. Two Coptic recipes mention anal discharge of blood (Till (1951) 25); cf. Worrell (1935) 192 for a possible reference to diarrhoea.

It is difficult to determine to which extent diarrhoeas and especially dysenteries posed a grave threat to adults in a pre-modern setting. Aretaios of Cappadocia ascribed diarrhoea to children up to puberty and dysentery to adults in the prime of life.[149] Accounts from before the late nineteenth century do not normally discuss the age-specific impact of these diseases. We can only assume that affections that were exclusively confined to infancy and early childhood would have been less likely to catch the eye of the occasional traveller than those which caused serious illness and deaths among grown men and women. Röser's statement in 1837 is a good example: he claimed that most of those Egyptians who suffered from acute and chronic diseases eventually succumbed to dysentery, which they contracted in addition to their existing conditions.[150] The assumption that diarrhoeal diseases also took their toll at more mature ages receives support from official statistics of causes of death from the third quarter of the nineteenth century. According to counts taken for 1859/60 and 1871, gastro-intestinal diseases reportedly caused around two-thirds of deaths in Cairo and slightly over half in Alexandria.[151] I will argue below (section 3.11) that if these classifications are anywhere near correct—and they are probably not very wide of the mark—, such diseases cannot have been confined to early childhood. Thus, a significant share of adult mortality would have been due to diarrhoeal diseases and related conditions, such as typhoid. By the 1920s, this picture had changed profoundly, possibly indicating a shift from an 'archaic' to a more 'advanced' disease environment in which adult mortality was dominated by pulmonary diseases. It therefore seems plausible that severe types of diarrhoea made a substantial contribution to seasonal mortality.

3.4. *Typhus, typhoid and relapsing fever*

Typhus and typhoid, albeit caused by different types of pathogens, were commonly conflated until the middle of the nineteenth century. Sandwith, in his standard work on the diseases of Egypt pub-

---

[149] Aretaios 4.9.15 (cf. 4.7.5). Celsus, *De Medicina* 2.8.30, states that diarrhoeal disease 'carries off mostly children up to the age of ten; other ages bear it more easily'. Pregnant women were also thought to be at risk.

[150] Röser (1837) 24. Cf. Frank (1820) 183 for its interaction with hepatitis.

[151] Based on Schnepp (1862b) 552–3 and Panzac (1982) 89 tab. 7 (1871). Cf. Pruner (1847) 217–23 for some fatal cases of dysentery among adults (although admittedly all of them foreigners).

lished in 1905, noted that until recently, different types of afflictions, which he called typhus, relapsing fevers, enteric and 'bilious' fevers, had been collapsed under the heading of 'typhoid fever'.[152] This confusion in early modern accounts makes it necessary to discuss these and related diseases in the same section. Epidemic louse-borne typhus is caused by *Rickettsia prowazeki* and invariably transmitted by the louse, *Pediculus corporis*. The disease, which attacks the blood capillaries in particular and causes rashes and spots (hence 'spotted fever'), headache, mental dullness, extreme weakness and sometimes delirium followed by stupor, coma and death, is not reliably attested prior to the twelfth century. There is a marked gradient in case fatality rates, varying from less than five per cent under age twenty to fifty per cent at age fifty and almost 100 per cent over sixty.[153] Endemic flea-borne typhus, or murine typhus, caused by *R. mooseri*, is currently endemic in Egypt. It is a disease of rats passed on to humans by the rat flea, *Xenopsylla cheopis*. Fatality rates are low, usually less than one per cent.[154]

Typhus has been described in Egypt since the sixteenth century. The last pandemic dates from 1815. In 1905, it was said that typhus could exist in any part of Egypt or Sudan during the spring months. In Alexandria and Cairo, deaths from typhus peaked from March to August. In keeping with its general properties, the disease struck and killed mainly adults aged twenty to fifty, and always spared children under the age of five. Sandwith associated the disease with overcrowding, deficient ventilation in the preceding winter, uncleanliness, faulty food conservation, and malnutrition.[155] From 1887 to 1900, 18,000 deaths from typhus were reported in Egypt; the actual tally remains unknown. The (recorded) death rate fell from half of all cases in the first decade of the twentieth century to one-quarter in the 1910s.[156]

In terms of its age distribution and seasonal incidence, typhus is readily consistent with the ancient mortality profile of Upper Egypt

---

152 Sandwith (1905) 16. See also Lancaster (1990) 160. For 'typhus' in Egyptian folk medicine, see Jagailloux (1996) 159.

153 Zinsser (1935) 215; Lancaster (1990) 160.

154 Lancaster (1990) 163.

155 Sandwith (1905) 17–19. According to Hirsch (1881) 401, typhus was well attested for nineteenth-century Egypt and Nubia. Wilson (1803) 263 comments on the abundance of lice in Egypt. For a link between rampant typhus and extreme filth, compare, e.g., Cooper (1965) 196–7.

156 Jagailloux (1986) 237–8. The *Infectious diseases handbook* (1922) 6 gives a thirty per cent death rate for 'typhus fever' in Egypt.

and Nubia. A disease that peaked from March to August, focused on adults from ages twenty to fifty and killed half of those infected might well have helped skew the seasonal distribution of deaths in the observed fashion. However, this possible interpretation faces serious obstacles. It is far from clear whether louse-borne typhus, which occurs in epidemic outbreaks and is frequently associated with conditions of severe disorder or deprivation, such as war or internment, could have been sufficiently powerful and widespread to leave a strong mark on the seasonal mortality pattern throughout the Nile valley (biased as our samples may be in favour of urban and monastic communities) over the course of a whole millennium. In this case, its apparent absence from the documented sites in Lower Egypt would also require explanation. An even greater problem arises from the fact that typhus is not identified in ancient sources. As long as we cannot even confirm the mere existence of typhus in antiquity, it is surely inadvisable to consider this disease a major killer in ancient and early medieval Upper Egypt and Nubia.

Typhoid is caused by *Salmonella typhi*, paratyphoid fevers by germs of the same genus (*S. paratyphi*). Typhoid is characterised by a protracted, debilitating febrile illness. The disease is acquired by ingestion of food or water that has been contaminated by a human who has acute disease, is recently convalescent, or is an asymptomatic chronic fecal shedder of typhoid bacilli. Contaminated water and milk are major sources of transmission of typhoid fever while paratyphoid preferably travels through food. Typhoid, however, is not only waterborne, and under conditions of primitive hygiene, direct personal transmission of infection may play an important role. Most deaths are caused by intestinal hemorrhage or perforation, which occur after about two weeks of untreated disease.

In countries where typhoid is still endemic, most cases occur in the hot season. Historically, the age group from fifteen to thirty was often particularly severely struck by typhoid.[157] In areas of low hygiene in developing countries throughout Asia and Africa, typhoid has been endemic, affecting most commonly people between ages five and thirty, while being rare under age two and over age fifty.[158] In such areas, the highest attack rate is now found from ages eight to thirteen.[159] In the early nineteenth century, typhoid fever could be as

[157] Biraben (1988) 438.
[158] Huckstep (1962) 49.
[159] Hornick (1982) 667.

lethal as smallpox, measles and scarlet fever. Prior to antibiotic treatment, case death rates ran from twelve to thirty per cent.[160] While figures of up to thirty or forty per cent are mentioned, death rates of eighteen to twenty per cent were reported as common for the nineteenth century. By the end of the nineteenth century in Germany, they had fallen to about nine to fourteen per cent.[161] In Sweden, from 1751 to 1830, on average 10.4 per cent of all deaths were attributed to typhus and typhoid fevers. In England and Wales from 1871 to 1880, typhoid accounted for 5.6 per cent of all deaths at ages fifteen to nineteen; mortality peaked from ages fifteen to twenty-four.[162] In earlier periods and in warmer climatic settings, the respective rates may have been considerably higher.

In 1861, Schnepp produced a study to the effect that various 'fevers', including 'typhus abdominal' (= typhoid) and 'typhoide bilieuse' (= relapsing fever), continued to spread through Egypt.[163] In that country, according to Sandwith, typhoid (which he refers to as 'enteric fever') found young adults most susceptible. Most fatalities occurred under the age of twenty-five. In Cairo, the disease thrived from October to March. This was somewhat atypical in that the hottest months were often the most favourable for this condition; it was, however, also prevalent in April and May. No global information on mortality seems to be available. Sandwith reported that seven of his ninety-one patients had died despite treatment, and estimated that three-quarters of all cases would recover without treatment.[164] The implied fatality rate of about twenty-five per cent for untreated typhoid is in line with other figures for the nineteenth century cited above. In the early twentieth century, reported cases of typhoid were associated with even higher mortality: between thirty and eighty per cent of the patients died.[165] In recent decades, Egypt was still a major

---

160 Ibid., 660.

161 Curschmann (1902) 382–3. See also Hirsch (1881) 441 (very high case fatality rates among British troops in India); Lancaster (1990) 71 (rates of eleven to seventeen per cent in the early twentieth century).

162 Sweden: Lancaster (1990) 404. England and Wales: ibid., 72 with tab. 6.5.1.

163 Schnepp (1862b) 527–8, with 527 n. 1. Antes (1801) 130 states that 'putrid and bilious fevers were common in spring among some classes of people, particularly in May and June'; this may be a reference to typhoid and relapsing fever. Volney's assertion that in the spring, eggs were 'a sort of poison in Egypt' ((1788) 251–2), points to food-poisoning and *Salmonella* infection. In 1840, the plague was preceded by 'abdominal typhus', i.e., typhoid, presumably around March.

164 Sandwith (1905) 49–87, esp. 52–3, 55, 68, 81.

165 Jagailloux (1986) 239–40. See also the *Infectious diseases handbook* (1922) 6 (thirty per cent death rate for 'typhus fever').

area of enteric fevers. In the early 1950s, typhoid and dysentery prevailed in the hot season.[166] Typhoid and paratyphoid continued to be endemic in all parts of the country, affecting not only children but also adults.[167]

Typhoid was known to ancient medicine,[168] and there can be no doubt that it was at least as common in ancient Egypt as in the more recent past. The fact that in the absence of modern public-health measures, communities which draw water from rivers have the highest rates of typhoid mortality, followed by those supplied by lakes, is of great relevance to the situation in Egypt.[169] Pollution levels in the river Nile itself are not the main issue.[170] Most Egyptians obtained their water not directly from the shore of the Nile but via canals, wells and cisterns. These primitive supply systems were particularly vulnerable to contamination. Again, the Fayum stands out because of its dependence on lake water and Nile water that had to be conveyed over a considerable distance in order to reach consumers. In fact, observers in periods as far apart as the thirteenth and the end of the nineteenth centuries were well aware of the health hazards inherent in the water supply of the Fayum.[171] The risk of contamination and infection must have peaked when the water levels were at their lowest, during the spring months prior to the onset of the inundation in late June.[172]

---

[166] Sakamoto-Momiyama (1977) 39.

[167] Huckstep (1962) 12 (for 1957); *Area Handbook* (1970) 125 ('acute gastroenteritis is widespread among the adult population').

[168] Grmek (1989) 89. An exceptionally meticulous case history in the Hippocratic Corpus deals with the death of a young woman from typhoid: Hippocrates, *Epidemics* 7.2 (vol. 5, pp. 382–6 ed. Littré), in Grmek (1989) 346–7.

[169] Lancaster (1990) 72. By the 1890s, the British had installed slow sand filters in Cairo to clear drinking waters of *Escherichia coli*: Curtin (1989) 119. This procedure reduced the number of microbes to not more than 100 per cubic centimetre, down from far larger amounts (250,000/cm^3 are attested for Calcutta in 1903).

[170] Rufus of Ephesus correctly praised the suitability of the Nile as a source of drinking water; however, his authority is undermined by his bizarre claim that *all* other rivers and lakes provided 'bad' water (in Oribasius, *Collectiones medicae* 5.3.6, *CMG* 6.1.1). Cf. Galen vol. 9, p. 389 ed. Kühn.

[171] In the thirteenth century, Nabulsi noted that the drinking water of the Fayum constantly mixed with the water of marshes and infiltration water: Zeki (1898) 268. Zeki himself described conditions in the city of Fayum in his own day thus: 'Les habitants de la basse classe buvaient l'eau même du canal où se déversaient tous les immondices de la ville. Les classes aisées se servaient d'eau de puits; malheureusement chaque puits était voisin de fosses d'aisances qui le contaminaient de pernicieuses infiltrations' (ibid., 282).

[172] John Campbell noticed that 'ordinary peasants (...) in the Summer Months

The attested prevalence of typhoid from October to May a century ago is consistent with the seasonal amplitudes for both Lower and Upper Egypt in antiquity. With its high fatality rates and concentration of cases under age thirty, the disease would have contributed to the documented distributions. Its effects must regularly have been exacerbated by its interaction with other infections. Thus, typhoid often concurs with bacillary dysentery.[173] Malaria may suppress some immune responses to unrelated pathogens, including salmonella infections.[174] In fact, typhoid and dysentery were generally found to be common in malarial areas in England and other European countries.[175] In the nineteenth century, this association prompted the invention of the phantom disease of 'typhomalarial fever', which often resulted from a misdiagnosis of typhoid.[176] That the combination of malaria, typhoid and other intestinal infections could have an impact on mortality rates at mature ages is illustrated by the example of Ravenna where at the end of the seventeenth century, these diseases (subsumed under the headings 'febbre' and 'febbre maligna') accounted for most recorded causes of death among adults and helped produce a mortality peak in October.[177]

In Egypt, typhoid infections would also coincide with outbreaks of relapsing fever. Louse-borne relapsing fever is caused by *Borrelia recurrentis*, and humans are its only host. Originally likewise confused

when the *Nile* is low, are constrained to use other water, which is not only unwholesome by Comparison with the *Nile*, but perhaps the most unwholesome in the World' ([Campbell] (1739) 402); his reference to low water levels is more consistent with the conditions in the late spring. In the early twentieth century, however, the number of *E. coli* bacilli in the Nile was found to be largest while the river was rising and before it had reached its maximum, i.e., in the early summer: Craig (1912) 250. Theophrastus, fr. 214A ed. Fortenbaugh, suggests a link between low water levels of the Nile and disease. One wonders what to make of a description given by Antes (1801) 91, presumably with reference to Cairo: 'From the beginning of March to the middle of June the river contains a vast quantity of little worms about one-fourth or one-third of an inch long, particularly near the shore; but they are quite inoffensive, even if drunk in great quantities with the water.'

[173] Curschmann (1902) 205. For other coincident diseases, see Huckstep (1962) 205–10.

[174] Gilles and Warrell (1993) 75. See also the references in Salmon (1992) 552 n. 51.

[175] Dobson (1997) 336, with reference to James (1920) 162, and also Whitley (1864) 452, as quoted by Dobson (1997) 335, on the co-existence of typhoid and malaria in England. See Smith (1982) 213, 305 (but cf. 319), on America.

[176] This pseudo-disease is discussed by Smith (1982); see esp. 182, 309, 317–18. Cf. Sallares (forthcoming).

[177] Bolognesi (1980) 271.

with typhus (and thus known in French as 'typhus bilieux' or 'typhus recurrent'), in about half of all cases it is accompanied by jaundice. The case fatality rate stands at five per cent but can rise as high as seventy per cent under crisis conditions such as war or famine. Tick-borne relapsing fever is caused by various species of *Borrelia* organisms and transmitted by ticks of the genus *Ornithodorus*. Fever is higher than in the louse-borne variety and paralysis occurs more often.[178] During the siege of Cairo in 1800, 260 of 600 infected French soldiers died.[179] Sandwith stated that around 1900, relapsing fever was more common in Lower Egypt because of its high population density and overcrowding in houses during the winter, and located the disease among the 'poorest natives'. In the same way as typhus, it never struck persons under the age of five or over the age of fifty. Epidemics occurred from February to May. Mortality varied greatly, but could be in excess of ten per cent.[180] In the early twentieth century, relapsing fever was also common among the poor of Upper Egypt. Death rates of six to eleven per cent were observed. An outbreak in Egypt in the 1940s affected more than 100,000 people.[181]

Infectious jaundice (Hepatitis A and B) was sometimes epidemic in the summer. Cases were concentrated from ages twenty to thirty, but also ranged from fifteen to forty. In Alexandria, the disease occurred from April to October, or in two peaks from May and June and from September to October. Observed mortality varied from ten to sixty per cent in localised outbreaks: 'The death rate is highest in the spring at the beginning of an explosion, and lowest in summer when the epidemic is waning.'[182] Given the seasonal characteristics of relapsing fever and infectious jaundice, a high incidence of these diseases is fully compatible with the mortality pattern for ancient Upper Egypt and Nubia.

The strongest evidence of the impact of typhoid and related conditions on the seasonal mortality distribution in Egypt comes from

---

178 Lancaster (1990) 183–4.

179 Jagailloux (1986) 238.

180 Sandwith (1905) 33–48, esp. 36. Mortality: ibid., 43, with reference to epidemic death rates of eighteen per cent in India and fifteen per cent in St Petersburg (1865). With reference to Egypt, the *Infectious diseases handbook* (1922) 6 puts mortality at ten per cent.

181 Jagailloux (1986) 239 (early 1900s); Lancaster (1990) 185 (1940s).

182 Sandwith (1905) 100–14, esp. 100, 102–03, 108 (quote). Coptic medicine was acquainted with jaundice: Kolta (1984) 159.

Schnepp's tabulation of reported causes of death in Cairo and Alexandria within a twelve-month period from July 1859 to June 1860. The monthly incidence of the three leading 'causes' has been plotted in Figures 1.39 and 1.40.[183]

Unfortunately, the classification could hardly be more vague: 'convulsions' in particular are a mere symptom, not a disease, and we must wonder to what extent the actual causes of death were or could be identified. We will return to this breakdown in section 3.11. What concerns us at the moment are the pronounced peaks of deaths attributed to 'fièvres typhiques' during the spring, from April to May in Cairo and from May to June in Alexandria. Because of the more central location of this city, the situation in Cairo is probably somewhat more likely to be representative of the whole country. As Schnepp employs 'fièvres typhiques' and 'fièvres typhoides' as interchangeable terms but distinguishes between 'typhus' and 'fièvres typhoides', it appears that the rubric 'fièvres typhiques' in the statistic was meant to cover typhoid as well as paratyphoid and relapsing fever.[184] Schnepp himself harboured no illusions about the reliability

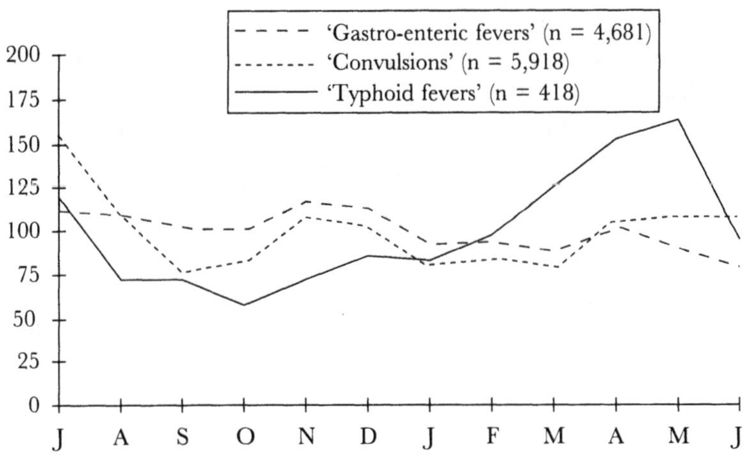

Figure 1.39 Seasonal incidence of causes of death in Cairo, July 1859 to June 1860

[183] Based on Schnepp (1862b) 552–3.
[184] Ibid., 559–60.

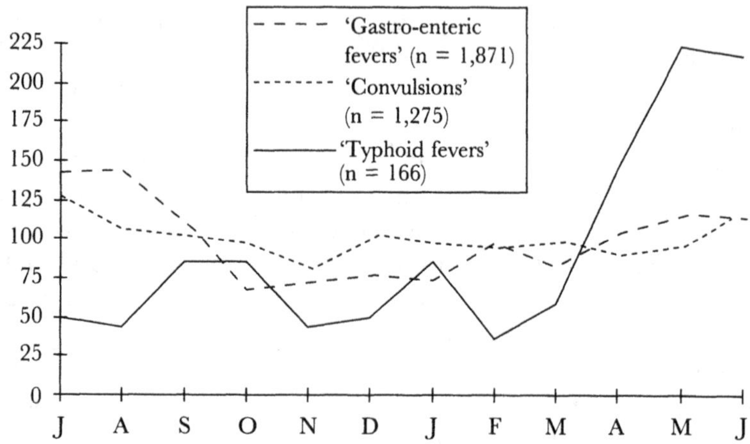

Figure 1.40 Seasonal incidence of causes of death in Alexandria, July 1859 to June 1860

of this taxonomy, which was established without the help of autopsies,[185] and it is very well possible that additional cases were subsumed under the broad category of 'fièvre gastro-entérique' that must have been associated with similar symptoms. Hence, the attested shares in the total death rate of 2.79 per cent in Cairo and 2.63 per cent in Alexandria should not be accepted at face value.

No age distribution is provided for this or other causes of death. However, since mortality from typhoid was largely confined to older children and young adults, it would account for a considerable proportion of all deaths in these age cohorts. If about fifteen per cent of all deaths occurred between ages five and thirty, typhoid could easily have caused in excess of fifteen per cent of these fatalities. If the actual incidence of cases was higher than attested, the disease could have been even more significant. In a medium of documentation that was as heavily biased in favour of teenagers and young and middle-aged adults as the ancient epitaphs of Egypt, a strong concentration of typhoid-related deaths in the early spring would inevitably cause a larger number of commemorative artifacts to be set up in that part of the year than in other seasons. This observation obviates the need to assume that a particular kind of disease,

[185] Ibid., 559: 'ces diagnostics offrent peu de garantie scientifique'.

in this case typhoid and other enteric fevers, had to be dramatically more frequent during the first millennium CE than in the nineteenth century in order to become instrumental in the shaping of the observed seasonality pattern.[186] Although the amount of variation in our samples is so considerable that it is unlikely to reflect the impact of enteric fevers and concurrent dysenteries alone, these diseases must have been a major factor in the underlying mortality regime.

3.5. *Malaria*

Malaria is contracted by humans through the inoculation of the saliva of female mosquitoes containing infective forms of the malaria parasites. These unicellular parasites, belonging to the genus *Plasmodium*, invade the erythrocytes in the bloodstream and cause to them to burst at the end of synchronised sporogenous cycles. This process triggers periodic paroxysms of chills and fever. *Plasmodium falciparum*, also known as malignant tertian malaria, the most pernicious type of malaria, not only causes fever of up to 41°C but may induce anaemias, malarial haemoglobinuria or 'blackwater fever' (the excretion of haemoglobin in the urine), splenomegaly, jaundice, renal dysfunction and pulmonary oedema. The other varieties of malaria found in Egypt, *P. vivax*, or benign tertian fever, and *P. malariae*, or quartan fever, are considerably less pernicious but likewise act as a contributing factor to morbidity and mortality. Maternal malarial infection is known to reduce the birthweight of infants, thereby increasing the incidence of stillbirths and neonatal mortality. Moreover, malaria readily coexists with gastro-intestinal infections. It tends to suppress immune responses to typhoid, and dual infection is common. In general, high levels of malaria infection render gastro-intestinal infections more dangerous. Malaria also raises the fatality rates from respiratory diseases, such as tuberculosis and pneumonia. Thus, while primary malaria infection, above all in the case of *P. falciparum*, may be lethal for small children or non-immune adults, endemic malaria has even greater *indirect* effects on morbidity and mortality. In this

---

[186] Any such idea, in addition to being impossible to substantiate, would also conflict with the fact that extremely high levels of exposure to typhoid (such as under tropical conditions) make adults less susceptible to the disease. Frequently reinforced immunity may arise from numerous subinfectious exposures to typhoid bacilli: Hornick (1982) 667. Cf. already Curschmann (1902) 67.

way, it represents a considerable health risk to the adolescent and adult population in general. The demographic impact of this disease will be considered in Chapter 2.2.[187]

The low incidence of sickle-cell anaemia in modern Egypt may speak against a long tradition of endemic malaria.[188] However, this will best be understood as a function of the fragmentation of the Egyptian disease environment: dangerously high levels of malaria infection appear to have been limited to certain parts of the country. Geology favours the spread of malaria in the marshy areas of the Nile Delta, above all in its northern stretch that is dominated by lakes and the estuaries of the various tributaries of the Nile. Owing to the presence of a large lake and the particular nature of its irrigation system, the Fayum was also particularly exposed to the hazards of malaria; this region will be discussed separately at the end of this section. Intermittent fevers were most common at the end of the inundation period in the autumn,[189] when the receding river had replenished existing marshes and left numerous small pools of stagnant water that would slowly contract or dry up over the following months. Seasonal wetlands of this kind provided perfect breeding grounds for mosquitoes. Moreover, permanent marshes are frequently attested in ancient Egypt, above all for the Delta.[190]

Evidence of malaria infection has been reported for Luxor in Upper Egypt around 1200 BCE. A recent study claims that six out of seven naturally desiccated Egyptian mummies under review, dating from 3200 to 700 BCE, show significant concentrations of a *P. falciparum* antigen in the skin, muscle, brain and lung tissue, suggesting that they were suffering from the most dangerous type of malaria at the time of their death. By contrast, only one of eleven individuals from North Argin in Nubia (350–550 CE) that have also been examined displays the same symptoms.[191] Herodotus claimed that Egypt was so heavily infested by swarms of mosquitoes that in some areas, people spent the nights on raised structures to steer clear

---

[187] Standard accounts of malaria include MacDonald (1957); Pampana (1963); Gilles and Warrell (1993). On malaria in antiquity, see, e.g., Grmek (1989) 275–83; Sallares (1991) 271–81 and (forthcoming). The synergistic interaction of malaria with other diseases is discussed in great detail in Sallares (forthcoming).

[188] Thus Butzer (1976) 93.

[189] Jagailloux (1996) 159.

[190] Traina (1988) 90–1, with references.

[191] Cockburn (1981); Miller *et al.* (1994) 31. Cf. Sallares and Gomzi (forthcoming) for further discussion.

of the low-flying insects. Until fairly recently, this custom was typical of heavily malarious regions such as the English marshlands, the Roman Campagna, the notorious Pontine Marshes, and similarly infested parts of Greece and the East Indies.[192] The advice given in a hieroglyphic text from a temple at Denderah not to leave the house after sunset in the weeks following the inundation of the Nile (i.e., when pools of stagnant water enabled mosquitoes to proliferate) also speaks volumes.[193] Magical texts of the Graeco-Roman period refer to various types of intermittent fevers. A charm from the village of Tebtunis in the Fayum asks to 'save Tais (. . .) from every shivering fit, whether tertian or quartan or quotidian fever, or an every-other-day fever, or [one] by night, or a mild fever'.[194] A similar text, which may also originate from the Fayum, again goes into some detail: 'Protect Touthous, whom Sara bore, from every shivering fit and fever: tertian, quartan, quotidian, daily, or every other day [it occurs]'.[195] A third magical spell comes from Hermopolis Magna on the Bahr Yussuf west of the Nile, evoking 'every shivering fit and fever, whether daily or intermittent by night or day, or quartan fever'.[196] A Christian amulet from the same region, from Oxyrhynchus, also differentiates between 'every kind of chill, quotidian, tertian, and quartan'.[197] Other texts contain briefer references to malaria.[198] The term 'tertian fever' covers *P. falciparum* and *P. vivax*, whereas 'quartan fever' surely describes *P. malariae.*[199] Some of the 'daily fevers' were also *P. falciparum* (given that the daily periodicity is commoner than the tertian periodicity), while others may have been caused by multiple infection with different strains of malaria as well as by unrelated diseases, such as typhoid.

---

[192] Herodotus 2.95. See Sallares (forthcoming) for references.

[193] Capasso (1985) 304.

[194] *P.Tebt.* 275 = *PGM* 33.1–25, in Betz (1992) 267.

[195] *P.Berol.* 21165 = *PGM* 106.1–10, in Betz (1992) 310–11 (Fayum?).

[196] *PGM* 18b.1–7, in Betz (1992) 255.

[197] *P.Oxy.* VIII 1151 (fifth century CE?).

[198] Esp. *P.Erlangen* 37 = *PGM* 87.1–11, in Betz (1992) 301 ('the headache, daily fevers, nightly, quartan, semitertian'); see also *PGM* 7.218–21, 104.1–8, 115.1–7 (Betz (1992) 122, 310, 314). Cf. Wilcken (1901) 425–6. Medical texts from ancient Egypt, by contrast, do not refer to intermittent fevers: Nunn (1996) 73. Burke (1996) ignores Roman Egypt.

[199] Given that *P. vivax* also produces 'tertian' fevers, this expression does not strictly speaking constitute unequivocal proof of the presence of falciparian malaria. However, the evolutionary history of the latter strongly suggests its early spreading into Egypt: see Sallares (forthcoming).

Prosper Alpinus, in the 1580s, also hinted at superinfection when he observed that assorted 'infectious fevers' were treated with baths, including intermittent fevers, one variety of which would recur daily. In the 1660s, Father Gonzales encountered tertian fevers in Lower Egypt.[200] As usual, more specific information is limited to the last two hundred years. In the nineteenth century, in keeping with the geological preconditions, malaria was endemic on the littoral and in parts of the interior of Lower Egypt, and also in Middle Egypt including Cairo and the Fayum.[201] In 1800, Savaresi distinguished between 'tertian', 'double tertian' and 'soporific tertian' fever in Damietta in the Delta. A 'double tertian' implies two generations of parasites whose cycles are not synchronised; 'soporific tertian' may be a way of referring to lethargy in falciparian malaria caused by brain infection. These phenomena were mostly confined to a few months: following isolated infections from September to November, these fevers emerged with great force in December and lasted until the onset of the winter rains in January or February. Locals were said to have reported this cycle to unfold in each year throughout the coastal region. The French noted that in Lower Egypt, gastro-intestinal disorders prevailed until August or September and were then replaced by 'remittent' and 'intermittent' autumnal fevers. This situation had not changed by 1862 when Schnepp identified the 'ravages of malaria' in the Delta as a result of the inundation that made malaria flourish in the late autumn.[202] In fact, Palladius had already stated in the early fifth century CE that at the time of the inundation of the Nile, 'many take sick'; he himself fell a victim to an unspecified disease that may have caused a spleen disorder.[203] It is perhaps not unreasonable to interpret this statement against the background of malarial infection at the end of the inundation period.[204]

In the early days of the Roman occupation of Egypt, the geographer Strabo commented on the salubrious climate of Alexandria:

---

[200] Alpin (1980) 320 (bk. III, p. 248); *Voyage* (1977) 492 (= 1673, bk. VI, p. 394).

[201] Jagailloux (1986) 260.

[202] Savaresi (1800b) 123–4 (Damietta); Bruant (1800) 52 (Lower Egypt); Schnepp (1862a) 193.

[203] Palladius, *Historia Lausiaca* 35.4, also cited by Bagnall (1993) 185. In addition, Palladius suffered from a stomach condition. His poor health eventually prompted him to leave Egypt and move to Palestine, 'where the air is lighter' (35.12).

[204] Dengue fever is said to have occurred annually, occasionally at epidemic strength, and always from the beginning to the end of the inundation. In the nineteenth century, it was not a prime cause of death: Jagailloux (1986) 244. Cf. Hirsch (1881) 41–2, for the eighteenth century.

> And this likewise results from the fact that the land is washed by water on both sides and because of the timeliness of the Nile's risings; for the other cities that are situated on lakes have heavy and stifling air in the heats of summer, because the lakes then become marshy along their edges owing to the evaporation caused by the sun's rays, and, accordingly, when so much filth-laden moisture rises, the air inhaled is noisome and starts pestilential diseases, whereas at Alexandria, at the beginning of summer, the Nile, being full, fills the lake also, and leaves no marshy matter to corrupt the rising vapours (17.1.7).

Strabo failed to tell his readers what happened when the waters began to recede, while other sources of the same period explicitly referred to marshland in close proximity to the city.[205] In the late sixteenth century, local physicians explained the annual spread of 'lethal pestilential fevers' in Alexandria during the autumn with reference to the propinquity of the lake Mareotis. This suggests that by then, at any rate, malaria had become a serious problem for the city. In the mid-nineteenth century, intermittent fevers began to appear in Alexandria as early as April and May. Many inhabitants then suffered from malaria but mostly died of dysentery and tuberculosis. Apparently, the fever would reduce their ability to withstand other diseases rather than act as a clinical cause of death: in 1871, 4.1 per cent of all cases of death in Alexandria to which a cause had been attributed were due to malaria. Fifty years later, this disease had been almost eradicated as a direct cause of death.[206]

---

[205] *Bellum Alexandrinum* 1 refers to a *palus* south of the city; according to Josephus Flavius, *Bellum Judaicum* 2.386, the city was protected by marshland. Galen (vol. 16 p. 363 ed. Kühn) claimed that the *héle* of Egypt were the only healthy marshes known to him. This view, however, seems to derive in the first instance from his general theory that continually stagnant water emitted noxious vapours that caused disease (pp. 358–62). In Egypt, by contrast, the annual inundation of the Nile 'flushed out the old water and brought in new water' (p. 363, see also Rufus of Ephesus in Oribasius, *Collectiones medicae* 5.3.6, *CMG* 6.1.1). Seen through the lens of the miasmatic concept of intermittent fevers, this cyclical reinvigoration could readily be expected to curb malarial infection. In reality, the annual inundation certainly did not have the effect of suppressing malaria (see above and below). Galen's concomitant reasoning that Egypt's marshes were healthy because their water did not become putrid in the winter and overheated in the summer (p. 363) is similarly unpersuasive. Even so, it is not inconceivable that Galen's favourable opinion of Egyptian marshes was reinforced by a low incidence of malaria in Alexandria, as implied by Strabo.

[206] Alpin (1980) 91 (bk. I, p. 51) (1580s); Dikaios (1862) 500–01 (mid-1800s); Panzac (1982) 90 (1871 to 1920s). Pruner (1847) 357 observed that in his days, malaria was endemic in the southwestern part of Alexandria (i.e., close to Mareotis) but almost absent from the northwest (i.e., at the sea).

During the nineteenth century, malaria was not regarded as a universal problem for the whole country. While Lower Egypt and the Fayum stood out as areas of endemic malaria, Upper Egypt would mainly experience temporary outbreaks. Because of such events, May and August were known as the 'months of Anopheles'. Similar seasonal crises are attested for the oases in the Libyan desert west of the Nile.[207] The background of such outbreaks remains obscure since it is difficult to correlate their timing with climatic or hydrological conditions. In a report issued in 1919, the Anti-Malarial Commission found malaria to be more generally present in the country. The authors referred to mosquito-breeding swamps in the unreclaimed marshlands of the northern Delta, and blamed defective drainage and canals for the spread of breeding grounds. Anopheles mosquitoes were known to breed all over Egypt with the result that in most districts, malaria had become endemic. Allowing for the phenomenon of anophelism without malaria, the study argued that the transfer of malaria-infected soldiers from the Western Oases, Greece and Mesopotamia during World War I had increased the danger of transmission.[208] This suggests that in the Ptolemaic period, the migration of thousands of Greeks and Macedonians to Egypt, especially to an area that must have been as rich in anopheline vectors as the Fayum (see below), may have had the effect of introducing new strains of malaria to their new homeland. Even if malaria was less widespread in the southern Balkans than is sometimes assumed, there can be little doubt that a considerable number of settlers would have carried *Plasmodium* organisms in their bloodstream. Local populations may be better able to cope with familiar, 'indigenous' infections than with newly introduced foreign strains.[209]

The commission noted that while malaria did not normally appear in epidemic form, it was endemic in the infected districts, and 'per-

---

[207] Hirsch (1881) 142; Jagailloux (1986) 260. Sandwith (1905) does not even include malaria in his survey of the major diseases of Egypt.

[208] Anti-malarial Commission (1919) VII, 1, 4. The same had happened in Kent during World War I, where new strains of malaria were introduced by soldiers arriving from abroad: see Dobson (1997) 349–50, 360.

[209] Bagnall (1997b) 18 estimates that about thirty per cent of the population of the Ptolemaic Fayum originated from outside Egypt. Corvisier (1994) contests the view that malaria was rampant in Hellenistic Greece. For malaria in Macedonia, see Borza (1979). In general, see Sallares (forthcoming). In Kent in the First World War, *vivax* malaria imported from Salonica provoked much more violent reactions than local strains: Dobson (1997) 360.

sistent or chronic in the individual attacked'. Although not an important clinical cause of death, malaria was found to lead 'to a general lowering of the vitality of the whole population and to a general increase in the death rate'. This assessment is surely correct and receives ample confirmation from the comparative material considered in the first chapter. During and for some time after the inundation, the area of possible breeding places expanded enormously. However, while the floods stretched from July to December, temperatures that were favourable to breeding were confined to the period from August to October. Two types of breeding grounds were singled out as the most important, namely marshes and lakes fed by the arterial drains of the Nile, and outcrops of infiltration water.[210]

According to a survey conducted in 1913, the inhabitants of a number of cities in the Delta showed relatively high rates of spleen enlargement suggestive of malaria infection. The Western Oases continued to be plagued by fevers in the summer and fall. New malaria infections were concentrated in the months from August to November, peaking in October.[211] Barber and Rice investigated the scale of malaria infections in 1936, an unusually warm year. Among children up to age fifteen, different levels of infection and spleen enlargement indices correlated with different ecological settings. The highest incidence was found close to rice fields that required perennial irrigation; this, of course, is of little relevance for ancient Egypt.[212] The next highest frequencies occurred in the vicinity of lakes. Malaria infection was moderate to high in the Delta in general, and low or absent in the Nile valley. In those parts of Alexandria that bordered on the lake Mariut (the ancient lake Mareotis), one-third of children who were examined carried parasites and two-fifths showed spleen enlargement; in about one-third of the cases, *P. falciparum* was the cause.[213] This shows that at least in particularly warm years, despite

[210] Anti-malarial Commission (1919) 3 (quote), 7–9.

[211] Spleen counts: Anti-malarial Commission (1919) 33–4. The survey yielded enlargement rates of 13.5 per cent in Mansura, 14 per cent in Damietta and 16.5 per cent in Benha. New infections: ibid., 43–7 (appendix III). Pruner (1847) 357 already reported that malaria rose after the floods had peaked.

[212] Considerable amounts of rice were grown in Roman Syria, Palestine, and also in western Asia Minor: Konen (1999) 29–33. By contrast, only four Egyptian papyri mention rice (34–6). However, in view of the lack of papyri from Lower Egypt, we cannot rule out the possibility that just like in the modern period, rice cultivation was then already more common in the Delta (cf. 36 n. 44).

[213] Barber and Rice (1937) 414, 418–19 tab. 1. *P. vivax* produced lower spleen rates: 429–31.

a general downturn in infections, Alexandria was still heavily exposed to malaria.

Anopheles pharoensis was found in most stagnant and semistagnant waters containing vegetation, and thrived in rice fields and in or at the borders of lakes. Tests have shown that this species has a strong avidity for human hosts, and greatly prefers them to animals. However, in the environmental conditions of Egypt it has a short lifespan and is therefore a less effective vector than *A. gambiae* in tropical Africa. In general, in 1936 malaria appeared to be widely distributed throughout the country, though dependent on local conditions and generally less so in Upper Egypt.[214] Again, the production of anopheline mosquitoes peaked in October since by that month, ponds, pools and ditches had become well filled with water from the inundation and the water in village cesspools rose.[215] In 1942, *A. gambiae* penetrated Upper Egypt as far as Asyut, probably causing thousands of additional deaths.[216]

In the nineteenth and early twentieth centuries, the most malarial region outside the northern Delta was the Fayum,[217] a large depression about sixty kilometres south-west of modern Cairo (Map 2). It covers an area of some 12,000 square kilometres, with a general slope to the north-west. That part of the province is dominated by a lake, known as Lake Moeris to Herodotus, simply referred to as 'the lake' during the Graeco-Roman period, and now called Birket Qarun. Its surface currently lies forty-five metres below sea level and covers an area of 214 km^2. It is fed by the Bahr Yussuf, which leaves the Nile at Dairut and runs parallel to the river until at Hawara it breaks through the range of hills west of the Nile valley into the Fayum. While some details of the hydrological history of the Fayum are still open to debate, there is no doubt that the size

[214] In 1942/3, *Anopheles gambiae* caused a malaria epidemic that spread from Upper Egypt: Butzer (1976) 93 n. 9.

[215] Barber and Rice (1937) 417, 423, 433. See also Kirkpatrick (1925), on the Egyptian mosquito species, and Barsoum (1938) for further discussion of malaria in Egypt. Morsy, el Kadery, Salama, Sabry, Kotb and el Sharkawy (1995) investigate mosquito species in the present Fayum.

[216] Shousha (1948). During the spring of 1942, the death rate in the Abu Simbil region increased more than tenfold: 313, tab. III; cf. 321 on the overall death toll. In principle, Upper Egypt south of Asyut provides almost ideal conditions for the spread of A. gambiae during the months of September, October and November when both temperature and humidity are high: 319.

[217] Nineteenth century: Pruner (1847) 356; Hirsch (1881) 142. For the twentieth century, see below.

of the lake and its water level have changed dramatically over the past few millennia.[218] It is now believed that the lake reached its maximum elevation (since the sixth millennium BCE) of twenty-three metres above the current sea level during the period of the Old Kingdom, around 2800 BCE. The Pharaohs of the Twelfth Dynasty regulated the flow of water from the Bahr Yussuf through the Lahun gap, establishing a lake at about eighteen metres above sea level. It appears to have covered an area up to ten times as large as today, and extended much farther to the east and south. Against this background, Herodotus' description of the large 'Lake of Moeris' in the Fayum, albeit inaccurate in detail, has again begun to seem acceptable.[219] Ptolemy I started to drain the lake by restricting the inflow of water until the water level dropped to about two metres below the current sea level. Continued under his successor Ptolemy II, this project added hundreds of square kilometres of fertile land to the Fayum and attracted settlers, many of them from abroad. At that stage, the lake may still have been up to three times as large as it is now. Unlike the rest of the country, the fields of the Fayum were not inundated but had to be irrigated by means a network of smaller canals. In the second century CE, the lake stood at seven metres below sea level, but by the end of the Roman period, the water level had dropped more dramatically, perhaps down to around thirty metres below sea level, and must have shrunk accordingly. The salinity of the water kept increasing: in the eighteenth century, its water was still sweet in the east but bitter in the west.[220]

Unsurprisingly, the presence of the lake and perennial irrigation conspired to turn the Fayum into one of the most malarial regions

---

[218] The stages of the development of Birket Qarun are discussed by Wendorf and Schild (1976) 155–226, esp. 223 fig. 159; Hassan (1986b), esp. 492 fig. 6. See also Ginter and Kozlowski (1986) on the prehistory of the Fayum.

[219] For the view that the lake was even larger in the Old Kingdom than later on, see Wendorf and Schild (1976) 226; Hassan (1986b) 491 (who reckons with sea levels of eighteen to twenty-two metres in the Old Kingdom, fifteen to eighteen metres in the Middle Kingdom, and *c.* twenty metres in the late Dynastic period). This interpretation supersedes the previous theory that the measures taken under Amenemhet I had increased its size (e.g., Ball (1939)). On Herodotus 3.149, see most recently Evans (1991). At twenty metres above sea level, the lake would have covered about 2,100 km^2 (Hassan, 493).

[220] This summary draws on Wendorf and Schild (1976) 161, Hassan (1986b) 491. Hewison (1989) 60–1 and Rathbone (1996) 52 also give brief outlines. For maps of the changing shape of the lake, see Wendorf and Schild (1976) 224 fig. 160; Hassan (1986b) 484 fig. 1; Hewison (1989) 58. I remain sceptical of the revisionist model of Davoli (1998) 339–40.

of Egypt. According to the first detailed account of the Fayum, composed by Abu Osman el Nabulsi el Safadi in the thirteenth century, the exceedingly numerous marshes of the region spoiled the air with miasmatic vapours. He also described the local population as lethargic, noting that resident outsiders would eventually adopt the same characteristics, commented on the perspiration of the locals and blamed their reputed unbalance, melancholy, absentmindedness and depravity on the contamination of air and water. All these features are strongly reminiscent of other pre-scientific descriptions of malarial areas and their inhabitants.[221] Quantitative evidence is inevitably confined to the twentieth century. In 1913, the city of Fayum—successor to the ancient city of Crocodilopolis/Arsinoe—counted as one of the nine most heavily malaria-infected municipal areas in the country, and was the only one of them that was located outside the Delta.[222] By 1922, the rate of spleen enlargement in this city had fallen from eight per cent nine years earlier to 2.3 per cent, an improvement that was due to intervening prevention measures.[223] Four observations help to put these figures into perspective. First, the spleen index was subsequently found to be an inaccurate measure of malaria infection in that it understated the actual incidence.[224] Second, the precipitous drop of the spleen count by two-thirds within a mere nine years (together with comparable successes in Lower Egypt) suggests that in preceding decades, and especially before the British takeover of Egypt in 1882 initiated the fight against malaria, rates of infection may have been substantially higher. Indeed, as early as 1898, Abu Zeki claimed, undoubtedly with some hyperbole, that the current governor of the Fayum had managed to remove most pestilential pools of water and to improve the sanitary conditions in the city of

[221] Zeki (1898) 264–9. For the notion of malaria as marsh miasma, see Sallares (forthcoming); and compare Dobson (1997) 53, 300–03, 338–42 on life style in English marsh parishes. Nabulsi's sweating, brutish Fayumites, whose appearance was that of 'dumb savages', who 'do not move unless pushed, like beasts', and who are given to idling their time away indoors (264–5), resemble the 'dull, sluggish, sordid, (. . .) deceitfull, malicious, disdainefull' inhabitants of the Kentish marshlands in the eighteenth century, who were 'soaked in debilitating sweat' and walked 'slowly and painfully' (quoted from contemporary sources in Dobson, 301, 303).

[222] Anti-malarial Commission (1919) 33–4.

[223] Anti-Malaria Commission (1928) 29. Similar improvements were achieved in the Delta: in Mansura and Damietta, the spleen rates fell from 13.5 and 14.0 per cent in 1913 to 4.1 and 5.5 per cent in 1923, respectively, and in Benha they were reduced from 15.5 per cent in 1913 to a mere 0.7 per cent in 1925: ibid., 27.

[224] Barber and Rice (1937) 416.

Fayum.[225] Third, regarding the situation in antiquity, we need to bear in mind that in the Roman period, the distance between the city of Arsinoe and lake Moeris was about one-third shorter than at present. The level of exposure to disease vectors would have been correspondingly higher. Finally, the modern city of Fayum was an early beneficiary of prevention measures that were only belatedly introduced to smaller settlements. Thus, even in the 1920s the villages of the Fayum were still lagging badly behind the provincial capital. Reports testified to the 'existence of a very considerable amount of Malaria in that province'. A sample of seven villages produced a mean spleen count of ten per cent which, however, concealed significant local variation: 'In those villages in the Faîyûm which have good elevation and good natural drainage there is no Malaria, where they are low-lying and the drainage bad (. . .) Malaria is prevalent'.[226] This observation is fully consonant with the general model of 'contours of death and disease' that predicts an inverse correlation between altitude and the frequency of malaria infection: this relationship has been discussed in detail by Sallares.[227] The commission noted that the desert had been subjected to perennial and controlled irrigation; in the presence of natural undulations of the country that were intersected by ravines running in the direction of Birket Qarun, all drainage gravitated to and discharged into the lake. Drainage, however, was imperfect, and had not kept up with irrigation: hence, the ravines, which were natural drainage channels, in many cases turned into swamps.[228] As we shall see in a moment, there is reason to believe that in antiquity, these inauspicious conditions had already existed on a magnified scale. In the city of Fayum at the end of the nineteenth century, the extraction of soil for brick production created wide and deep pits which filled with infiltration water and so turned into pools of stagnant water that exuded 'des miasmes délétères' (i.e., triggered malaria infection).[229] A more recent report found that drainage water also sometimes stagnated in the

[225] Zeki (1898) 283: 'aujourd'hui, presque toutes ces mares pestilentielles ont disparu et les conditions hygiéniques et sanitaires de la localité se sont progressivement ameliorées.'

[226] Anti-Malaria Commission (1928) 37–8.

[227] Sallares (forthcoming). This is also a central theme of Dobson (1997), esp. 81–187, 223–8, with the figures on pp. 85, 148, 158.

[228] Anti-Malaria Commission (1928) 37.

[229] Zeki (1898) 283. Pruner (1847) 357 noted that in the Fayum, the incidence of malaria was correlated with the presence of hollows filled with stagnant water.

villages, inviting mosquitoes to commence breeding. It further referred to the practice, said to be common among villagers, of throwing refuse into drainage canals, which could cause diseases.[230] In the mid-thirties, the Fayum was still one of the most malarial parts of Egypt.[231] In 1936, in the locality of Ezbet El Sham-ekh Masoud in the Fayum, near the Birket Qarun which even then was bordered by fresh-water swamps, one-third of the children were infected by malaria (almost entirely by *P. vivax*) and one-fifth showed spleen enlargement.[232] The *British National Formulary* still advises visitors to Egypt that the Fayum is the only part of the country with a risk (albeit only a 'low risk') of malaria infection from May to November.[233]

Under Ptolemaic and Roman rule, the hydrography of the Fayum was even more conducive to the spread of malaria. In the early twentieth century, excepting rice fields (which were uncommon in antiquity), the highest incidence of malaria in Egypt was encountered in the vicinity of lakes. In all freshwater lakes or freshwater areas of lakes, the warm season saw a great output of anopheles mosquitoes.[234] Two thousand years ago, assuming that the lake was deeper than at present, a larger share of the Fayum bordered on its shores and a larger proportion of the population was potentially exposed to infection. At that time, the large village of Karanis, one of the main sources of surviving Roman census returns from the rural Fayum, was situated close to the lake instead of several miles away as it is today. A second smaller lake which later disappeared, *Mikra Limne*, lay south-east of the main lake. Moreover, papyrological evidence repeatedly refers to 'shore land' in the territories of villages that were not located anywhere near currently existing lakes, above all in the south-western Fayum.[235] Rathbone has therefore ventured the guess that in that area, in the central depression of the Gharaq basin and at the south end of the Wadi Nezla, two small

---

230 Anti-Malarial Commission (1933) 4–5.

231 Anti-malarial work (1939) 3 tab. I.

232 Barber and Rice (1937) 418 tab. 1.

233 *British National Formulary*, no. 29 (March 1995) 261; confirmed by Morsy, el Kadery, Salama, Sabry and el Sharkawy (1995). Thirty years ago, *Area Handbook* (1970) 126 considered malaria to be 'mildly endemic' in the Nile valley.

234 Barber and Rice (1937) 414. Archaeological evidence of certain fishes and molluscs shows that the ancient Fayum lake was a freshwater lake: Hassan (1986b) 493.

235 The historical topography of this area, known in the classical period as the '*meris* of Polemon', is currently studied by members of the International Workshop for Papyrology and Social History: see Rathbone (1996).

lakes were allowed to form.[236] They may have been subject to seasonal fluctuation, expanding in the summer and fall and contracting after the inundation period. The territory of Ibion Argaiou, for instance, included some marshland and uncultivated shore-land, presumably to the south of one of these small lakes. A considerable number of other villages appear to have been situated in close proximity to marshes. It is doubtful whether these locales had been created by ill-managed irrigation. In view of the many abortive or incomplete drainage projects of antiquity, the efforts of the first Ptolemies would almost certainly have fallen short of clearing the entire area previously covered by the lake. Later on, under Roman rule, the elongated marsh in the *meris* of Themisteos on the western fringe of the Fayum appears to have been deliberately maintained in order to grow papyrus.[237] Bonneau has argued that the swamps of the Fayum showed a tendency to dry up between the third century BCE and the early Roman empire; in some cases, agricultural exploitation expanded onto what had previously been marshland. This development, however, must not be exaggerated: some local wetlands are known to have persisted throughout the Roman period, and even in the thirteenth century, by which time desiccation had progressed much further, Nabulsi was impressed by the ubiquity of marshes in the Fayum.[238] In fact, the apparent early Roman imperial advance of farming into imperfectly reclaimed areas—quite possibly the result of mounting population pressure—may well have exposed increasing numbers of people to malaria. After all, marshy spots need not be large to have an impact: Ross reported in 1903

[236] For this and the local data from the southwestern Fayum that follow at the end of this paragraph, see Rathbone (1996) 53–6.

[237] In the early first century CE, according to Bonneau (1982) 188 (on *P.Mil.* 6), this marsh was some thirty kilometres long; see the map 189, fig. 38. For its water management, see *P.Wisc.* 31, 34–5 (= Sijpesteijn (1967)): *P.Wisc.* 34 (144 CE) records a protest that 'the usual amount of water should flow to the above-mentioned *drymos*, until it is filled (*héos plésethei*)'; otherwise it would be without yield for three years (lines 4–6, 12–13). *Drymos*, here and elsewhere, is a '(marshy) pool' (Sijpestein (1967) 126). The marshland in question was expected to produce a rent (*P.Wisc.* 31); in addition to papyrus production, Sijpestein (1967) 126 draws attention to the potential of fishing in such locales.

[238] Desiccation and agricultural use: Bonneau (1982) 183–5, 188, 190. Substantial marshes appear to have survived in particular in the south-west: ibid., 187–8, and below. Reclaimed plots, although usually secured by dikes, could again be rendered marshy by an excessive influx of irrigation water; papyri refer to accidents caused by breaches of dikes: Bonneau (1982) 183–4. On Nabulsi, see above, n. 221.

that in Ismailia on the Suez Canal, the primary cause of malaria infection were *small* marshes in immediate proximity to the town.[239] In the Tutun basin to the north of Tebtunis (another major source of rural census returns), the territories of no fewer than four villages—Kerkeesis, Ptolemais Melissourgon, Tebetenu and Oxyrhyncha—are known to have comprised tracts of marshland. Livia owned papyrus marshes near Theadelphia in the northwestern Fayum (*P.Mil.* 6), yet another important source of rural census documents. An elaborate network of irrigation canals extended into peripheral parts of the region which are only now being reclaimed from the desert. Kom Talit in the south-western Fayum, for instance, was occupied from the Ptolemaic period to the eleventh century. Recent excavations have revealed large numbers of wells and cisterns, connected with water-channels, and a series of water-supply and drainage channels.[240]

All in all, there can be no doubt that in antiquity, the Fayum was considerably moister than in the more recent past. Because of the higher water-level of the lake, areas that in the early twentieth century derived some degree of protection from mosquitoes from a somewhat elevated position may previously have been lowlands that were more heavily exposed to infection. It is interesting to learn that the easternmost fields of the territory of Kerkeosiris were occasionally flooded by water bursting in from the fields of Talei and Theogonis, whose irrigation canals must therefore have been higher. Small seasonally fluctuating lakes, tracts of marshland and an extensive system of irrigation and drainage canals all favoured high levels of malaria infection. Even if malaria had not already been endemic in the region, it would have been introduced by the Greek and Macedonian settlers of the Ptolemaic period. And indeed, as we have seen above, one or even two of the known magic spells that were designed to ward off quotidian, tertian and quartan fevers originated from the Fayum.[241] These texts form only one of several different strands of evidence—hydrographic conditions, traces of malaria in parts of ancient Egypt where it had not been particularly prevalent in the more recent past, and pertinent comparative data from the early twentieth century—that all point to the same conclusion: that

---

239 Ross (1903) 12.

240 Crawford (1971) 109; for Kom Talit, see Kirby and Rathbone (1996) 29–30.

241 Another of these documents comes from Oxyrhynchus, where marshland is also attested: *P.Oxy.* XIV 1687.11 and 20.

malaria was probably an important factor in the disease environment, and thus in the mortality regime, of the ancient Fayum.[242]

This, in turn, has serious implications for any demographic study of Roman Egypt that primarily depends on evidence from that part of the country (see below, Chapter 2). Moreover, it is at least conceivable that malaria may have contributed to the apparent decline of many of the best-known settlements of the Fayum after the second century CE.[243] This development seems to have been precipitated or accompanied by the neglect of the irrigation system. Sometimes associated with a drop in population size, perhaps due to the severe epidemics of the late second and mid-third centuries CE, a failure to maintain irrigation and drainage canals would also have favoured the spread of malaria. Thus, neglect of the irrigation works prompted at least in part by disease could easily have resulted in a further aggravation of the disease environment, this time (or perhaps also again?) caused by malaria, which would then have deepened any existing crisis. Up to a point, the decay of the canals and the impact of malaria may have reinforced each other.

In Egypt in general, malaria infections coincided with the inundation, peaking in the month of October. To judge from the Egyptian mortality statistics of the 1920s, this failed to have an appreciable impact on the seasonal incidence of deaths in most parts of the country, including the Fayum (above, Figs. 1.26–27). This can be explained in several ways. By that time, eradication measures had already made significant progress, possibly changing what may have been a somewhat different seasonal pattern for previous generations. It is worth remembering that the data for 1859/60, which are probably biased in favour of Lower Egypt, produce a mortality plateau from October to January (above, Fig. 1.37). Moreover, the available statistics up to the 1920s are clearly deficient; among the cases they conceal, the deaths of infants may well be particularly numerous.[244] Among small children, malaria was more likely to be a clinical cause of death than for adults. Malaria often interacts with other diseases and therefore more commonly becomes a contributing cause of death.[245]

---

[242] Future biomolecular analysis of ancient bone samples from the Fayum may enable us to corroborate this view through physical evidence. Cf. Woodward (1996).

[243] See most recently van Minnen (1997) 15, with further references.

[244] See above, p. 49.

[245] See Sallares (forthcoming), and this chapter, section 3.4.

The Greek tombstone inscriptions from Upper Egypt document elevated mortality from November to January as well as a stronger peak in the spring (see Figs. 1.1–2). In theory, the former might reflect the direct effects of primary infection, while the latter could have been boosted by the overlap of continuing fevers with a surge in other infections. In practice, however, it is impossible to substantiate this scenario, all the more so as it lacks firm support from comparative evidence. The extreme rise in mortality in the early spring suggested for the ancient Fayum (above, Fig. 1.11) occurred too early in the year to be caused by primary malaria infection. Springtime recrudescences of previous infections, while possible, can hardly explain that peak. In the Fayum today, the winter is cool, with a maximum of 10 to 15°C and a minimum of 5 to 10°C from December to February. February brings cold, northerly gales, followed by the southwesterly *khamseen* from March to May that drives up the temperature.[246] Although climatic conditions need not have been identical in antiquity, they cannot have been sufficiently different to permit high levels of malaria infection as early as March and April. Again, this does not preclude the possibility, entertained in the previous section, that lingering intermittent fevers may have exacerbated infections that were typical of that season, such as enteric fevers.[247]

The continuous rise of the death rate during October, November and December attested for Terenouthis and Leontopolis (above, Fig. 1.17) is perhaps more readily consistent with the seasonal incidence of malaria, and in this case, a possible parallel can be found. As I have shown above (Fig. 1.37), the Western Oases in the Libyan desert, uniquely in 1920s Egypt, produced a seasonal mortality pattern that closely resembles the distribution for Roman Lower Egypt. At that time, rates of spleen enlargement were exceptionally high in the oases, ranging from one-half to three-quarters of the juvenile population.[248] Hyperendemic malaria of this kind may well have had a more immediate effect on the death rate than under less extreme circumstances. Once more, it may seem bold to explain the match

[246] Hewison (1989) 3.

[247] Pruner (1847) 360 reported, with reference to Egypt, that malaria infection could last for several months, if not years, and interacted with 'gastric' and 'bilious' fevers.

[248] Jagailloux (1986) 262; and see already Hirsch (1881) 142. As noted above, the transfer of malaria-infected soldiers from the oases was considered to pose a risk to the rest of Egypt. Malaria is still a problem in this region.

between two seasonal mortality patterns—in this case between two sites in the ancient Delta and the Western Oases of the early twentieth century—with reference to a shared disease environment. We cannot be sure whether Terenouthis and Leontopolis were exposed to malarial marshland, and we must not discard the possibility that different pathogens may have generated comparable seasonal manifestations. Nonetheless, it is tempting to identify malaria at least as a contributing factor in the mortality regime of these two communities.[249]

3.6. *Tuberculosis*

High rates of pulmonary tuberculosis have a significant impact on death rates and in particular on the age-specific distribution of mortality. Young adults are heavily affected. In England from 1851 to 1860, for instance, 44.4 per cent of all men who died aged fifteen to twenty-four were killed by tuberculosis, as were 51.3 per cent of the women. In Norway, in the years from 1921 to 1925, seventy per cent of all deaths from ages fifteen to twenty-nine and fifty per cent from ages thirty to thirty-nine were caused by this disease.[250] Its well-proven capacity to dominate early adult mortality is potentially of great relevance to a study of attested seasonal mortality in ancient Egypt. If deaths from tuberculosis are sufficiently frequent and concentrated in a given season, they may become an important factor in determining the shape of the monthly mortality distribution for teenagers and adults. In northern Europe, consumption was primarily a phenomenon of the winter season.[251]

Although there can be little doubt that tuberculosis reached back into the distant past, its incidence in either ancient or early modern Egypt is far from clear. It has been argued that in the early dynastic period, tuberculosis had become common owing to population growth, urban crowding and the domestication of cattle that enabled the pathogen, *Mycobacterium tuberculosis*, to evolve from *M. bovis*.[252] Osseous tuberculosis can sometimes be identified in ancient bones.[253] Thus, two Egyptian mummies show focal areas of calcification and fibrosis consistent with mycobacterial disease, possibly spinal tuberculosis.

---

249 See below, at the end of the following section.
250 Lancaster (1990) 361 tab. 35.3.1 (England); 95 (Norway).
251 E.g., Landers (1993) 209–11 (from December to April in early modern London).
252 Zimmermann (1979).
253 E.g., Ortner and Putschar (1981) 141–76.

Skeletons from Abydos are marred by vertebral lesions and periostitis that provide evidence of tuberculosis, also among small children.[254] Other cases have been reported but often remain ambiguous.[255] An ancient Egyptian medical text refers to persons who spit blood, which may be interpreted as a reference to pulmonary tuberculosis.[256] We know that in the Roman period, the dry climate of Egypt was prized among consumptives, who were advised that a stay in that country would improve their condition. However, as Grmek has pointed out, this practice could also have had the undesirable effect of facilitating the dissemination of tuberculosis in the local population.[257] Considered rare by Clot Bey in 1840, in 1862 tuberculosis could nevertheless be called worse than dysentery—a tall order—and a deadly disease of Egypt.[258] Schnepp observed that the hot winds of the early spring troubled consumptives, especially in Upper Egypt: the *khamseen* was credited with doubling their fevers and precipitating violent oral discharge of blood.[259] It seems that from then on, it accounted for a rising share of total mortality.[260] In the years from 1886 to 1890, eight per cent of deaths in Cairo and 5.5 per cent in Alexandria were attributed to tuberculosis, and as recently as 1970 it was found to be endemic, especially among urban adults.[261]

Taken together, the existence of physical evidence of tuberculosis from ancient Egypt, its focus on young adults, who are overrepresented in the funerary texts from which the seasonal mortality pattern is derived, and the association between the early spring in Upper

---

[254] Mummies: Walker *et al.* (1987) 47–8. Skeletons: Baker, Kealhofer and Richards (1989).

[255] Sandison (1972) 217; Zimmermann (1979); Macke and Macke-Ribet (1993) 301; Nunn (1996) 73–4. See Grmek (1989) 179–80, for previously discovered evidence; he notes that the traces of osseous tuberculosis point to the presence of pulmonary, intestinal and glandinal tuberculosis also (180). For a critical discussion, see Buikstra, Baker and Cook (1993) 27–98, 38–45, esp. 42–5 on recent findings. Examination of bone lesions that are indicative of tuberculosis can now be supplemented by DNA analysis targeting *M. tuberculosis* (e.g., Mays *et al.* 2001).

[256] Manniche (1989) 67.

[257] Celsus, *De Medicina* 3.22; Plinius, *Epistulae* 5.19.6. Grmek (1989) 194. With reference to the 1830s and 40s, Pruner (1847) 283 observed that the assumption that Egypt was free of tuberculosis mostly applied to western immigrants, not to the native population.

[258] Clot-Bey (1840) I 373 (preceded by Frank (1820) 158); Jagailloux (1986) 245–6.

[259] Schnepp (1861) 643.

[260] This may in part have been a function of decreasing mortality from gastrointestinal diseases: see below, section 3.11.

[261] 1880s: Jagailloux (1986) 248. In 1906–10, the rates were 5.3 and 6.8 per cent, respectively. Cf. also ibid., 246 n. 44. I have not seen Valassopoulo, Parodi and Lévy (1912). 1970: *Area Handbook* (1970) 125–6.

Egypt and a seasonal aggravation in the condition of patients in the mid-nineteenth century suggests that tuberculosis may have contributed to the pronounced surge of the death rate documented for the Nile valley of the first millennium CE. The main problem with this interpretation lies in the fact that the known seasonal patterns of mortality in the nineteenth and early twentieth centuries do not reflect any such surge, even though tuberculosis appears then to have been a significant cause of death. We would be forced to speculate that in antiquity and the early Middle Ages, tuberculosis was far more widespread in Egypt than in the more recent past. This idea is impossible to substantiate but deserves some attention. In the Roman period, Upper Egypt was more heavily urbanised than at any time until well into the twentieth century; tuberculosis is most easily transmitted in an urban setting. The Coptic monasteries from which most of the later evidence is drawn, with their concentration of adult men in what must have been crowded living conditions, also created an environment favouring a continual presence of tuberculosis. In view of the provenance and age bias of the ancient data, tuberculosis may well have influenced the seasonal mortality patterns found in Upper Egypt.[262] As for ancient Lower Egypt, the people of Alexandria, around 1860, were said to suffer from malaria but die of other diseases, including tuberculosis. A similar seasonal convergence of malaria and respiratory illnesses, above all tuberculosis, provides a reasonable explanation for the mortality peak from October to February, and from November to January in particular, that is so conspicuous among adults and, to a lesser extent, children in the epitaphs of Terenouthis and Leontopolis.[263] In this context, it deserves attention that according to Hirsch, in the third quarter of the nineteenth century the highest the incidence of tuberculosis in Egypt was found in the north.[264]

---

[262] Alternatively, deaths from tuberculosis in the winter may have been more common in the Nile Delta where that season was generally colder and wetter than farther south, perhaps even more so in antiquity than at present (cf. above, p. 54). This would fit the seasonal patterns of Terenouthis and Leontopolis. However, it seems hard to imagine that such a massive discrepancy could have existed between the conditions in the Nile valley and at two locations in the southern half of Lower Egypt.

[263] On the interaction between malaria and respiratory diseases, see, e.g., North (1896) 273 and Collari (1932) (Rome); Del Panta (1989) 48–9 (Italy); Balfour (1936) 119 (Greece); Giglioli (1972) (Guyana); Gilles and Warrell (1993) 56; and the discussion in Sallares (forthcoming). For the possibility of malaria in Lower Egypt, see above, section 3.5.

[264] Hirsch (1886) 132.

3.7. *Smallpox*

In populations in which smallpox is constantly present or reintroduced at brief intervals by recurrent epidemics, infants, small children, and immigrants who had not previously been exposed are its most common victims.[265] Under such conditions, this disease may significantly raise the overall death rate.[266] Seasonal fluctuations are well attested, although hard to explain.[267] In London, from 1670 to 1819, deaths from smallpox were concentrated in the second half of the year.[268] In Geneva in the late sixteenth and throughout the seventeenth centuries, repeated outbreaks of smallpox determined the overall pattern of seasonal mortality: this disease caused fatalities in such numbers and so predominantly during the late summer that years of smallpox were characterised by substantial mortality peaks that were largely absent from other years (Fig. 1.41).[269] Perrenoud rightly calls this particular pattern 'archaique, contemporain des grandes crises démographiques, [qui] ne laisse émerger qu'une forte surmortalité estivale d'origine épidémique'.[270]

In early modern Egypt, where smallpox had long been endemic, it killed small children.[271] Volney described how the malnourished children of Cairo fell a victim to this disease.[272] Without vaccination, the death rate stood at forty to fifty per cent of all cases.[273] In

[265] E.g., Benenson (1976) 438: in areas of endemicity, smallpox strikes from ages zero to four, otherwise from ages five to fourteen. For age-specific death rates in populations that are not accustomed to this disease, see below, Chapter 2, p. 162. Fenner *et al.* (1988) offer a comprehensive study of smallpox.

[266] E.g., Mercer (1985) and (1990) 46–73. In England in the early eighteenth century, perhaps ten to fifteen per cent of all deaths were caused by smallpox, although estimates as high as twenty per cent have also been put forward: Brunton (1992) 404. Mercer (1990) 73 refers to rates from eight to twenty per cent in different parts of Europe. See also below, Chapter 3, p. 197, with special reference to early modern Egypt. Clot Bey's claim that in the 1820s, smallpox was killing 50,000 to 60,000 children per year (Panzac (1985) 278, (1987) 17–18) is, however, grossly inflated.

[267] Benenson (1976) 437.

[268] Landers (1993) 209–10.

[269] Based on Perrenoud (1979) 429 tab. 99, 475 tab. 109.

[270] Ibid., 429. Omran (1971) 516 defines this as the first stage of the epidemiologic transition in history, 'the age of pestilence and famine', described in his tab. 1. On Omran's model, cf. Riley and Alter (1989).

[271] Jagailloux (1986) 69. See in general Sandwith (1905) 122–38.

[272] Volney (1788) 246–7.

[273] Sandwith (1905) 129. The history of smallpox eradication in nineteenth-century Egypt is described by Jagailloux (1986) 69–72, Kuhnke (1990) 111–21. See below, Chapter 3, pp. 198–9.

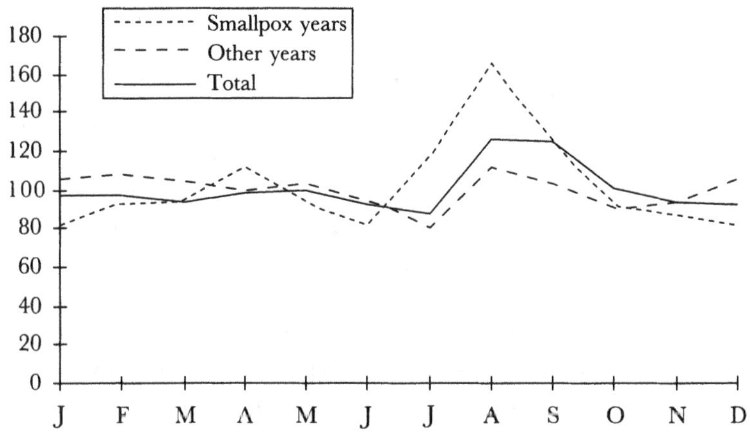

Figure 1.41 Seasonal mortality in Geneva, 1617 to 1649

the late sixteenth century, according to Prosper Alpinus, smallpox would rage from March to May. In the words of John Campbell, 'young People especially at *Cairo* and *Alexandria*, are in Danger every Summer from a malignant kind of Small-Pox which rages excessively'. In the nineteenth century, it could be present from September to May but was most prevalent at the end of autumn and at the beginning of spring.[274]

The early history of smallpox in Egypt is obscure. Some evidence points to its presence in dynastic Egypt (with Pharaoh Ramses V as its most prominent victim).[275] It would usually appear in epidemic form: the infectious disease that struck Athens in 430 BCE, famously described by Thucydides, and which is now commonly identified as smallpox, had ravaged Egypt before reaching Greece, and the 'Antonine plague' of 166 CE also hit the country.[276] In the early seventh century CE, Ahrun of Alexandria described a smallpox epidemic in Alexandria. To judge from the account given by the Persian physician

[274] Alpin (1980) 97 (bk. I, p. 55); [Campbell] (1739) 402; Pruner (1847) 128; Sandwith (1905) 122–3.

[275] Regöly-Mérei (1966); Ebbell (1946) and (1967) 7–39. Cf. Hopkins (1983) 14–16, 164.

[276] See Sallares (1991) 244–62, with references and a discussion of previous scholarship. On the Antonine epidemic in Egypt, see Rathbone (1990) 114–9, and in general Duncan-Jones (1996); see also below, Chapter 2, p. 162. Catastrophic mortality in Alexandria in the 260s, as insinuated by Dionysius of Alexandria (Eusebius, *Historia Ecclesiastica* 7.21.9–10; cf. Delia (1988) 289; Parkin (1992) 63–4), cannot be linked to a specific disease.

Al-Razi around 900 CE, smallpox had by then become endemic in the Middle East.[277] It is, however, impossible to tell whether smallpox permanently established itself in parts of the Mediterranean after the Antonine pandemic;[278] it had apparently failed to do so in 430 BCE. The lack of sufficiently populous cities in the fifth century BCE may help to account for this failure. In the Roman period, by contrast, Alexandria and other densely settled parts of Egypt would have offered an exceptionally favourable ground. Smallpox was, after all, endemic in Egypt at a time when its population was smaller or at any rate not larger than under the Romans and also less urbanised.[279] We therefore cannot rule out the possibility that smallpox was present in that country for much or most of the period covered by our funerary evidence of seasonal mortality.

A peak from March to May, as reported for the sixteenth century, might be in keeping with the ancient data from Upper Egypt. However, problems abound. If smallpox had indeed been endemic in significant parts of Egypt for much of the first millennium CE, deaths would have been heavily concentrated in the first years of life and thus almost invisible in the epigraphic record. In this case, the observed seasonal patterns could not be related to smallpox. Conversely, had the disease only emerged at substantial intervals (radiating from a stronghold of fully endemic smallpox such as Alexandria), the resulting mortality crises might to some degree have disrupted funereal rites and stifled epigraphic commemoration. Again, it would hardly have had a major effect on the attested distribution of deaths. It seems doubtful whether an intermediate scenario of serial epidemics, which one might call the 'Geneva model', could reasonably be applied to an entire millennium and a variety of different sites spread out over a large area.[280] Smallpox outbreaks at the end

---

[277] Al-Razi in Greenhill (1848) 28–30, who described it as a disease of infancy and childhood: 'hardly anyone escapes it' (28); 'children (...) rarely escape being seized with this disease' (29); 'as to young men (...) this disease only happened to a few individuals among them' (30), such as those who experienced merely a 'weak smallpox' in childhood (30 n. 2), and thus failed to acquire lasting immunity; 'as for old men, the smallpox seldom happend to them' (30). This pattern is completely incompatible with the age distribution of epidemic smallpox.

[278] Cf. Sallares (1991) 230, 255, who doubts any such development. The history of smallpox is discussed by Fenner *et al.* (1988) 209–44.

[279] See below, Chapter 3, p. 197.

[280] However, in his forthcoming Ph.D. thesis at Columbia University, Yan Zelener argues in favour of continuing periodic smallpox outbreaks in the centuries following the 'Antonine plague', especially in Italy and Egypt.

of the autumn and at the beginning of spring, as in the nineteenth century, are perhaps more readily consistent with the seasonal mortality patterns for Terenouthis and Leontopolis. Here, the evidence is more narrowly focused in time and space. However, as we have seen above (section 2.5), the mortality rise of the cool months appears to have been concentrated among adults. Nothing could be less typical of smallpox. The documented seasonality patterns in antiquity cannot be explained with reference to smallpox.

3.8. *Plague*

Plague, caused by *Yersinia pestis*, was one of the deadliest scourges of early modern Egypt. Following the catastrophic mortality of the Black Death, the disease persisted well into the nineteenth century. Plague is reported for 133 years between 1517 and 1894. Between 1571 and 1835, thirty-three serious epidemics can be identified, at a mean interval of no more than eight years. It became increasingly more common over the course of the eighteenth century, and severe crises in 1718, 1758/9, 1783/4, 1791 and 1835 cost the lives of hundreds of thousands of people. By the 1780s, plague had become fully endemic in Egypt: during the first half of the nineteenth century, on average, the disease struck every other year.[281]

Outbreaks frequently conformed to a broad pattern implying a gradual northward spread of the disease, presumably as a function of rising temperatures (Table 1.12).[282]

Table 1.12 Seasonal incidence of plague in early modern Egypt

	Onset	Peak	End
Upper Egypt	March	April	May
Middle Egypt	April	May	June
Delta	April	June	July
Littoral	May	July	October

[281] Black Death: Dols (1977). Subsequent outbreaks: Dols (1979) 175–6, 184–9; and see Raymond (1972) 204–7. Severe crises in the eighteenth century: Raymond (1972) 205–9. Plague of 1835: McCarthy (1976) 12–15; Panzac (1985) 348–52. Endemic plague up to 1844: McCarthy (1976) 12; Panzac (1987) 18. Chapter 3 provides a more detailed overview.

[282] Pollitzer (1954) 33.

Pertinent reports by European travellers go back to the sixteenth century. While individual accounts may disagree on the typical duration of outbreaks, they all share the belief that the plague ceased at the first sign of the inundation. According to Prosper Alpinus, the disease was active from March to May and disappeared in June. Pococke stated that it usually broke out in February, peaked during the *khamseen* season, and ended in June. In Volney's opinion, the plague was most violent in the winter, and always stopped in June. Sonnini claimed that it always emerged in April and never failed to cease at the summer solstice. According to Antes, it was most common from February to June, and 'it seldom remains after the 24th of June'. This pattern, he asserted, 'has always been observed in Egypt'. In the 1830s, Lane also noted that the plague arrived in the spring and was severe during the *khamseen*. Even a few years before its eventual exit from the country, in 1841 plague reappeared lightly in that season.[283] In any case, the plague would not always depart on time, especially in the North; Sandwith noted that it often continued into July.[284] The impact of a plague outbreak in Cairo in March and April 1801 was recorded by French observers (Fig. 1.42).[285]

The spring-time peak of the plague in Upper and Middle Egypt is readily compatible with the ancient seasonal mortality pattern. Moreover, it was claimed that whereas the elderly were little affected by the plague, 'the most vigorous and the strongest appear to be most subject to it'.[286] John Hatcher's study of Christ Church Priory in Canterbury in the fifteenth century has shown that recurrent outbreaks of plague may indeed create a substantial seasonal peak in the overall mean mortality distribution of an adult population.[287] Hence, the importance of the disease in antiquity deserves closer scrutiny. For plague to have had a noticeable impact on the mor-

---

[283] Alpin (1980) 107 (duration), 125 (disappearance) (bk. I, pp. 60, 71), with an extensive discussion of the latter (126–40 = bk. I, pp. 71–9). In 1581, Forésien claimed that the plague lasted for three months and stopped when the Nile began to rise: *Voyage* (1971) 49. George Sandys also wrote that the plague ceased with the inundation: *Voyages* (1973a) 42 (= *Sandys Travels*, London 1673, 76); so did [Campbell] (1739) 403. Pococke (1743) 196 (cf. also Norden (1757) vol. I, 86); Volney (1788) 255; Sonnini (1799) 18; Antes (1801) 38, 47, 49; Winter (1992) 235 (Lane); Yates (1843) 136 n.*.

[284] Sandwith (1905) 158; and see also Frank (1820) 22.

[285] Desgenettes (1813), in Panzac (1982) 96 tab. 9. On this event, see ibid., 95–8.

[286] Antes (1801) 52.

[287] Hatcher (1986), esp. 26 tab. 1, 28–9, 36. Cf. Scheidel (1996a) 144–5.

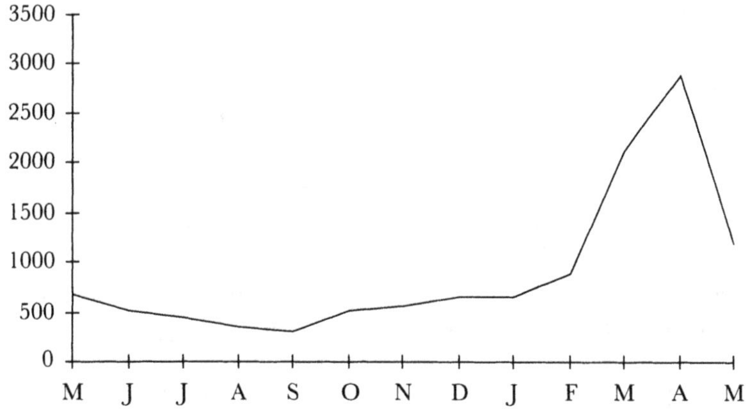

Figure 1.42 Monthly mortality figures in Cairo, May 1800 to May 1801

tality regime of ancient Upper Egypt and Nubia, it had to occur on a fairly regular basis for about forty consecutive generations. Neither occasional and weak isolated outbreaks nor rare catastrophic epidemics would have left a strong mark on the existing record.

For much of the first millennium, there is no evidence to the effect that plague was common in Egypt, although the disease itself was known. An outbreak of bubonic plague is first reported for 'Libya'—presumably a generic term for North Africa—in the Hellenistic period. In the early second century CE, the physician Rufus of Ephesus regarded this disease as prevalent in Libya, Egypt and Syria.[288] This statement is consistent with the geographical distribution of plague among rodents today.[289] The two main carriers, rat and flea, were both present in Roman Egypt. In general, the black domesticated rat (*Rattus rattus*) is attested in the Mediterranean at least from the Hellenistic period, while the brown rat (*Rattus norvegicus*) appears to be have been known in Iran and Mesopotamia. A number of Egyptian mummies of birds of prey contain half-digested remains of the Egyptian Rat, *R. rattus alexandrinus*. Fleas must also have been common.[290]

[288] Rufus of Ephesus (in Oribasius, *Collectiones medicae* 44.14, *CMG* 6.2.1); see Sideras (1994) 1195. For discussion and further ancient references, see Thüry (1977) 275 with 279 nn. 1–7, Sallares (1991) 266 with 466–7 n. 375. The scepticism in Marasco (1998) 46–7 seems ill-founded.

[289] Mollaret (1989) 104 map 1.

[290] See Thüry (1977), and his articles 'Floh' and 'Ratte' in *Der Neue Pauly*. Armitage (1994) 232–3 contemplates the possibility that the black rat reached the Near East

However, plague is essentially unstable among rats. In Africa today, it remains endemic among species of wild rodents other than rats. In antiquity, this may have reduced exposure of humans.[291] Even if we accept that the disease regularly appeared in Egypt, we are completely ignorant about the severity of these plague events. Not a single reported epidemic of the Roman period can be associated with bubonic or pneumonic plague, and its symptoms are never described in medical papyri.[292]

The first known plague pandemic began under Justinian in 541 CE and lingered for over two hundred years.[293] Egypt was struck by three major waves in 541/2, 639/40, and 686.[294] Further outbreaks are reported for the years 698, 703, 705, and 746/7.[295] Around 750, it disappeared from the Middle East. The documented seasonality patterns for the first millennium do not reflect this series of mortality crises. All mummy labels and many of the Greek inscriptions predate the Justinianic plague, while most of the relevant Coptic texts were set up from the eighth to the tenth centuries. Moreover, the victims of major epidemics must have been less likely to receive proper tombstones: the depletion of families and general disorder tend to suppress the 'epigraphic habit'.[296]

---

from India as early as the second millennium BCE, concluding that it had become permanently established in the eastern Mediterranean by the Roman period. Fleas are mentioned in *P.Lond.* 121.149ff., and evidence of them has been found in northwestern Roman Europe (Thüry (1977) 276). When the plague was at its height around 1800, Wilson (1803) 263 emphasised that in Egypt, rats occurred 'in extraordinary abundance' and fleas 'in such quantities, that in twelve hours clean linen was covered with thousands of spots of blood'; he concludes that 'many of these disagreeable animals the Egyptians may say are also inmates of Europe, but in no other country are they so numerous or so voracious as in Egypt.'

[291] E.g., Lancaster (1990) 98. See Hinnebusch (1997) on the sudden emergence of the plague bacillus (*Yersinia pestis*) through minor mutation.

[292] Leca (1971) 207.

[293] See Russell (1968); Biraben and Le Goff (1969); Dols (1974); Biraben (1975) 25–48; Patlagean (1977) 87–91; Bratton (1981); Conrad (1981) (*non vidi*); Durliat (1989); Congourdeau (1993); Conrad (1994); McCormick (1998) 52–65; Alston (2001) 182–91. Cf. Maddicott (1997) for its spread in seventh-century northwestern Europe.

[294] Biraben and Le Goff (1969); Dols (1974). Allen (1979) 14 states that Egypt was also affected in 673/4. The so-called 'plague of al-Jarif' of 688/89 may also have spread to Egypt: Dols (1974) 378. Around 600 CE, the Alexandrinian physician and priest Ahrun described bubonic plague: Conrad (1982) 294.

[295] See Dols (1974) 378 n. 79 for references. Cf. Biraben (1975) 31.

[296] Compare Thucydides 2.52.4; *Historia Augusta, Life of Marcus Aurelius* 13.3; Procopius, *Bella* 2.22–3. Cf. above, n. 49.

The extent to which less severe but more regular local outbreaks in the preceding centuries, which seem to lie behind the accounts given by Rufus and his sources, helped shape the seasonal mortality pattern in the long term remains unclear. It is probable that even at low levels, plague could have exacerbated other diseases. In 1840, for instance, the plague was preceded by 'marsh fevers' and 'abdominal typhus' (i.e., typhoid) which struck with much greater force than usual. Schnepp noted later that due to the disappearance of the plague in the 1840s, it was no longer possible to describe this kind of interaction, but referred to comparable epidemics of 'typhus de misère' in the Levant.[297] In antiquity, repeated moderate exposure of this kind could certainly have contributed to the marked surge in mortality during the spring.

3.9. *Cholera*

Cholera (*Vibrio cholerae*) originates in India, where it has been most prevalent in the hot season with increased humidity, although a wide range of seasonal variation is also on record. In the modern age, cholera first reached Egypt in 1831.[298] The seasonal incidence of the major cholera epidemics in that country again reveals a preference for the hot season. While the first wave in 1831 ravaged the country from July to October, the outbreaks of 1848, 1850 and 1865 were confined to the months from June to August, May to July, and May to June, respectively.[299]

The antiquity of cholera is unclear. Cholera-like diseases are described by various classical authors, but whether any of these diseases were genuine cholera is impossible to decide. Severe diarrhoeal diseases accompanied by dehydration were also recorded by early Chinese and Hindu sources. Dysenteric types of dehydrating illness were not uncommon in the more distant past, but it seems that cholera proper was largely confined to India.[300]

---

297 Schnepp (1862b) 563–4, with reference to Pruner.

298 For a discussion of cholera in nineteenth-century Egypt, see Panzac (1985) 411–45.

299 Jagailloux (1986) 231.

300 Cook (1996) 19. Cf. Lancaster (1990) 68.

3.10. *Other diseases*

In the nineteenth century, measles were very common in Egypt as a fatal disease of children. It was dangerous in the first instance under the age of five. Sandwith estimates that in Lower Egypt, one-third of all deaths under the age of five were caused by measles.[301] Existing statistics are useless, but a more cautious estimate suggests that in the nineteenth century, death rates from measles were similar to those found in tropical Africa, where between two and ten per cent of patients would die in rural areas.[302] Broncho-pulminary complications would occur in the winter months. Greek and Roman texts contain no reference to measles.[303]

Schistosomiasis, or bilharzia, is known to have been endemic in Egypt since before the Pharaohs.[304] It has traditionally been common in the countryside: in the nineteenth century, *Schistosoma haematobium* was found all over the country, whereas *S. mansoni*, which causes bloody diarrhoea and dysentery, was limited to the northern Delta.[305] The incidence of schistosomiasis has greatly increased with perennial irrigation.[306] Around 1900, it was generally unknown in infants but attested from ages four to seventy; most cases occurred from ages fifteen to forty-five. It affected individuals who worked on flooded land, including peasant women. At that time, the average mortality rate was unknown owing to the lack of statistics: in one hospital, 5.8 per cent of all cases ended fatally.[307] In the early twen-

---

[301] Sandwith (1905) 119–22. This is reminiscent of the previous scale of small-pox mortality at the same ages; see below, Chapter 3, p. 197.

[302] Jagailloux (1986) 241–2. This, again, makes it a principal cause of death in the early years of life.

[303] Grmek (1989) 336.

[304] For predynastic evidence of schistosomiasis, see Deelder *et al.* (1990); Miller *et al.* (1993). Pharaonic Egypt: Adamson (1976); Lippi and Lippi (1985); cf. Leca (1971) 214–16; Sandison (1972) 216. Late antiquity: Miller *et al.* (1992). It was common in the Dakleh Oasis: Dzierzykray-Rogalski (1980). A comprehensive study of Egyptian schistosomiasis from *c.*2686 BCE to 641 CE is currently underway: Contis and David (1996).

[305] Jagailloux (1986) 256–7. The Nile Delta and eastern Brazil between Recife and the lower Sao Francisco are now the two main areas of hyperendemic *S. mansoni* in the world: Lancaster (1990) 195 fig. 19.2.1. In the nineteenth century, Hirsch (1883) 207 singled out Lower Egypt and the Cape region as the two foci of *S. haematobium* in Africa.

[306] Rivlin (1961) 248; Toledano (1990) 20. The transition from basin irrigation to perennial irrigation could raise the incidence of *S. haematobium* infection from ten to ninety per cent in the same area (Wilcocks (1962) as cited by Lancaster (1990) 194).

[307] Sandwith (1905) 214–40, esp. 221, 226. The contribution of schistosomiasis to mortality is generally difficult to quantify: Lancaster (1990) 195.

tieth century, forty per cent of over 1,000 Egyptians aged five to sixty who underwent necropsy in a Cairo hospital showed evidence of schistosomiasis. In 1937, it was estimated that almost half of the Egyptian population was infected, and local rates, above all in the Nile Delta, could be much higher.[308] In 1970, it was still considered a most serious health hazard. Today, about one in five Egyptians is thought to be infected with schistosomiasis, with prevalence rates as high as eighty-five per cent in some villages. It thrives in areas of stagnant water, such as portions of the Delta and the Aswan Dam area.[309] In the context of manual agricultural labour, infections would peak in the early winter and symptoms began to arise after three months of incubation in the spring and summer.[310] Even so, schistosomiasis is unlikely to contribute to seasonal mortality: although transmission rates vary with the seasons, the heavy worm-burden affects the body continually. It may, however, help render other illnesses more dangerous or lethal, and causes liver fibrosis, renal damage, bladder calcification and abdominal swelling.[311]

Dracunculiasis or dracontiasis (guinea-worm disease) in second-century CE Egypt was described by Rufus of Ephesus; according to Paulus of Aegina, it was well established in that country in late antiquity.[312] Ankylostomiasis is another common worm-disease. Around 1900, hookworm infection was widespread in both Lower and Upper Egypt, as opposed to schistosomiasis which favoured the Delta. Most patients, usually peasants, were aged twenty to forty. Its symptoms, sleepiness, debility and wasting, contribute indirectly to mortality by preventing sufferers from working and through interaction with other diseases.[313]

There is no doubt that these and related conditions were endemic in the Roman period. A number of ancient Egyptian medical recipes

---

[308] Sandison (1980) 30. 1937; Lancaster (1990) 195. See in general Scott (1937).

[309] *Area Handbook* (1970) 125; Contis and David (1996) 253. On schistosomiasis in modern Egypt, see DeWolfe Miller *et al.* (1978); Abdel-Wahab (1982).

[310] Sandwith (1905) 222. Bradley in Chambers, Longhurst and Pacey, eds. (1981) 127–9, discusses seasonal aspects of schistosomiasis.

[311] In the words of Abdel-Wahab (1982) 89, 'Schistosomiasis rarely exists as the sole infection or disease-state in many areas of Egypt. Malnutrition, enteric diseases, viral hepatitis, malaria, filariasis, amebiasis, and other diseases and states of ill-health, more often coexist in schistosome-infected individuals than not.'

[312] Rufus of Ephesus, *Quaestiones Medicinales* 12.67 ed. Gärtner (*CMG Suppl.* IV, p. 44, with commentary pp. 100–1); Paulus of Aegina 4.58.1 ed. Heiberg (*CMG* IX 1, p. 387). Guinea-worm infestation in Egypt appears to date back to the Pharaonic period: Adamson (1988). For its eradication in recent times, see Watts (1998).

[313] Sandwith (1905) 233–80, esp. 244, 254, 260, 264–5; also Hirsch (1883) 219.

include remedies against worms.[314] Frequent osteological signs of malnutrition in ancient Egypt, such as stunting, Harris lines and *cribra orbitalia*, may suggest low levels of food intake but are also consistent with parasitic infection, such as by *S. haematobium* and hookworm.[315] In this connection, it is particularly interesting that the discovery of schistosome antigen in mummies from the twelfth century BCE points to worm infection even among the elite.[316]

According to Aretaios, diphtheria was particularly common in Roman Egypt and was thus known as 'Egyptian (and Syrian) ulcers'. The physician gave what Grmek calls a 'masterful description' of this disease, which he regarded as lethal and widespread among children up to the age of puberty.[317] By the nineteenth century, syphilis had become an important cause of neonatal and infant death.[318] In 1800, a French observer found rachitis to be a major attrition factor in Cairo, prevalent in malnourished children aged one to three. Asthma was also very frequent in that city, as was blindness, the commonest cause of which would have been trachoma. Blindness had already been noted by Johann Wild at the beginning of the seventeenth century and by Father Gonzales in the 1660s; Volney found it to be common to every month and age, especially in Cairo and the Delta, less so among bedouins, foreigners and the upper classes. Sonnini also stressed the ubiquity of eye disorders.[319] Such conditions were endemic and not strongly seasonal, but occurred most frequently during the hot months.[320] Scorpion stings must have posed

---

314 Manniche (1989) 66, 80, 86, 104, 134, 140. See also Nunn (1996) 69–73, and cf. Leca (1971) 211–12, for a possible reference to ankylostomiasis in *P.Ebers*. For Coptic recipes against worms, see Till (1951) 24; Kolta (1984) 161.

315 Brahin and Fleming (1982) 79. Chronic anaemias caused by parasites also resulted in skull defects: Hillson (1980). Evidence of chronic malnourishment, e.g., enamel hypoplasia, is common in ancient Egypt: Rose, Armelagos and Perry (1993) 65. See also Mittler and van Gerven (1994) on Coptic Nubia, and cf. in general Garnsey (1999). For a large number of skeletons with *satisfactory* nutritional and health status from a predynastic Egyptian cemetery (3900–3300 BCE), see Podzorski (1990).

316 Deelder *et al.* (1990).

317 Aretaios 1.9.3–5; Grmek (1989) 338.

318 Jagailloux (1986) 248–9. Cf. Grmek (1989) 133–51, on the antiquity of syphilis; also Baker and Armelagos (1988) 706, 710. The latter favour the thesis that syphilis was introduced to the Old World from the Americas after Columbus.

319 Renati (1800) 187–9; *Voyages* (1973b) 20; *Voyage* (1977) 267–9 (= 1673, bk. IV, p. 141); Volney (1788) 241–2; Sonnini (1799) 25–6. Frank (1820) 157 cited Olivier to the effect that in Damascus, Baghdad and Mossul, ocular inflammations were less common than in Egypt.

320 Clot-Bey (1840) I 360–1. Eye afflictions were already reported in the second century CE in *O.Claud.* 174, 212–13 (July), 217 (August).

a serious hazard on the fringe of the desert.[321] It is unnecessary to prolong this survey.[322] For the sake of completeness, however, one might add that a claim that AIDS was already known in ancient Egypt has failed to find favour.[323]

3.11. *Early statistics of causes of death*

In nineteenth-century Egypt, statistics that detailed causes of death invariably rested on shaky foundations. Contemporary observers found it particularly difficult to distinguish between different gastro-intestinal disorders. When sources of that period identify 'fièvres gastro-enteriques' as the leading cause of death among children, this term must be taken to cover a whole range of (non-typhoid?) diseases.[324] The loose terminology of Schnepp's statistics for 1859/60 highlights the diagnostic shortcomings of his day (Table 1.13).

Table 1.13 Principal causes of death in the Egyptian populations of Cairo and Alexandria, July 1859 to June 1860 (in per cent)[325]

Cause	Cairo	Alexandria
Convulsions	39.5	20.2
Gastro-enteric fevers	31.2	29.6
Tuberculosis	14.0	3.1
Pulmonary diseases	0.1	11.5
Wasting	4.5	9.3
Typhoid fevers	2.8	2.6
Scrofula	0.2	0.3
Not stated	7.7	23.3

The conspicuous discrepancies in the relative incidence of tuberculosis ('phthisie') and other lung diseases ('maladies de la poitrine') in the two cities may hint at some amount of confusion in the diagnosis of pulmonary illnesses. 'Convulsions' could have been caused by a variety of medical conditions from gastro-intestinal infections

[321] *O.Claud.* 212 and 223 refer to such cases in the desert environment of Mons Claudianus.

[322] R. Sallares is preparing an extensive discussion of leprosy in the ancient Mediterranean, including Egypt. This disease has no obvious seasonal dimension.

[323] Ablin, Gonder and Immerman (1985).

[324] Cf. McCarthy (1976) 7. See above, section 3.3.

[325] Based on Schnepp (1862b) 552–3. See above, Figs. 1.39–40.

to tetanus and appendicitis. Hence, all gastro-intestinal diseases combined must have accounted for more than one-third but fewer than three-quarters of all deaths in Cairo, and for between one-third and one-half of all deaths in Alexandria. The actual rates are impossible to determine, and we are reduced to guesswork. However, the fact that de Regny's statistics for 1871 attribute a much larger proportion of all deaths to gastro-intestinal diseases (see below) strongly indicates that they also caused most of the mortality from 'convulsions' reported for 1859/60.

The records of the European Hospital in Cairo for the years from 1844 to 1861 provide somewhat more detailed information but are also seriously deficient: no fewer than 44.1 per cent of all cases and 38.2 per cent of all deaths are attributed to unspecified 'maladies diverses' (Table 1.14). 31.6 per cent of all deaths were caused by what must have been gastro-intestinal infections. This figure is lower than for the indigenous population, which suggests that even limited treatment, such as was at the disposal of European physicians of the mid-nineteenth century, could reduce the impact of these diseases. Even so, death rates remained high: dysentery and enteric fevers would kill from one-sixth to one-fifth of those affected.

Table 1.14 Reported cases of disease and causes of death in the European Hospital in Cairo, 1844 to 1861 (in per cent)[326]

Disease	Proportion of all cases	Proportion of all deaths	Death rate
'Gastric' and 'bilious' fevers	17.2	10.4	4.5
Dysentery	6.6	14.7	16.7
'Fièvre typhique'	2.1	6.5	23.1
Malaria	6.4	2.8	3.2
Liver disorders	6.0	13.6	17.1
Tuberculosis	1.5	9.1	44.1
Pulmonary diseases	3.1	3.4	8.2
Scrofula	0.4	0.2	2.9
Syphilis	7.2	1.0	1.0
Eye inflammations	5.7	0.2	0.2
Other diseases	44.1	38.2	6.5

[326] Based on Schnepp (1862b) 561: 8,195 cases and 617 deaths. The subtotals in Schnepp's tabulation do not always add up.

A comparison of data from 1859/60, 1871, and 1920 to 1925, shows a shift from gastro-intestinal to pulmonary diseases (Table 1.15). In the 1920s, causes were named for eighty-six per cent of all deaths; in 1859/60, this rate must already have been similar.[327] Even so, owing to intervening progress in diagnostics and possible differences in recording practices, these sets of data cannot be put on exactly the same footing. At the same time, the differences between the third quarter of the nineteenth century and the 1920s are so pronounced that to some extent they are bound to reflect actual change. The data presented in Tables 1.16 and 1.17 reveals the static character of child mortality between 1889 and 1922. This suggests that the observed shift primarily occurred at higher ages.

Table 1.15 Principal causes of death in Cairo and Alexandria, 1859/60, 1871 and 1920/25 (in per cent)[328]

Diseases	Cairo			Alexandria		
	1859/60	1871	1920/25	1859/60	1871	1920/25
gastro-intestinal	<73.5	68.7	34.9	<52.5	55.5	37.4
pulmonary	14.1	14.0	28.3	14.6	11.3	24.1

Table 1.16 Causes of death from ages one to five in Cairo and Alexandria, 1889, expressed as a share of all causes (in per cent)[329]

Disease	Cairo	Alexandria
gastro-enteric	47.3	35.5
respiratory	26.4	20.9

[327] Schnepp (1862b) 552 gives a total of 14,986 deaths in Cairo during a twelve-month period; causes of death are stated for 13,831 cases (92.3 per cent). Although according to McCarthy (1976) 30, in 1859/60 the population of that city totalled 290–295,000, the actual figure was at least 340,000. (This estimate is derived from the fact that his population figures for the whole country in these years need to be raised by about one-sixth: see below, Chapter 3, p. 208. The same method is here applied to his figures for Cairo.) A Crude Death Rate of 45 per 1,000 (cf. ibid., and Panzac (1985) 369) would consequently have resulted in 15,300 deaths per year. In this scenario, nine out of ten deaths would have been associated with a specific cause. It is, however, hard to imagine that a mere two per cent of all metropolitan deaths went unrecorded, and it seems more reasonable to reckon with a somewhat larger population total. Even so, the proportion of deaths that were not classified as to cause is unlikely to have been much larger than twenty per cent.

[328] Based on Schnepp (1862b) 552–3 (1859/60); Panzac (1982) 89 tab. 7 (1871), 85 tab. 2 (1920/25).

[329] Based on Jagailloux (1986) 275.

Table 1.16 *(cont.)*

Disease	Cairo	Alexandria
pneumonia	0.5	3.2
neurological	13.3	20.9
developmental	9.1	16.6
measles	0.9	2.6
smallpox	0.5	0.3

Table 1.17 Principal causes of death in Cairo, 1920 to 1925, expressed as a share of all causes (in per cent)[330]

Diseases	1922		1920/25
	Age 0–1	Age 1–5	All ages
gastro-intestinal	65.1	54.9	34.9
pulmonary	24.5	29.1	28.3

Table 1.18 Principal and unknown causes of death in Cairo, 1922, expressed as a share of all deaths (in per cent)[331]

Diseases	1922		1920/25
	Age 0–1	Age 1–5	All ages
gastro-intestinal	43.7	49.8	32.1
pulmonary	16.4	26.4	20.7
unknown	32.9	9.2	14.1

In Cairo in 1922, thirty-five per cent of all deaths occurred under the age of one, and another twenty-eight per cent during the subsequent four years of life.[332] Thus, most deaths from gastro-intestinal diseases must have been confined to early childhood. In the 1920s, fewer than ten per cent of deaths from these causes occurred above age five, compared to over one-third of all deaths from pulmonary diseases. These calculations are corroborated by reports that in 1930, in Egypt as a whole, twenty-six per cent of mortality under age two

[330] Based on Panzac (1982) 86 tab. 3 (children), 85 tab. 2 (total).
[331] Ibid.
[332] Panzac (1982) 86. Cf. below, Chapter 3, p. 214, for further evidence of mortality.

but only 6.4 per cent of deaths at higher ages were caused by diarrhoeal and enteric diseases. In the 1960s, when the population was growing more rapidly than in the early twentieth century and deaths in early childhood therefore accounted for a larger share of total mortality, about forty per cent of all deaths were attributed to diseases of the digestive system.[333]

The statistics from the third quarter of the nineteenth century paint a different picture. Back then, two-thirds rather than one-third of reported deaths in Cairo, and at least one-half in Alexandria, were ascribed to gastro-intestinal diseases. Even if about fifteen per cent of all deaths went unclassified, and had all been due to other factors, more than half of all deaths in Cairo would have been associated with a single type of disease. Since many deaths in early childhood must have been caused by different infections, such as tetanus, malaria, syphilis and measles, fatalities from gastro-intestinal diseases must also have been prevalent beyond age five.[334] In that period as well as in previous centuries, gastro-intestinal diseases appear to have had a significant impact on juvenile and adult mortality.[335] Hence, owing to seasonal variation in infection rates, they would also have helped shape the seasonal pattern of deaths at more mature ages.

4. *Conclusions*

From the sixteenth into the nineteenth centuries, European visitors to Egypt unanimously described the spring as the season of disease and death. In this respect, their accounts, however sketchy and unscientific, tally well with early medical studies from Napoleon's army doctors to Sandwith. Drawing on evidence discussed in sections 3.2 to 3.9, Table 1.19 offers a crude illustration of this broad

[333] 1930: Cleland (1936) 177 tab. C. 1960s: El Baz and Orabey (1975) 10. Omran (1973b) 59 fig. 9, considers changes in the leading causes of death in the early twentieth century.

[334] As noted above, Sandwith (1905) attributed one-third of all deaths under age five to measles. A similar rate had been typical of endemic smallpox until the middle of the nineteenth century. In the third quarter of the nineteenth century, with an annual rate of population growth between 1.0 and 1.5 per cent and low life expectancy, up to fifty-five or even sixty per cent of all deaths may have occurred under age five (cf., e.g., Coale and Demeny (1983) 57).

[335] Panzac (1982) 90 also concludes that diarrhoeas, dysenteries and enteric fevers, despite their focus on early childhood, affected all age groups.

consensus. In this tabulation, each of the principal seasonal diseases of Egypt is recorded for those months of the year in which it was considered to be prevalent. (Local anomalies, such as conditions in Alexandria, have not been taken into account.)

Table 1.19 Seasonal contours of infectious disease in Egypt from the sixteenth to the early twentieth centuries

JAN	FEB	MAR	APR	MAY	JUN	JUL	AUG	SEP	OCT	NOV	DEC
				dia							
				dys							
			dia	typ							
			dys	toi							
			typ	rel							
		typ	toi	jau	dia	dia					
		toi	rel	mal	dys	dys	dia				
		rel	jau	tub	typ	typ	dys	dia			
	toi	tub	tub	sma	sma	sma	typ	dys			
toi	rel	sma	sma	pla	pla	pla	mal	mal	mal	mal	
sma	sma	pla	pla	cho	cho	cho	cho	sma	sma	sma	sma

Key: dia = diarrhoea; dys = dysentery; typ = typhus; toi = typhoid; rel = relapsing fever; jau = infectious jaundice; mal = malaria; tub = tuberculosis; sma = smallpox; pla = plague; cho = cholera

Not all of these diseases were simultaneously active. The incidence of plague, smallpox and cholera in particular fluctuated heavily over the course of the nineteenth century. Even so, there can be no doubt that the range of serious diseases greatly expanded with rising temperatures in the early spring, peaking before the onset of the inundation. The contours of this distribution are strongly reminiscent of the seasonal mortality patterns from the ancient Nile valley, but fail to hint at the secondary surge in the death rate during the cool season.

No single factor can be held accountable for the high index of seasonal mortality variation produced by the evidence of tombstones and mummy labels from ancient and early medieval Upper Egypt and Nubia. Rather, a high incidence of a number of pathogens must have been required to skew the seasonal pattern in the observed fashion.[336] Statistics from the third quarter of the nineteenth century

---

336 Unfortunately, the 'sick lists' from Mons Claudianus (second century CE) are insufficiently well preserved to permit a reconstruction of the seasonal distribution

are consistent with the assumption that gastro-intestinal diseases contributed to juvenile and adult mortality. Typhoid, paratyphoid, relapsing fever and hepatitis would all spread in the early spring, focussing on older children and young adults. In the absence of preventive measures and effectual medical intervention, the seasonal convergence of these infections could not fail to raise the death rate at that time of the year. Other agents would also come into play. The Greek epitaphs point to elevated mortality in the late autumn and early winter, a phenomenon that is readily compatible with the autumnal peak of malaria infections and respiratory diseases precipitated by the drop in the temperature, especially among the elderly. In the months that followed, tuberculosis was exacerbated by the heat and the sand storms of the *khamseen*, and those who had been weakened by intermittent fevers since October or November would find themselves dangerously exposed to the infections of the spring. High levels of malaria in the preceding season and the sudden emergence of diarrhoeal and enteric diseases around March, perhaps facilitated by the falling levels and increasing contamination of the water in the canals, may have concurred to trigger the exceptional mortality crises of the early spring that we find attested for the Fayum.

We cannot tell with certainty whether these factors were sufficiently potent to generate the observed seasonality patterns. It is certainly conceivable, albeit impossible to demonstrate, that local outbreaks of plague added to adult mortality in the spring. Moreover, we are not necessarily aware of all seasonal causes of death in ancient Egypt. Over four hundred years ago, Prosper Alpinus referred to a springtime disease, known as 'Dem el muja' among the locals, which was supposedly capable of killing a grown man within hours, as were inflammations of the brain at the same time of the year. In 1739, John Campbell likewise wrote about 'pestilential Fevers, which are mortal in twenty-four hours'.[337] Finally, the bias of the funerary record in favour of teenagers and young and middle-aged adults inevitably distorts our vision: diseases that caused only a moderate proportion of all deaths overall but focused on these age groups would have a disproportionately strong impact on the shape of the documented

of disease (Cuvigny (1992) 78–82, esp. 81); moreover, these lists only rarely identify the underlying diseases.

[337] Alpin (1980) 93–4, 97 (bk. I, pp. 53, 55); [Campbell] (1739) 402. Cf. Pruner (1847) 367–73 for a possible parallel.

seasonal mortality distribution. Typhus (which may not have existed in ancient times), typhoid, relapsing fever and plague all belong in this category.[338]

In our discussion, prominence has been given to the ancient evidence from the Nile valley which covers a wider range of space and time than the data from Lower Egypt. As for the apparent lack of seasonal variation in ancient Alexandria, it deserves notice that this city, already praised by Strabo, has also more recently been considered to be healthier than Cairo.[339] Its seaside setting may have sheltered its inhabitants from the worst effects of some of the seasonal infections that ravaged the shores of the Nile. The mortality patterns for Terenouthis and Leontopolis are rather more difficult to reconcile with more recent information on disease and death. It is however reassuring that data from the third quarter of the nineteenth century point to a similar, albeit much weaker, rise in the death rate towards the end of the year (cf. above, Fig. 1.37). As neither site need have been 'typical' of the interior of the Delta—if 'typicality' were a legitimate concept at all—, it would be inadvisable to put too much weight on these samples. Local pockets of endemic disease could have transformed the demographic structure of individual communities. A high incidence of tuberculosis and respiratory disases might go a long way in explaining adult mortality maxima in the cool season. In this case, however, comparative evidence from the Western Oases in the 1920s may point to a background of hyperendemic malaria in the two ancient towns. It would kill the young and weaken adults, rendering them more vulnerable to other infections. According to early modern accounts, typhoid, for instance, could occur from the beginning of the year, and thus interact with intermittent fevers. The same is true of respiratory diseases. All the same, any interpretation of the data from Terenouthis and Leontopolis must needs remain exceedingly speculative.[340] This prob-

---

[338] If certain diseases were more lethal under conditions of very high, i.e., urban, population density, the urban emphasis of our evidence might also amplify seasonal amplitudes.

[339] Strabo 17.1.7, quoted above, section 3.5. See Panzac (1982) 88 tab. 6, for a comparison of the death rates of Cairo and Alexandria; cf. in general Panzac (1978).

[340] Scientific analysis of the skeletal evidence from the large cemetery of Terenouthis unearthed by a team from the University of Michigan in 1935 could have shed some light on the local disease environment. Unfortunately, the failure of the excavators to preserve this material spoilt a unique chance of conducting osteological studies of an ancient population with a known seasonal mortality pattern. This loss

lem, however, does not detract from their relevance to the study of ancient demography. The true value of these texts lies in the fact that by illustrating the potential for difference and the scope of regional variation, they underscore the hazards of deriving broad generalisations from local samples of evidence. I will return to this problem in the next chapter.

With few exceptions, the ancient seasonality patterns of Egypt have no parallel in the early modern period. By contrast, in terms of the *timing* of seasonal mortality peaks, the late antique data from the city of Rome and southern Italy are consistent with more recent evidence, even though they indicate higher *levels* of variation at mature ages. In Egypt, the ancient patterns differ from their modern counterparts in both respects. This, however, cannot be taken to imply that the Egyptian documentation is necessarily flawed or intrinsically implausible. The data for Upper Egypt and Nubia in particular fall into a smooth unimodal distribution that can be related to pre-twentieth century accounts of the seasonal incidence of disease. The contrasting evidence from Lower Egypt, whilst more difficult to interpret, at the very least cannot be dismissed out of hand. Although the biases inherent in the ancient funerary record to some degree impede straightforward comparisons between ancient and modern data, the very scale of the observed differences is strongly suggestive of a considerable amount of intervening *change*.

When Shaw, in his brief aside on seasonal mortality in Roman Egypt, introduced evidence of seasonal mortality from the 1920s for comparative purposes, he justified this step with the claim that at that time, 'the Egyptian population was still firmly pre-modern in type'.[341] This is correct to the extent that these data describe a pre-transitional population, characterised by high mortality and even

is particularly deplorable for a number of reasons: the burial district of Terenouthis offered a rare chance to study funerary texts, physical remains and other features of the burial process *in context* (cf. Morris (1992) 156–7); the epigraphic evidence of seasonal mortality in Terenouthis constitutes both the second largest and the earliest published homogenous local sample of pertinent data from antiquity proper (there are twenty times as many data from Rome, and the mummy labels, though roughly from the same period, do not reflect a single local population); the fact that it is now possible to identify malaria infection in bones of that age might have enabled us to test our hypothesis against the physical record. To judge by Hawwass (1979) 82–4, further excavations from 1969 to 1976 likewise led to the discovery of skeletons, but their fate remains unclear. A large new canal, the Nasser Canal, now cuts right through the site (ibid., 75–7).

[341] Shaw (1996) 123.

higher fertility. It would, however, be wrong to assume that until one or two generations ago, Egypt was subject to a single, uniform 'pre-modern' demographic regime or to stable, immutable seasonal patterns of disease and death. On the contrary, the disease environment, and hence the demography, of 'pre-modern' Egypt have evolved through a series of transformations that can still be traced back over more than two thousand years. For no other country in the world, with the possible exception of China, is it possible to identify broad shifts and changes across such an extended period of time. The ancient, medieval and modern evidence from Egypt affords us a unique chance of glimpsing the true *longue durée* of population history.[342]

As we have seen in the previous section, the disease environment underlying the relative incidence of leading causes of death documented for the 1920s could not lay claim to great antiquity. Two generations earlier, gastro-intestinal diseases took a much heavier toll on the population and more frequently posed lethal risks beyond early childhood. By then measles had begun to take over the role of smallpox in decimating the very young. This scenario, in turn, was itself the result of very recent changes.[343] During the first half of the nineteenth century, endemic smallpox rivalled diarrhoeal diseases as the major killer of infants and small children, while a sizeable share of deaths among adults was caused by the relentless onslaught of the plague. With this, we encounter the 'archaic pattern' of mortality evoked by Perrenoud which Europe had by then long left behind, and which stands apart from the two (or more?) more recent 'pre-modern' types of late nineteenth- and early twentieth-century Egypt. In the long run, even this earlier pattern was far from stable. While smallpox appears to have been endemic in the country since the Middle Ages, plague had had a more chequered history. Re-introduced

[342] This study has mainly drawn on funerary records from the first millennium CE that were composed in ancient Greek and Coptic, and on western accounts of Egypt commencing in the sixteenth century. Arabic sources (which are not normally available in translation) may well provide additional information for the intervening period and indeed up into the nineteenth century. It is hoped that the present study will encourage colleagues with the required linguistic expertise to elaborate on my discussion. For China, cf. briefly Lee and Campbell (1997) 217–18. Documentary evidence has survived from as far back as the Han period; for medical sources, see Dong, Xi and Thann (1996).

[343] All these changes predate the 'epidemiologic transition' from death from infectious diseases to death from chronic and degenerative diseases discussed by Omran (1971). Here, we are dealing with significant transformations within a pre-transitional context.

on a grand scale as the Black Death of the 1340s, it seems to have first abated after the early fifteenth century and then gradually regained momentum, intensifying in particular during the eighteenth century. Louse-borne typhus must have joined the canon of Egypt's scourges by the end of the Middle Ages. As we move further back in time into the first millennium of the Christian era, the picture inevitably blurs. Although we know that smallpox hit the country in the late second and in the early seventh centuries, it is impossible to tell when precisely it permanently established itself as as an endemic disease of early childhood. Evidence of plague is equally tantalizing: ravaging Egypt in successive epidemic waves from the sixth into the eighth centuries, it was already known in pre-Christian times and vaguely considered common under the early Roman empire. Leprosy appears to have spread greatly in the Roman period.[344] The incidence of tuberculosis remains unknown, and needs to be considered in conjunction with the development of leprosy.[345] The early history of malaria is similarly obscure. Although its presence is not in doubt, its demographic impact as well as the relative share of its various branches are difficult to gauge from isolated bits of evidence. Malaria does, however, seem to have been more widespread in antiquity than in the more recent past, with potentially serious consequences. In particular, the transformation of the Fayum into a marshy hunting ground of the Pharaohs followed by the large-scale drainage efforts of the Ptolemies and progressive desiccation during the Roman and later periods must have resulted in dramatic upswings and downturns in the regional prevalence of malaria.

Some general points ensue. Pre-modern Egypt had long been regarded as a strikingly unhealthy region. Given a population density that was exceptionally high by pre-modern standards—with a mean ratio of about 300 people per square kilometre of arable land in the early Roman period—, this unhappy state of affairs does not come as a surprise. Under these circumstances and in the absence of modern sanitation and public health measures, infectious diseases both endemic and epidemic were bound to thrive. A high rate of urbanisation could only have made matters worse. In fact, as the rates of urbanisation attained under Roman rule were unparalleled until

[344] As R. Sallares will argue in forthcoming work. See esp. Galen vol. 11, p. 142 ed. Kühn.

[345] E.g., Manchester (1986).

well into the the twentieth century, we lack comparative evidence to determine their likely effects in antiquity.[346] From that perspective, Egypt could hardly be less 'typical' of the ancient Mediterranean in general, even if 'typical' were at all a meaningful notion. For all their individual differences, most of the other parts of the Roman world shared lower rates of urbanisation and much lower levels of population density. In terms of health and life expectancy, Egypt, much like the city of Rome itself, may well have found itself at the bottom of the league. The problems inherent in extrapolations from certain conditions in certain localities of Egypt to the demographic regime of the Roman empire as a whole are necessarily compounded by the possibility of considerable local and regional variation within Egypt, as suggested by our evidence of seasonal mortality and consideration of specific ecological contexts.

Furthermore, the fundamental shifts in Egyptian disease patterns over the course of the past two millennia—some of them delineated above, others, perhaps, still hidden from our view—cast doubt on the applicability of demographic models derived from recent populations to a much more distant past. It is not at all obvious that ancient populations ought to have been defined by those age distributions which in modern models are associated with levels of life expectancy that are considered appropriate for such early societies. This potentially unrealistic premise stems from a static view of population history according to which different disease environments can invariably be accommodated within a set framework of age-specific mortality rates. Needless to say, it is impossible to infer actual death rates from seasonal patterns alone. As a general rule, however, high amplitudes of seasonality tend to coincide with high mortality *per se*. Hence, strong seasonal mortality variation between early childhood and old age implies high mortality among juveniles and adults. With respect to the late antique city of Rome, a scenario of this kind could be explained with reference to massive urban crowding and incessant immigration of adults who had failed to acquire immunity earlier in life. Modern observers might be inclined to concede that in a seemingly exceptional case like this, age-specific mortality rates

---

346 In Chapter 3, I argue for maxima of approximately six million inhabitants and 20,000 km^2 of arable in early Roman Egypt. In his forthcoming Leiden doctoral thesis, L. E. Tacoma discusses levels of urbanisation in Roman Egypt. See below, Chapter 3, p. 247.

need not have conformed to the predictions generated by model life tables. It now seems, however, that Rome was not quite as exceptional in this respect as one might have expected. Evidence from Egypt and Nubia, as well as Palestine, reveals comparable levels of fatal seasonal infection at mature ages. This finding raises an important question about the probable age structure of the Egyptian population. If seasonal mortality variation was very high across different age groups, adult death rates, in urban settings at any rate, may also have been uncommonly high relative to mortality in childhood and old age. This hypothesis will be explored in the next chapter.

CHAPTER TWO

AGE STRUCTURE AND LIFE EXPECTANCY

1. *Life tables from census returns?*

From the beginning of the first to the middle of the third century CE, the Roman authorities conducted a census of the population of Egypt at regular intervals of fourteen years.[1] On these occasions, each declarant had to draw up a list of the members of his or her household, including lodgers and slaves, with their names, filiations, ages, location within the family, and distinguishing characteristics. Over 300 of these census returns (or copies thereof), preserved in various states of completeness on papyrus, have so far been published. Long recognised as valuable evidence for the demographic structure of Roman Egypt, this material has recently been assessed in a sophisticated book-length study by Roger Bagnall and Bruce Frier. Their aim is to explore all aspects of this material, 'the size and structure of Egyptian households, the population's age and sex distribution, and the patterns of mortality, fertility, and migration that are likely to have prevailed in Roman Egypt'.[2]

In this chapter, I will focus on the relation of the attested age structure of the census population to the 'patterns of mortality, fertility and migration' of the actual population behind these texts. By now, 747 ages have become known, 351 for females, 372 for males, and 24 for individuals of unknown gender. 403 of these figures come from villages (*komai*), 344 from district capitals (*metropoleis*). The age distribution of the raw data highlights the need for smoothing procedures as a necessary precondition of any meaningful demographic analysis (Fig. 2.1).[3]

---

[1] For a comprehensive description of the census process and the format of the census documents, see Bagnall and Frier (1994) 1–30.

[2] Bagnall and Frier (1994) 1. For further demographic studies of the census returns, see above, Chapter 1, n. 4. More recently, additional evidence has come to light in the form of a long list of data copied from census returns, preserved in *P.Oxy.* 984A, which has been published and discussed by Bagnall, Frier and Rutherford (1997). However, these records suffer from various deficiencies and cannot be put on a par with the data exploited in the 1994 study: see Frier (1997) 90–4.

[3] Based on Appendix 2. This database contains the 710 data presented in Bagnall

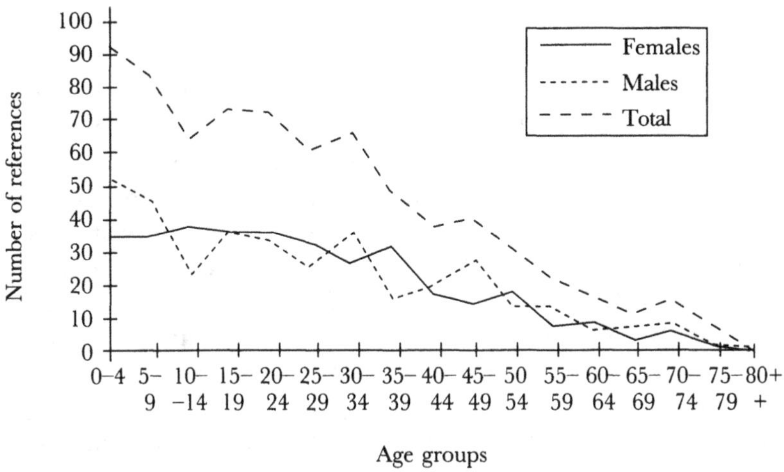

Figure 2.1 Ages in the census returns of Roman Egypt (raw data)

Bagnall and Frier consequently subject the raw data to a number of adjustments. Ages of women and men are treated separately, in keeping with the fact that modern model life tables distinguish between 'female' and 'male' patterns, and allowing for the possibility of sex-specific reporting biases. Starting from age five, the raw data are smoothed by converting them into seven-year moving averages in an attempt to neutralise random fluctuations as well as deliberate age heaping.[4] Excluding the first five years of life, which are particularly prone to careless reporting, these smoothed data are then consolidated into five-year brackets. In a second step, the village data for each sex are weighted against the urban data. This manipulation is meant to counterbalance the predominance of urban ages, which account for forty-six per cent of the record. In reality, the share of city-dwellers in the total population must have been smaller than that: Bagnall and Frier reckon with a level of urbanisation of around thirty-seven per cent, a rate that still seems far too high.[5] Schematically re-set at two-thirds of the total, the age-specific percentages for the village data are given twice the weight of the urban

and Frier (1994) 334–6 tab. A together with 37 new data. The 110 data from *P.Oxy.* 984A (Upper Egypt) will be considered separately: see below, pp. 153–4.

[4] For the latter, which is the result of cultural preference for certain digits, mostly multiples of ten, and of avoidance of others, such as seven, see Duncan-Jones (1979); Bagnall and Frier (1994) 44–7, and in greater detail Scheidel (1996a) 53–91, esp. 63–70.

[5] Bagnall and Frier (1994) 56. See below, section 4.

data.[6] Female and male ages are interpreted separately in terms of goodness of fit with Coale and Demeny's model life tables of the 'West' family.[7] The smoothed and weighted female data are shown to conform closely to the patterns predicted by Coale-Demeny models. The best fit is with Model West Level 2 Females with an annual growth rate of 0.2 per cent. The age distribution of the male data is somewhat more erratic, pointing to a higher life expectancy of the order of Model West Level 4 Males ($r = 0.2$), although Level 3 is also considered likely. On that basis, Bagnall and Frier reconstruct the profile of an aggregate population for the entire country with slightly different Crude Death Rates for each sex and a mean life expectancy at birth of close to twenty-four years.[8]

Thus, two major points form the core of their argument: that mean life expectancy at birth was in the lower twenties, 'probably between 22 and 25 years', and that the attested age patterns are consonant with the predictions of standard Coale-Demeny models. While the first result is intrinsically unsurprising and hardly wide of the mark,[9] the other has important implications well beyond the study of Roman Egypt. The high mortality models used for comparison are not based on empirical evidence but extrapolated from populations with significantly higher life expectancies: therefore, the census data might conceivably be viewed as offering a rare opportunity to check and validate these projections against empirical evidence.

This perspective, however, would reverse the position taken by Bagnall and Frier. Their approach to the census returns has to be interpreted within the wider context of Frier's long-term project to identify quantifiable ancient age data whose distribution conforms to model life tables. Life tables have commonly been taken as extrinsic to and independent of the record. For Hopkins, they underscored the unreliability of attested age distributions from antiquity.[10] The

---

[6] For the weighting ratio, see Bagnall and Frier (1994) 82, with reference to 53–6. This will be discussed below, sections 3.1 and 4.

[7] These model life tables are discussed below, section 2.

[8] Female data: Bagnall and Frier (1994) 75–90, esp. 87–90, males: 91–103, esp. 101–2, and 108 n. 49 for Level 3; total: 103–6, 109–10.

[9] Quoted from Bagnall and Frier (1994) 109. Similarly low levels of life expectancy at birth still appear to have prevailed in Egypt in the early twentieth century (see below, Chapter 3, p. 214 n. 136), although infant mortality rates are notoriously hard to determine. Cf. Bagnall and Frier (1994) 88 with nn. 36–7, for further comparative evidence.

[10] Hopkins (1966), esp. 251–8 (on Roman epitaphs). Cf. below, p. 123.

same way of using model life tables has been advocated for paleodemography.[11] As recently as 1992, Tim Parkin used them as a default position for want of anything as plausible, let alone better, in the ancient record: 'in effect, the cautious and informed use of model life tables can help us gain a greater understanding of the population and of the society of the ancient world, in ways that have hitherto been unattainable because of the lack of direct and realistic data on ancient populations'.[12]

By contrast, Frier's position has been to employ model life tables as heuristic devices in helping him to determine which empirical evidence has some *prima facie* claim to coherence and validity, and to accord some measure of credibility to such evidence from the classical world that can be shown to fit the predictions of these models. This is an important conceptual step. For instance, Frier found that a legal text known as Ulpian's life table, a schedule for calculating the tax value of annuities, appears to give figures for adult life expectancy that are broadly consistent with Model West Level 2, and drew on this source in constructing a schematic life table for the population of the Roman empire.[13] Meanwhile, his comparatively favourable assessment of this text has been criticised from different angles—among other things, because of peculiarities of the suggested pattern, the question of whether the jurists intended this schedule to reflect life expectancy, and the problem of how the Romans could have established mean age-specific mortality rates to begin with.[14] In another case, Frier identified cemetery populations

---

[11] E.g., Howell (1976) 25–6; see 28: 'Tools like the series of model life tables (. . .) are convenient reminders of what the common contemporary human population processes are, and can be seen as null hypotheses of what we should expect to find in an unknown situation, leading to interest, surprise or disbelief in accounts which do not fit the models.' Cf. also Howell (1986).

[12] Parkin (1992) 90. Model life tables have been used in this way in a number of recent studies, e.g., Hansen (1985); Saller (1994) 22–5; Scheidel (1996a) 117–37. In this connection, Saller 23 rightly stresses that although in the absence of proper empirical evidence, reference to model life tables 'allows the historian to understand the implications of a demographically realistic mortality distribution', there is no compelling reason to believe 'that the data from the Roman empire are good enough to justify reliance on any particular life table', all the more so as we need to allow for 'variation in time and location'.

[13] *Digest* 35.2.68 pr., analysed by Frier (1982).

[14] See above all Parkin (1992) 27–41, on the demographic value of this text, and 75–8 and 82–3 for a critique of the life table derived by Frier. See also Hopkins (1987) 120–1; Duncan-Jones (1990) 98–100; Saller (1994) 13–15; Golden (2000). In reaction to this, Frier (2000) 790 now takes a more cautious stance, conceding that

in fourth-century CE Pannonia that seem to mirror the age distribution of model life tables. Some other skeletal samples also resemble model life table patterns at adult ages, such as a few late Roman and early medieval cemetery populations from Lower Normandy.[15] Even so, the problem remains that for each burial population that conforms to the Princeton or UN models there are many more that do not. In fact, non-standard model life tables that are largely based on archaeological evidence differ conspicuously from more conventional projections.[16] Paleodemography has long been a discipline under siege, struggling to overcome potentially insurmountable obstacles to the reconstruction of actual populations from the mortuary record, obstacles among which the difficulty reliably to ascertain adult ages and the cultural bias of burial practices loom particularly large.[17] As long as the feasibility of skeletal demography remains in doubt, we have little reason to put much weight on apparent 'fits' between evidence and models. The same is true for age distributions derived from Roman tombstones, a few of which happen to tally reasonably well with segments of model life tables.[18] Like others, Frier now

---

'the peculiarities of Ulpian's schedule are so obvious that a degree of continuing scholarly caution may well be justified'.

[15] Frier (1983). In Normandy, see esp. Fénouville (Gallo-Roman) and Giberville-le-Martray: Pilet and Alduc-Le Bagousse (1987) 26 fig. 7.

[16] Weiss (1973) serves as a repository of paleodemographic samples and life tables, for which see below, section 2.

[17] Hassan (1981a) 96 considered it 'unfair to dwell on the difficulties involved in palaeodemographic analysis, for it is our only means of developing some understanding of the vital statistics of prehistoric populations'. The understandable reluctance of many of his colleagues to abide by this disturbing premise has spawned a series of critical assessments, such as Bocquet-Appel and Masset (1982); Buikstra and Konigsberg (1985); Greene, van Gerven and Armelagos (1985); Johansson and Horowitz (1986); Boddington (1987); Walker, Johnson and Lambert (1988); Lanphear (1989); Milner, Humpf and Harpending (1989); Paine (1989); Piontek and Weber (1990); Siven (1991); Jackes (1992); Konigsberg and Frankenberg (1992); Roth (1992); Johansson (1994b); Konigsberg and Frankenberg (1994); Saunders, Herring and Boyce (1995); Bocquet-Appel and Masset (1996); Hoppa and Saunders (1998); Paine and Harpending (1998); Aykroyd *et al.* (1999). See Sperduti (1995) for a recent paleodemographic approach to Roman population history; contrast Parkin (1992) 41–58, for a sobering review of some studies of Roman data, and also Morris (1992) 72–91.

[18] In Frier's view, such 'fits' may lend credibility to some of the epigraphic data from Roman North Africa: Frier (1982) 236, 238 (but cf. 236 n. 58), (2000) 791–2. This need not be the case: see now Scheidel (2001) 17–19. Given the wide range of epigraphic samples, some coincidental matches are only to be expected: see Hopkins (1966) 257–8, who exposes a spurious fit (in North Africa!), and Clauss (1973) for detailed documentation of the scope of local and regional variation. See also Duncan-Jones (1990) 102 and n. 26, and cf. above, Chapter 1, n. 2. It deserves notice that Frier's approach can also be reversed: thus, discrepancies between epi-

regards the census returns as the best demographic data from antiquity:[19] once again, their demographic value is corroborated through comparison with model life tables.

This perspective brings to mind Hopkins' cautioning against our accepting ancient 'evidence which confirms the hypothesis merely because it confirms it'. Although he refers to the funerary record, his warning *mutatis mutandis* also applies to other types of sources: 'We have to show instead some other grounds for its validity; for example, that in Africa all people who died were commemorated, hence the reasonable demographic levels of mortality at certain ages. But clearly we do not have enough evidence for such an assertion.'[20] In the Egyptian census, every member—or the same proportion of members—of each age cohort would have had to be registered for our comparison of model and data to be of any practical use. It is far from self-evident that this crucial precondition was indeed fulfilled. Moreover, it is likewise far from self-evident that at very low levels of life expectancy, model life tables provide a reliable objective standard for validation. When comparing census data with life tables, we may also wonder whether we are justified in privileging gender over other criteria of differentiation, such as place of residence. These issues will be discussed in the following two sections. Bagnall and Frier find a close match between evidence and model. But is this match genuine, and what does it mean?

2. *Model life tables and the age structure of high-mortality populations*

Model life table rates for high-mortality populations are mere extrapolations from conditions attested for historical populations with lower mortality. This fact is well documented in the first chapter of Coale and Demeny's *Regional model life tables and stable populations*, in which

taphs and model life tables have sometimes been explained with reference to disease, such as tuberculosis (Russell (1985) 93–110) or unspecified 'catastrophic mortality' (Paine and Storey (1997)). Such attempts are as unrewarding as the search for positive matches.

[19] Frier (2000) 790. Cf. Hopkins (1980) 320: 'far from perfect, but (. . .) the best data we have'; Parkin (1992) 21: 'far more representative than the figures from the tombstone inscriptions', yet 'far from perfect'; 59: 'the relative paucity of the returns and the rather irregular nature of the data produced from them mean that such data are of very restricted applicability'. See also Saller (1994) 19–20.

[20] Hopkins (1966) 264.

they set out the foundations of their models. First, they distinguish between three types of historical life tables. All known early collections of pertinent data were transmitted through continuous registration systems, such as births or baptisms, deaths or burials. Because of their various shortcomings, all databases of this type 'were barred from further consideration for constructing model life tables'. This procedure protects their models from contamination with misleading data but at the same time eliminates unique evidence from early high-mortality populations. This dilemma cannot be resolved.[21] A second source category, censuses from countries without a tradition of reliable vital registration, is defective, too, especially with respect to child mortality, and would require 'drastic adjustments'; Egypt and India are expressly named as examples. These data were also excluded. Again, this principle keeps out less developed populations with correspondingly higher mortality rates. Instead, Coale and Demeny's models are based on populations for which both continuous registration and censuses are available. Data of this kind began to flow in the nineteenth century and expanded over the past century; but they are still missing from large parts of the world. What is more, these samples were pruned even further; thus, only tables 'representing the experience of whole countries' are used in order to smooth regional peculiarities (with some exceptions, notably south Italy). These successive stages of elimination left 326 male and 326 female life tables, sixty-three per cent of them originating from Europe and only 7.1 per cent predating 1870, all of them European. However, hardly any of these preciously few pre-1870 data were eventually utilised in the construction of the model life tables.[22] Coale and Demeny stress 'the uniqueness of the accurate records—mostly those of European countries before World War I—that reflect relatively high levels of mortality'. As a consequence, populations characterised

[21] Quote: Coale and Demeny (1983) 4. They note that the deficiencies of the collections 'exclude the possibility of using these life tables for the purposes of generalizing on mortality conditions unless the validity of each table is carefully analyzed'. Yet what standards could possibly be applied to the analysis of such tables? Model life tables derived from more modern populations?

[22] Coale and Demeny curtly state that for Model West, 'tables before 1870 were eliminated because most of those examined (. . .) had irregular patterns that appeared to arise from faulty data' (12). Again, later age distributions are the only means of identifying such 'irregularities'—a vicious circle. To judge by their account, only the Swedish data from 1851 onward were included in the final database (for Model North).

by levels of life expectancy at birth of less than 33.4 years are entirely missing from these records.[23]

Coale and Demeny themselves are fully aware of these problems: 'We must concede that this use of the four families is far from satisfactory, because there is no strong reason for supposing that the age patterns of mortality exhibited in these four families cover anything like the full range of variability in age patterns in populations under different circumstances. (. . .) The question of what is the pattern of mortality in a population of an underdeveloped area is essentially unresolvable (. . .). By the time a population has reached the stage where age-specific mortality rates can be measured with confidence, the level and age pattern of mortality may have changed, so that the pattern of mortality during the underdeveloped period may never be known.'[24] This guarded judgement by the creators of today's most commonly employed model life tables may seem hard to reconcile with the confidence ancient historians have increasingly come to place in these projections.

The extrapolations behind model life tables are grounded in the assumption that different human mortality patterns are conditioned by pervasive structural similarities. It is possible to distinguish between two types of this uniformitarian principle. According to what we might call the 'weak' uniformitarian position, mortality will normally be higher at the beginning and close to the end of the life cycle than at adolescent and adult ages. This premise is hardly controversial: while infants are particularly vulnerable to infection and malnourishment, the elderly are put at risk by progressive degenerative disorders. By comparison, teenagers and young adults form the most resilient age cohorts, primed for sexual competition and reproduction.[25] The 'strong' principle of uniformitarianism holds that as overall mortality varies, age-specific mortality rates co-vary at predictably synchronised rates. Without this presupposition, straightforward extrapolation from

---

[23] Coale and Demeny (1983) 5, 24–5; Preston, McDaniel and Grushka (1993) 149 and 159 n. 1.

[24] Coale and Demeny (1983) 25. Other families of models, esp. United Nations (1982), with models for Latin America, Chile, South Asia, the Far East and General, register only minor variations. The lowest value of $e(0)$ in the database used to construct these models is 37.6 (males, Trinidad 1920–22); there are no models below $e(0) = 35$. Cf. also Ledermann (1969); Petrioli (1982).

[25] The resilience of these age groups is an essential precondition for the evolution of parental care: cf., e.g., Clutton-Brock (1991) 86–7.

known to unknown mortality patterns would be impossible.[26] Put very crudely, on this theory mortality in one age group changes by x if mortality in another age group changes by y, enabling us to determine the appropriate age structure of a given population.

In actual populations, the amount of deviation from these normative predictions is necessarily correlated with population size and levels of development. Small populations are more readily affected by migration or mortality crises that skew age-specific mortality and fertility and hence the overall age distribution. Excepting major wars (primarily the two World Wars), modern societies are less exposed to severe mortality crises than underdeveloped, 'traditional' societies. While 'tables covering years in which a country was in a major war were eliminated' from their database,[27] Coale and Demeny's recent western data are also free from fallout from catastrophic epidemics and famine.

But even in pre-modern societies, the demographic impact of famine is usually moderate, especially when compared to the death toll of epidemics.[28] It is true that only massive, and therefore infrequent, epidemic outbreaks of lethal disease are capable of heavily skewing the age structure. This is well brought out by a comparison of the dramatic local distortions of the age pyramids for Prato (1372–1470) and Florence (1427–70) caused by the the plague with the less significantly affected age pyramid for Tuscany as a whole (1427).[29] For Herlihy and Klapisch-Zuber, these data 'reveal the obstacles involved in utilizing for historical purposes model life tables which are based on stable or stationary populations. (. . .) The age pyramid of 1427 does not fit any of the theoretical distributions closely. (. . .) The assumption behind the model tables, that death and birth rates have remained constant over the life of the oldest members, is unrealistic when applied to a population molded by catastrophes.'[30] This observation holds generally true for local or regional

[26] E.g., Howell (1986) 219: 'When the parameters are known (. . .), the population structure that will result is highly predictable and can be projected backward and forward in time to examine the implications of sets of parameters'. However, Howell (1976, 1986) does not distinguish between different degrees of uniformitarianism.

[27] Coale and Demeny (1983) 5.

[28] See Watkins and Menken (1985), esp. 665. More recently, it took the Chinese population only three years to regain its 1959 size following the disastrous famine of 1960: Kane (1989) 236 tab. 12.4. For India, see Maharatna (1996).

[29] Herlihy and Klapisch-Zuber (1978) 373 fig. 20, 376–81 (figs. 21.A–B), also in iid. (1985) 175, fig. 6.3, 188–95 (figs. 6.7–11).

[30] Quoted from Herlihy and Klapisch-Zuber (1985) 195.

epidemics that were characteristic of the 'archaic pattern' evoked by Perrenoud. At levels of development where such events recurred with sufficient frequency (Omran's 'first epidemiologic stage'), they could have a lasting impact on local age distributions.[31]

Clark's calculations of the effects of various crises on chances of survival in North India offer an instructive example. She shows that in times of crisis, 'adult mortality slopes downwards more steeply than in the non-crises tables' (Fig. 2.2).[32] It deserves attention that this was the consequence of a series of smaller crises across a large area rather than of a single catastrophic event, such as the Black Death.

With regard to Roman Egypt, the census data are probably little affected by distortions of this kind because of their relatively wide spread over time. This is best illustrated by the apparent lack of any serious impact of the smallpox epidemic of the Antonine period (see below, section 3.2). For my present purposes, therefore, I are more interested in the possibility that historical populations may have differed from model life table patterns *on a regular basis.* Any such differences could primarily arise from two factors, migration and deviant mortality levels in certain age cohorts. Migration poses a particularly unpalatable problem, given that even at their best, census

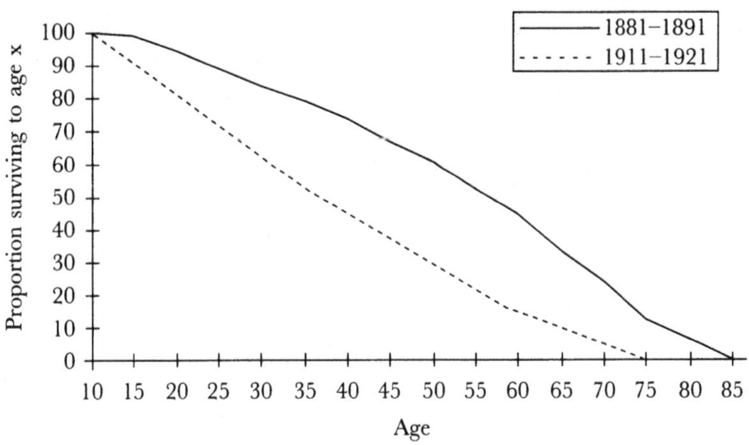

Figure 2.2 Comparison of proportions surviving by age in 'good' and 'bad' decades, United Provinces (North India), Females, 1881 to 1891 and 1911 to 1921

[31] For Perrenoud and Omran, see above, Chapter 1, p. 94 and p. 114.
[32] Clark (1989) 134. Fig. 2.2 is based on 135 fig. 5.

data only portray the existing population without revealing the ways in which it was constituted. As Coale and Demeny point out, only the combination of data from continuous registration and periodical enumerations (censuses) of a population enables us to reconstruct reliable model life tables.[33] On their own, census data do not strictly speaking tell us about the intrinsic mortality regime. Multifactorial model life tables that control for variables such as migration cannot be devised for poorly documented populations. Again, the geographical spread of the Egyptian census returns across much of Middle Egypt can be taken to mitigate this problem, although the small size of the samples and the urban bias of the record may well obscure migrational patterns. I will return to this issue in the next section.

Concerning the second possible source of variation, age-specific mortality rates, attention has focussed on the relationship between infant and adult mortality rates as predicted by model life tables. Early modern English data suggest that mortality in infancy or early childhood could vary independently of the adult death rate, thus exposing the risk of extrapolating (unknown) infant mortality rates from (attested) mortality at mature ages. This also impinges on the credibility of model life tables that are predicated upon fixed ratios of infant to adult mortality. Woods concludes that mortality rates in infancy and adulthood move at different levels depending on variables including the prevalence of breastfeeding and of tuberculosis among adults.[34] Other studies find that by adhering to the matrix of standard model life tables, adult mortality rates may underpredict life expectancy at birth by as much as ten years by overestimating the scale of infant mortality relative to mature death rates.[35]

Preston, McDaniel and Grushka have developed a new type of model life table for use in high-mortality populations, drawing on data for African-Americans who moved to Liberia between 1820 and 1843 where they faced a very high burden of infectious disease to which they had not become immune. In this model, with life expectancy at birth at twenty-two years, life expectancy at age five is 33.55, compared to 38.35 years in Model West Level 2 Females ($e(0) = 22.5$)

[33] Coale and Demeny (1983) 4.

[34] Woods (1993), esp. 200, 206–8, 215. For additional evidence, see Imhof (1990) 199–216, esp. 199, 202. Cf. also Scheidel (2001) 22–3.

[35] Summarised by Smith (1991) 59, who also criticises some inflated estimates of the Crude Death Rate in fourteenth-century England (70–75 per 1,000) resulting from this method (57–9).

(Fig. 2.3).[36] Thus, the new model deflates exaggerated predictions of infant mortality and allows for higher mortality up into middle age. Fewer people survive from ages fifteen to forty-five than envisaged by standard models.[37]

An analogous need for adjustment is suggested by Mari Bhat's research on colonial India. The Indian mortality regime was characterised by unusually heavy adult mortality relative to deaths at lower ages, a feature that is not well reflected in most modern demographic models. Mari Bhat maintains that from 1881 onward, life expectancy at birth was between one and two years higher than previously estimated, whereas life expectancy at age five was one year lower. Mere extrapolation overstates mortality during the first five years of life, especially in infancy, but underestimates adult mortality.[38] Age patterns among Chinese peasants (1929–31) diverged even

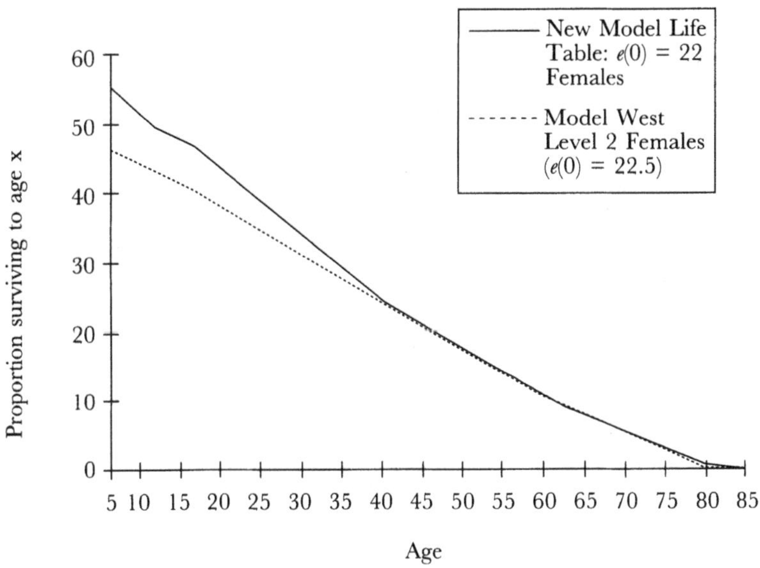

Figure 2.3 Age-specific survivorship according to different model life tables

[36] Preston, McDaniel and Grushka (1993). Fig. 2.3 is based on 156 tab. 4. Cf. John (1988) 76–120, esp. 111–13 tabs. 6.1–2, who calculates life tables for Trinidadian slaves with very low life expectancy.

[37] These discrepancies are much larger at very low levels of life expectancy ($e(0)$ = 18–20) than at higher levels ($e(0)$ = 28–30): ibid., 158, and cf. 157 fig. 3.

[38] Mari Bhat (1989). He criticises the way in which child mortality was calculated by Coale and Demeny (1983), arguing that their procedure fails at very low levels of life expectancy (103–6).

more from standard model life tables than the Indian data: early child mortality was lower, adult mortality higher still. He concludes that to judge from these data, 'Coale and Demeny model life tables may give an erroneous picture of the age pattern of mortality at very low levels of life expectancy. From this it is tempting to conclude that high mortality regimes are characterised not so much by high child mortality, as model life tables indicate, but by extraordinarily high adult mortality.'[39]

Demographic data from three villages in the province of Mino in central Japan, covering the years from 1751 to 1869, likewise indicate considerably higher mortality from ages fifteen to forty than envisaged by standard models (Fig. 2.4).[40] Age-specific rates of probability of dying (q_x) fluctuate within a broad range flanked by Model West Levels 6 ($e(0)$ = 31) and 12 ($e(0)$ = 46).

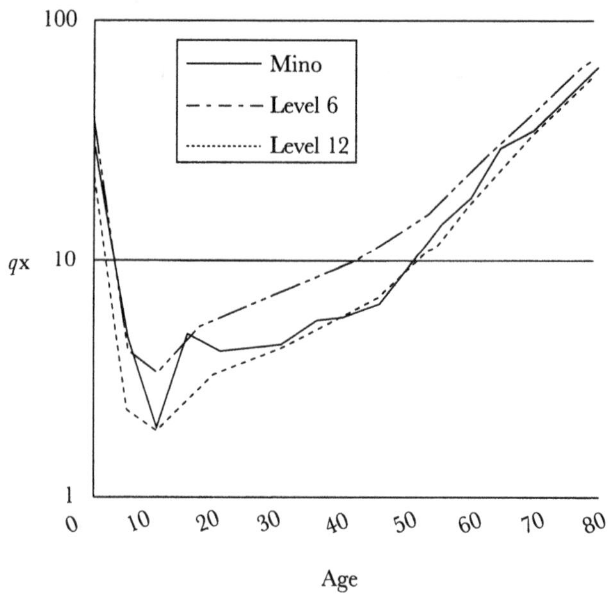

Fig. 2.4 Age-specific probability of dying for Mino villages, 1751 to 1869, compared to model life table schedules (both sexes combined; logarithmic scale, in per cent)

[39] Ibid., 113. For China, see 111 tab. 13, and below. See also Goldman (1980) and Gragnolati, Elo and Goldman (1999) for elevated adult mortality in the Far East, and below, p. 134.

[40] Saito (1997) 143 tab. 8.4; cf. 144 fig. 8.3.

Disproportionately high death rates at mature ages can be explained with reference to endemic disease. Coale and Demeny excluded from the final database those of their 326 pairs of life tables which originated from populations with a high incidence of tuberculosis. In the case of Hungary, for instance, tuberculosis affected the age distribution from ages five to thirty-five; in Scandinavia, it caused distortions between ages five and thirty-five or forty.[41] As a consequence of this omission, the age structure of tuberculosis-ridden populations cannot be matched with model life tables. In principle, survivorship curves ought to be 'steeper' down to the middle of the life cycle and the proportion of survivors beyond ages thirty-five or forty ought to be smaller than predicted by standard models.[42] The authors of the study of Chinese peasants that reveals high probabilities of dying between ages five and twenty note that since vital statistics from Scandinavian populations severely affected by tuberculosis were excluded from the Coale and Demeny projections and since tuberculosis was prevalent in China at that time, tuberculosis is a plausible explanation for this discrepancy between evidence and model. In this case, 'spliced' life tables (i.e., composites of different life tables for different age cohorts) yield the best results. The Chinese mortality pattern appears to be 'different from the structure of any model life tables in the collection presented by Coale and Demeny'.[43]

Recent studies show that malaria could be an even more serious factor.[44] The Princeton models are unaffected by this disease because the available south Italian data were judged to be of insufficient quality to be used in the construction of life tables and also because malaria is of minor significance in datasets for entire nations.[45] At the same time, the local and regional impact of malaria on demographic structure has been all the more conspicuous. Under conditions of hyperendemicity, mortality is generally more frequent at

[41] Coale and Demeny (1983) 11–12. They do not elaborate on the results of experimental modelling based on life tables for tuberculosis populations (11).

[42] Age-specific death rates for tuberculosis can be found in Woods (1993) 213 fig. 13. For Scandinavian tuberculosis mortality, see Puranen (1991), esp. 84 fig. 4 (with a peak in the early twenties); cf. White (1999) 290 tab. 1 for the United States (with a peak in the late twenties and early thirties).

[43] Barclay *et al.* (1976), esp. 621, cf. 623 fig. 2. Quote: 624.

[44] See esp. Del Panta (1989) and Dobson (1997). Sallares (forthcoming) provides further discussion, drawing on the same body of evidence.

[45] *Contra* Shaw (1996) 133, whose focus on national statistics leads him to conclude that malaria does not appear to have been a significant cause of death in pre-modern Italy. Regional data paint a very different picture.

mature ages. In nineteenth-century Grosseto in the malaria-ridden Maremma of Tuscany, for instance, death rates from ages five to nine and from thirty to sixty were much higher than predicted by any standard models. Mean life expectancy at birth was as low as twenty years (Table 2.1).[46] In this locality, hyperendemic *P. falciparum* almost halved life expectancy at birth relative to unaffected communities of the same period, produced much higher mortality across the life-cycle, and distorted the age-specific distribution of deaths.[47] Since direct mortality from malaria among adults was low, adult excess deaths must be explained in terms of synergistic interactions with respiratory and gastro-intestinal diseases. The same is true for the Crotonese where fifteen per cent of all deaths occurred between ages twenty and forty.[48]

Table 2.1 Probability of dying ($_nq_x$) between ages x and $x + n$ and life expectancy at birth ($e(0)$) in Grosseto, Italy, in the 1840s, and according to model life tables (in per cent)

Interval	Grosseto	Coale and Demeny Model		
		South 2	South 1	East 1
$1q0$	31.7	31.1	33.6	50.5
$4q1$	34.0	31.6	34.7	24.7
$30q20$	60.0	43.1	46.0	46.3
$e(0)$	20	22.3	19.9	17.4

In the marsh parishes of Essex two hundred years ago, when *P. vivax* was still endemic in the coastal lowlands of south-east England, less severe but structurally similar deviations are attested beyond age ten, especially for adults from twenty to sixty (Table 2.2).[49] Despite a close fit with Coale and Demeny's Model West Level 6 up to age twenty, these data progressively deviate from any standard model with increasing age (Table 2.3). Standard models life tables clearly

[46] Source: Del Panta (1989) 22.

[47] See ibid., for a comparison with the age structure in Treppio, a contemporaneous Appennine community at high altitude that was free of malaria: life expectancy at birth stood at thirty-seven years, and age-specific mortality corresponded closely to the predictions of Model South Levels 8 (Females) and 9 (Males).

[48] Arlacci (1983) 182. The only comparable proportion of deaths from ages twenty to forty is offered by Model West Level 1 Males with a negative growth rate of one per cent per year.

[49] Dobson (1997) 133–59. Source: 169 tab. 4.2.

cannot be applied to populations with a high prevalence of malaria: adult mortality will be much higher than predicted, especially beyond age thirty.[50]

Table 2.2 Incidence of deaths per person-years lived between ages *x* and *x* + *n* (m_x) in four Essex marsh parishes, 1780s to 1812, compared to a model life table (in per cent)

Age group	Marsh parishes	Model West Level 6 (Females)
0–4	9.5	10.0
5–9	0.9	0.9
10–14	**1.1**	0.7
15–19	**1.3**	1.0
20–29	**2.0**	1.3
30–39	**2.7**	1.6
40–49	**4.2**	1.9
50–59	**4.7**	2.9
60–69	5.9	5.7

Table 2.3 Proportion of individuals aged twenty dying between ages twenty and *x* in four Essex marsh parishes, 1780s to 1812, and according to model life tables (in per cent)

Interval	Marsh parishes	Coale Demeny Model West		
		Level 6	Level 2	Level 1
20–29	18.3	14.1	**19.1**	20.7
20–39	36.8	28.8	**37.7**	40.4
20–49	58.6	44.1	53.5	**56.7**
20–59	75.9	61.2	69.9	**73.0**
20–69	87.4	80.3	**87.0**	89.1

A recent study of the genealogical data of 33,000 members of the imperial Qing lineage born in Beijing between 1700 and 1840 has shed new light on the impact of endemic smallpox on age-specific life expectancy.[51] In 1700, when mean life expectancy at birth ($e(0)$) stood at close to twenty-two years, one child in eight would die during the first year of life ($1q0$ = 12.5, a rate equivalent to Model West Level 14 Males, where $e(0)$ is as high as 49.5). The probability of

[50] Petrioli (1982) uses data from African malarial populations to devise alternative life tables.

[51] Lee, Wang and Campbell (1994) 398 fig. 1, 401 fig. 4.

dying between ages one and five of forty per cent, by contrast, far exceeded the most pessimistic rate envisaged by standard models.[52] Endemic smallpox, as a disease of early childhood, is most active within this particular age bracket. From age five onwards, age-specific life expectancy fairly closely tracked the predictions of Model West Level 1 Males. By 1800, by which time smallpox mortality had abated, the picture had changed quite dramatically. Mean life expectancy at birth had risen to thirty-six years, while the infant mortality rate had declined to ten per cent (equivalent to Model West Level 16 Males, $e(0) = 54.1$) and mortality from ages one to five had dropped precipitously from forty to nine per cent (equivalent to Model West Level 11 Males, $e(0) = 42.1$). At the same time, average death rates had changed little in adolescence and not at all at mature ages. As a consequence, age-specific life expectancy dropped relative to standard model predictions as people aged, from a value close to Model West Level 8 Males all the way to one slightly below that for Model West Level 1 Males (Figure 2.5). Thus, even after the conquest of smallpox, the disease environment of Beijing continued to shape the age distribution in a way that rendered it incompatible with standard models.

Ratios of early to mature mortality rates that are impossible to reconcile with any Coale-Demeny tables are likewise attested for rural Manchuria in the late eighteenth and much of the nineteenth centuries (Figs. 2.6–7).[53] For men, age-specific mortality rates oscillate between fairly low rates in early adulthood (equivalent to Model North Level 12 Males, $e(0) = 44.2$) and much higher rates later in life (equivalent to Model North Level 3 Males, $e(0) = 22.3$). Conversely, women experienced extraordinarily high mortality in their teens (equivalent to Model North Level −8 (!) Females, a negative level extrapolated from the existing tables) but were better off in old age. The reasons for these fluctuations are difficult to ascertain: tuberculosis, the burdens of childbearing, and general neglect have been blamed for the observed 'excess female mortality in adolescence and young adulthood', whereas male excess mortality at later ages appears to have been a distinctly Chinese phenomenon, perhaps associated with a disease known as *laozheng*, most likely tuberculosis, which was

[52] The highest value for $4q1$ is twenty-six per cent in Model West Level 1 Males ($e(0) = 18$ years).

[53] Lee and Campbell (1997) 63 tab. 4.2.

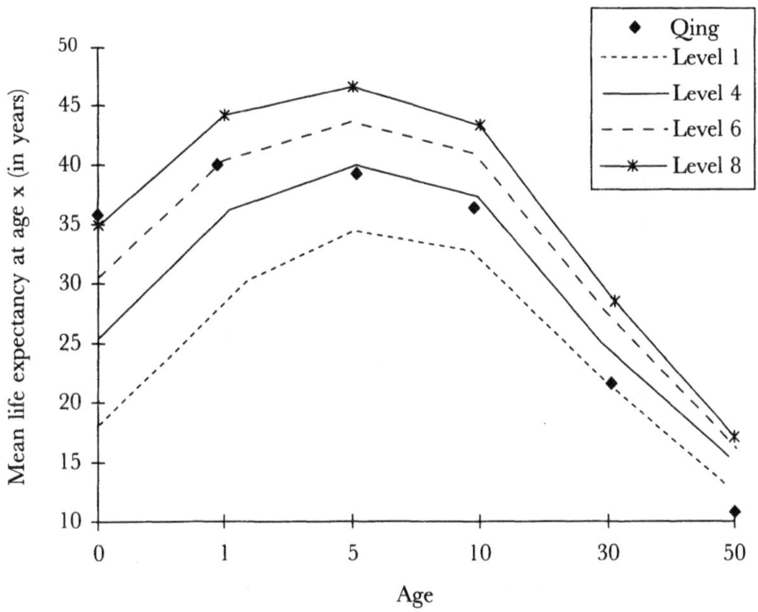

Figure 2.5 Age-specific life expectancy among the Qing of Beijing in 1800 and according to model life tables (Model West)

highly prevalent among men.[54] Again, it was local ecological and socio-economic conditions which determined local patterns of death.

Another but very different set of data suggesting non-standard age distributions is provided by cemetery populations. Aggregate osteological evidence frequently points to more considerable mortality at mature ages relative to juvenile mortality than predicted by model life tables. As a result, the elderly are often almost missing from these samples. However, owing to persistent difficulties in establishing the age of adult bones, this impression may largely be a function of the consistent underestimating of age at death. The inherent unreliability of paleodemographic findings is made particularly vexing by the unique status of skeletal remains as primary evidence from a very distant and otherwise largely impenetrable past. In principle, given the genesis of standard model life tables, it is certainly not inconceivable that such populations exhibited demographic characteristics that differed significantly from those documented for the

[54] For discussion, see ibid. 71–6.

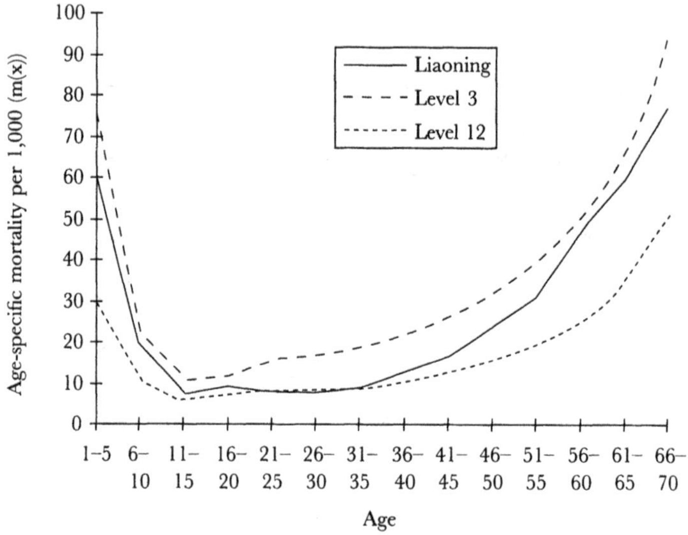

Figure 2.6 Age-specific male mortality rates in rural Liaoning, Manchuria, from 1792 to 1867, and according to model life tables (Model North Males)

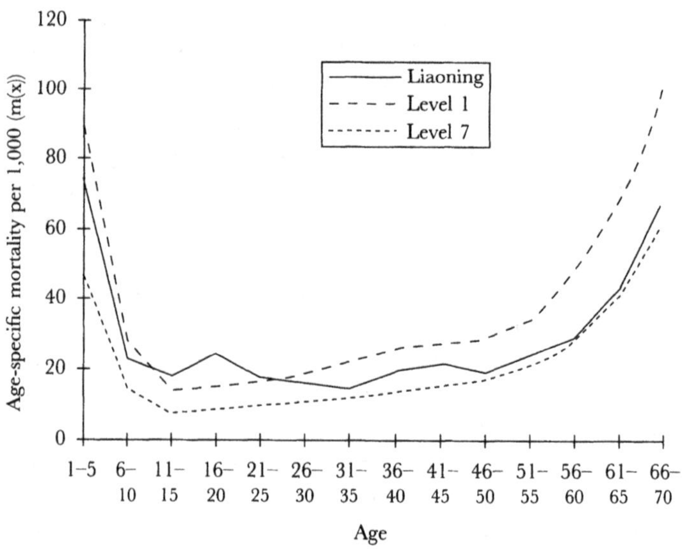

Figure 2.7 Age-specific female mortality rates in rural Liaoning, Manchuria, from 1792 to 1867, and according to model life tables (Model North Females)

more recent past. Anthropologists therefore need not be mistaken in considering alternative models that unlike the Princeton tables do 'not impose a fixed age pattern or set of age patterns of mortality on the data'.[55] Even so, the credibility of any such alternative models depends on our ability to distinguish misrepresentation, as through the underageing of bones, from the genuine demographic impact of attrition factors, such as certain diseases.

The failure to address, let alone solve, this problem mars the most widely known family of anthropological model life tables. Kenneth Weiss' projections are based on fifty population counts made up of fourteen censuses of living populations (mainly aboriginal groups with limited age-awareness) and thirty-six skeletal samples ranging from Australopithecines to medieval Europe. As usual, the osteological data required some massaging to be of any use. The prehistoric samples in particular show a broad range of variation and high attrition rates among adults. Inevitably, the various life tables derived from this material reflect shared features of the underlying paleodemographic analyses, above all high mortality at mature ages. Looked at more closely, these models inspire little confidence. In all skeletal populations used by Weiss, all reconstructed ages from age fifteen are arbitrarily raised by ten years in order to control for consistent underageing. His tables are based on data for age cohorts from ages ten or fifteen to fifty or sixty (depending on idiosyncracies of presentation in different reports), most commonly from ages fifteen to fifty-five. The model age distribution beyond age fifty-five is supplied by the Coale-Demeny models, a procedure apparently made necessary by the almost complete lack of old individuals in the available samples, presumably an artifact of misageing beyond the scope of Weiss' ten-year correction. Survival rates for the first fifteen years of life—which are of course crucial for estimates of overall life expectancy and fertility rates—are based on probabilistic assumptions and thus in effect simply made up.[56] As a consequence, the Weiss tables consist of three unrelated segments: a speculative section from birth to age fifteen; a centrepiece related to massaged source material; and a final leg on the elderly borrowed from the standard models these projections are

[55] Gage (1988) 439.

[56] Weiss (1973) 21–2 (samples), 114–86 (tables), 59 (ten-year correction), 13 (central age range), 23 (transfer from Coale and Demeny), 59–61 (comments on misageing), 26–9 (survival rates from birth to age fifteen: 'their internal structure (. . .) is arbitrary' (29)).

meant to replace. Any level for the first fifteen years of life may be combined with any level for mature ages, resulting in the pattern shown in Figure 2.8.[57]

The marked discrepancy between the Princeton and the Weiss tables, especially for teenagers and young adults, is surely intriguing, and compatible with the above observation that severe environmental stress can significantly reduce survival rates after childhood. However, given the difficulties of judging the validity of the underlying skeletal age patterns (all of them analysed before the 1970s), we would probably be ill-advised to put these projections on the same footing as standard model life tables.

By contrast, tightly focussed case-studies hold considerably greater promise. A recent study of 334 crania from two diachronic cemeteries from the medieval site of Kulubnarti in Upper Nubia (modern northern Sudan), dating from 500 to 1500+ CE, reveals a striking correlation between the prevalence of cribra orbitalia and mortality patterns. Cribra orbitalia, like other kinds of porotic hyperostosis, are

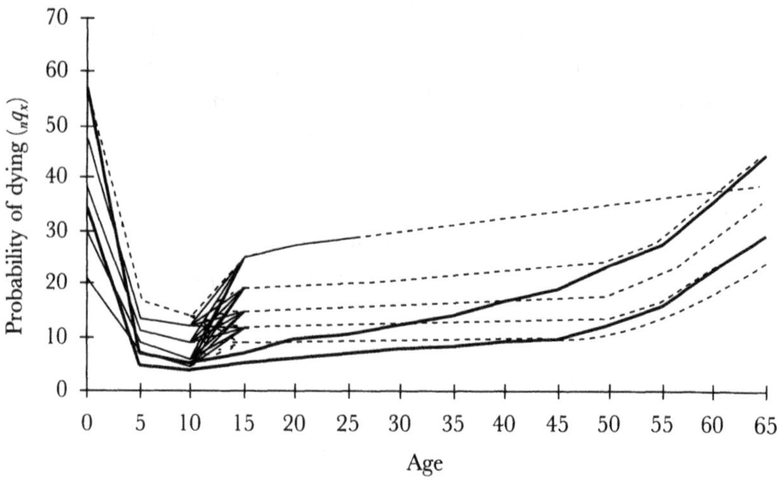

Figure 2.8 Probability of dying between ages x and $x + n$ according to Weiss's model life tables (in per cent)

[57] Fig. 2.8 plots the rates of every other life table in the categories MT 15-j, 20-j, 25-j, 30-j and 35-j, and so covers the whole range of variation envisaged by Weiss (see 36 for his system of notation). The lower bold line represents Model West Level 6 Females, the upper one Model West Level 1 Males.

strongly associated with iron deficiency anemia, mainly caused by malnutrition and parasitism. These bone lesions are typically a childhood condition. In the Nubian sample, cribra orbitalia can be observed in forty-five per cent of the crania. Its frequency peaks at seventy-eight per cent from ages four to six, and remains higher than seventy per cent up to age thirteen. The mean rate from age seventeen onwards stands at thirty per cent. These findings forcefully demonstrate that the condition(s) that caused cribra orbitalia greatly reduced the chances of survival to maturity. As a result, mean life expectancy differs dramatically between those with and those without bone lesions. At ages four to six, average life expectancy for children with cribra orbitalia is 15.5 years lower than for their unaffected coevals. Only sufferers managing to survive to the end of their teenage years were then no longer at a relative disadvantage (Fig. 2.9).[58]

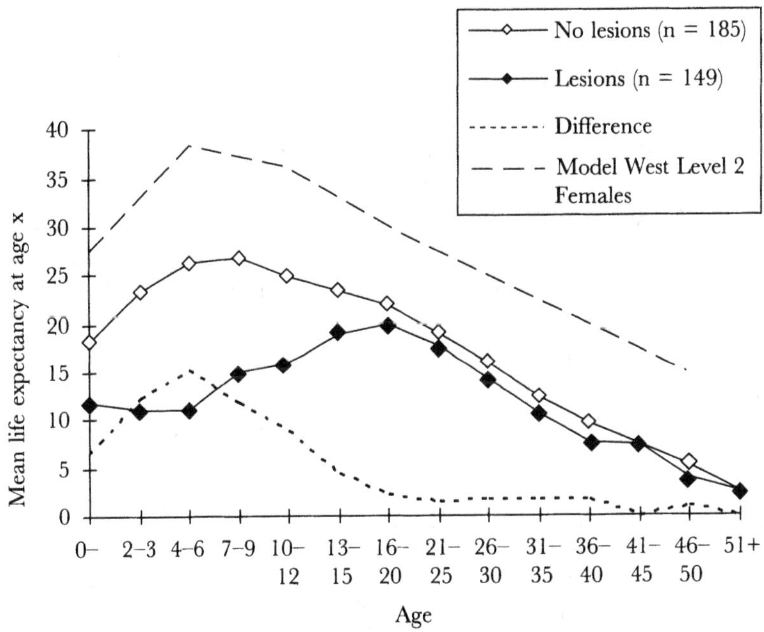

Figure 2.9 Age-specific life expectancy in the cemetery population of Kulubnarti, Nubia

[58] Mittler and van Gerven (1994), esp. 289–91. Compare in general Saunders and Hoppa (1996) for a discussion of the different properties of survivors and non-survivors in skeletal samples. On porotic hyperostosis as a childhood condition, see, e.g., Stuart-Macadam (1985).

It ought to be emphasised that in this context, the numerical values for mean life expectancy at particular ages are of no relevance.[59] What matters here is (1) that the *shape* of the curve representing age-specific life expectancy for unaffected individuals is perfectly consistent with the predictions of standard model tables, and (2) that the difference between the two subsets is so pronounced. The age-specific incidence of cribra orbitalia in the Nubian sample is consistent with that found in other skeletal populations. We must conclude that in populations with a substantial incidence of cribra orbitalia, mortality during the first fifteen years of life was much higher relative to adult mortality than predicted by any standard model life table. Even in the high-mortality variants of the Coale and Demeny models, the chances of dying are always considered lowest from ages five to twenty. This assumption is clearly at variance with the evidence of this and comparable osteological samples exhibiting high rates of bone lesions that keep falling with rising age.[60] If high rates of parasitism and bone lesions were not characteristic of the populations on which Coale and Demeny's extrapolations are based, as seems likely, their models would necessarily fail to reflect conditions under this kind of grave environmental stress. A strong prevalence of cribra orbitalia is not uncommon in ancient bone samples, including recent finds in the vicinity of imperial Rome.[61] Further differential studies of the demographic implications of bone lesions may therefore well result in a radical re-appraisal of the applicability of standard model life tables to ancient populations.

All in all, the demography of underdeveloped populations increasingly turns out to be more complex than the Coale-Demeny models allow for.[62] There is now little doubt that at low levels of life

[59] Suggested life expectancy is clearly too low at any age, presumably as the result of consistent underageing of bones: this is underlined by the apparent collapse of the population over age fifty.

[60] Mittler and van Gerben (1994) 289. Cribra orbitalia do not simply fade with age: cf., e.g., 292 fig. 5. For the age-specific incidence of bone lesions in Greece and Asia Minor from the Paleolithic to the nineteenth century, see Grmek (1989) 276 tab. 2: in samples from the Early Iron Age to the Byzantine period, 14.3 per cent of the skeletons of infants and children and 11 per cent of those of adults show traces of porotic hyperostosis.

[61] Cf. briefly Garnsey (1998) 149. Additional material comes from largely unpublished finds from Portus, Vallerano and Osteria dell'Osa. For Portus, see Sperduti and Manzi (1990), and in general Rossi *et al.* (n.d.). Sperduti (1995), on Portus, does not correlate bone lesions with mortality.

[62] For the sake of completeness, elevated adult mortality caused by endemic violent conflict also deserves mention. Keeley (1996) documents the importance of this

expectancy, their life tables tend to exaggerate infant and early child mortality compared to adult mortality. Mortality crises have been shown to cause more serious deviations from the predicted pattern. Although often limited in time and space, such events can have a significant impact on local or regional samples. Long-term distortions of the age-distribution may arise from endemic disease, such as tuberculosis and malaria. Again, this factor will primarily be visible at the local level. Although more conspicuously non-standard features of many skeletal populations, as mirrored in the Weiss models, remain difficult to interpret, the study of bone lesions reveals a strong correlation between a high incidence of parasitism and age-specific life expectancy.

These observations raise an important methodological point. Judging by recent scholarship in the field, students of antiquity are inclined to accept, however reluctantly, standard model life tables as a predictive standard and to evaluate ancient evidence accordingly: from that perspective, the model is used to validate the data. On the other hand, demographers concerned about the general applicability of standard models derived from recent experience may be particularly interested in historical evidence that matches their retrapolations: in that case, the data would be taken to corroborate the model. Thus, while Bagnall and Frier assess the reliability of the Egyptian census data through the lens of standard model life tables, others might then marshal these supposedly reliable data in support of the models themselves. In view of emerging doubts about the representative value of the standard models, this possible inversion of the ancient historian's approach greatly adds significance to the alleged match between evidence and model. The question is not so much whether the average age composition of the dozens of millions inhabitants of the Roman empire deviated significantly from standard predictions. After all, there can never be an answer. The real question is whether local or regional samples of Roman population data can reasonably be expected to reflect genuine differences between such local or regional populations and model life tables. Recent research surveyed in this section suggests that this is indeed the case. It is true that demographic data, such as the Egyptian census returns, may produce

factor in simple, tribal populations. Though arguably of little relevance for the study of Roman provinces, violent death must repeatedly have been instrumental in shaping (male) age distributions in belligerent Greek *poleis*.

non-standard patterns for reasons unrelated to mortality proper, and that alternative attrition factors need to be considered where appropriate. It is, however, no longer possible to dismiss the mere possibility that observed discrepancies between evidence and model are rooted in the mortality regime of ancient populations.

3. *Age structure in the census population of Roman Egypt*

3.1. *Evidentiary biases*

In case the age composition of the aggregate population of Roman Egypt had indeed been shaped by age-specific mortality rates in keeping with the predictions of standard model life tables, would the existing sample of demographic data necessarily reflect this underlying pattern? The sample is tiny: a bit over three hundred census returns are the (published) survivors of up to twenty-four million documents that may once have existed, a ratio of one to 80,000.[63] This would not be a problem if the sample were truly random. In geographical terms, however, the existing data are heavily biassed in favour of Middle Egypt. As we have seen in the previous chapter, the ecology of this region in some respects differed from that of the Nile valley. The Nile Delta, probably home to more than half of the total population, is almost entirely missing from the record, and no documents from Alexandria are available. As Bagnall and Frier themselves acknowledge, the census returns in the first instance support a study of the demography of Middle Egypt.[64] The representative value of these data is open to doubt: the fact that levels of development and standards of living must generally have been low—and life short—throughout Roman Egypt does not rule out the existence of significant regional variation. The demographic impact of malaria is only one possible variable.[65]

[63] If average household size is put at 4.3 (Bagnall and Frier (1994) 67) and every Egyptian had to be registered (ibid., 12), and the total population fluctuated between between five and six million (see below, Chapter 3, and in this chapter, section 4), the nineteen known censuses from 11 to 257 CE would have produced a maximum of 24.3 million returns. Allowing for incomplete coverage or larger household size, the actual figure may well have been considerably lower.

[64] Bagnall and Frier (1994) 51.

[65] Variation in seasonal mortality patterns has been documented in Chapter 1. For malaria in the Fayum, see above, Chapter 1, section 3.5. I will return to this issue at the end of this chapter.

Within the limited remit of the extant documentation, we encounter additional biases in favour of cities and even certain households. A few families were recorded in different censuses, whereas a random sample so small would virtually never feature any given person more than once.[66] As already noted, the urban population is heavily over-represented. Bagnall and Frier's adjustment that assigns the village data twice the weight of the urban records, implying an urbanisation rate of one-third, sits uneasily with comparative evidence of urbanisation in pre-modern societies. An overall rate of one-fourth, or of under one-fifth excluding Alexandria, may still seem high but less implausible.[67] It is, however, interesting to see that even an urban-rural ratio as high as one to four does not greatly change the weighted age distribution (Fig. 2.10).

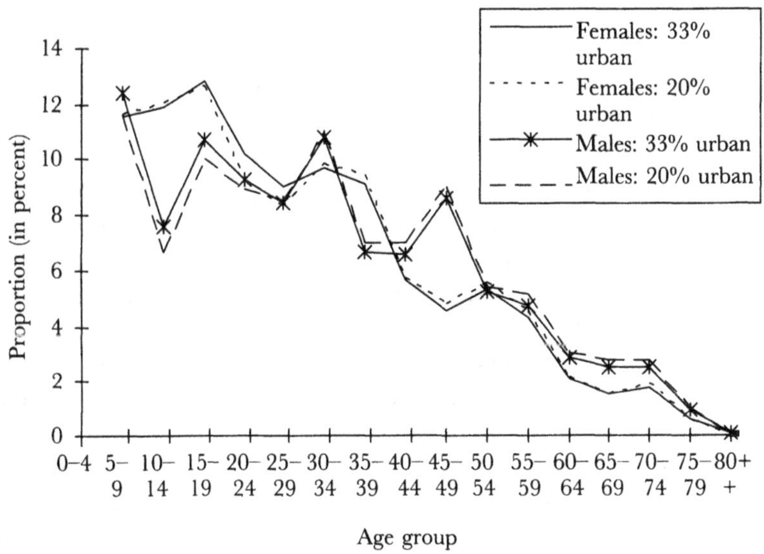

Figure 2.10 Weighted age distribution in the census returns of Roman Egypt (seven-year moving averages)

[66] Cf. Bagnall and Frier (1994) 41, 43. This bias arises from the preservation of many returns in the context of archives.

[67] See below, Chapter 3, p. 247, with discussion; cf. below, section 4. It is hard to say whether the Fayum, which dominates the record, was disproportionately urbanised.

3.2. *Cities and villages*

Bagnall and Frier's reconstruction of the average age distribution in Roman Egypt is predicated upon the implicit premise that a simple combination of the (weighted) urban and rural data yields a representative approximation of the aggregate underlying population. This premise, however, is only valid in the absence of significant age-specific misreporting or concealment and of significant differences in the age composition of city-dwellers and villagers. None of these conditions can be taken for granted. Bagnall and Frier note differences between two out of three types of subsamples. The different patterns for men and women are explained with reference partly to sex-specific mortality regimes, as predicted by model life tables, and partly to the underreporting of juvenile males. Their discussion of differences between two chronological subsets (before and after the 'Antonine plague') will be considered below (section 3.2).

However, the data also reveal significant differences between the age patterns for cities and villages. Moreover, neither distribution matches the patterns predicted by model life tables (Table 2.4 and Fig. 2.11). These discrepancies have so far failed to attract attention. In principle, there are four different ways of explaining deviations of either the urban or the rural datasets from the normative model: (1) these deviations are not statistically significant but merely a function of small sample size and random fluctuation; (2) they are caused by temporary migration between city and countryside; (3) they are the result of selective underreporting; (4) they reflect genuine differences in local mortality patterns. While the first two explanations do not conflict with Bagnall and Frier's principal premise, the latter two make it impossible to infer a general average from collapsing all subsamples into a grand total. In the following, I will argue that the observed deviations are caused by a combination of these latter two factors.

The first of these four options must be discarded. In the cities, 71.1 per cent of the inhabitants aged five and over are between five and thirty-four years old, compared to 64.7 per cent in the model ($p < 0.0208$). If the lower age-limit is raised to fifteen in order to control for deficient reporting at immature ages, the deviation is even more pronounced: 62 per cent of those fifteen and over are aged fifteen to thirty-four, compared to 53 per cent in the model ($p < 0.0066$). In the villages, 58.7 per cent of the population older than five belong to the age bracket from five to thirty-four, as opposed to 64.7 per cent in the model ($p < 0.0182$). 48.1 per cent of those aged fifteen

Table 2.4 Age structure of discrete subsamples of the census population of Roman Egypt (in per cent; figures in parentheses give numbers based on seven-year moving averages)[68]

Age	Model	Villages		Metropoleis	
(1) Total					
5+	100	100	(353.8)	100	(299.5)
5–34	64.7	58.7	(207.6)	71.1	(212.9)
35+	35.3	41.3	(146.2)	28.9	(86.6)
15+	100	100	(281.7)	100	(227.8)
15–34	53.0	48.1	(135.5)	62.0	(141.2)
35+	47.0	51.9	(146.2)	38.0	(86.6)
(2) Females					
5+	100	100	(192.4)	100	(127.6)
5–34	65.5	61.6	(118.6)	71.8	(91.6)
35+	34.5	38.4	(73.8)	28.2	(36.0)
15+	100	100	(146.4)	100	(98.8)
15–34	53.6	49.6	(72.6)	63.6	(62.8)
35+	46.4	50.4	(73.8)	36.4	(36.0)
(3) Males					
5+	100	100	(153.7)	100	(163.4)
5–34	64.3	53.0	(81.5)	71.6	(117.0)
35+	35.7	47.0	(72.2)	28.4	(46.4)
15+	100	100	(129.6)	100	(116.5)
5–34	53.0	44.3	(57.4)	60.2	(70.1)
35+	47.0	55.7	(72.2)	39.8	(46.4)

and over are fifteen to thirty-four years old, against 53 per cent in the model ($p < 0.1$).[69] The differences between evidence and model are statistically significant, and therefore warrant close scrutiny.

The second alternative requires us to assume that large numbers

[68] The 'Model' columns are based on Bagnall and Frier (1994) 88 fig. 4.3 (females), 101 fig. 5.3 (males), 105 fig. 5.5 (total). All other data are derived from Appendix 2 (raw data converted into seven-year moving averages).

[69] When applied to our data arranged in ten-year age brackets, Pearson's chi-square test of goodness of fit is less sensitive to the general focus or direction of deviation (i.e., young vs. old) than the *z*-test as employed in the text, and therefore yields lower levels of significance: in three cases (urban ages 5+ and 15+, and rural ages 5+) there is roughly a one in ten chance than the observed deviation from the model distribution is fortuitous. As we will see below, the much weaker level of significance for rural ages over fifteen of three chances in ten, and of one in ten according to the *z*-test in the text, is a function of the fact that only the male half of the village data differ conspicuously from the proposed model.

of villagers of both sexes under the age of twenty migrated to the cities and gradually returned to the countryside from their late teens onwards.[70] That way, the 'missing' young adults of the villages would be counterbalanced by the adolescent 'peak' in the cities (cf. Fig. 2.11). This raises the question of the location and identity of this transient population: which of the 'surplus' young city-dwellers may have belonged to this group? For this second explanation to apply, temporary immigrants had to be recorded in the census; otherwise, their (*eo ipso* uncontroversial) presence could not skew the *attested* urban age distribution. Lodgers are obvious candidates for this group. Twenty-seven of 344 urban ages, or 7.8 per cent of the total, belong to lodgers. Slaves and ex-slaves may also be considered mobile outsiders, accounting for forty urban ages (11.6 per cent). Together, lodgers and slaves provide close to one-fifth of the urban data. If all of them had originally hailed from outside the cities and eventually returned to the countryside (surely an unrealistic assumption) and if they had been concentrated in the age cohorts that are overrepre-

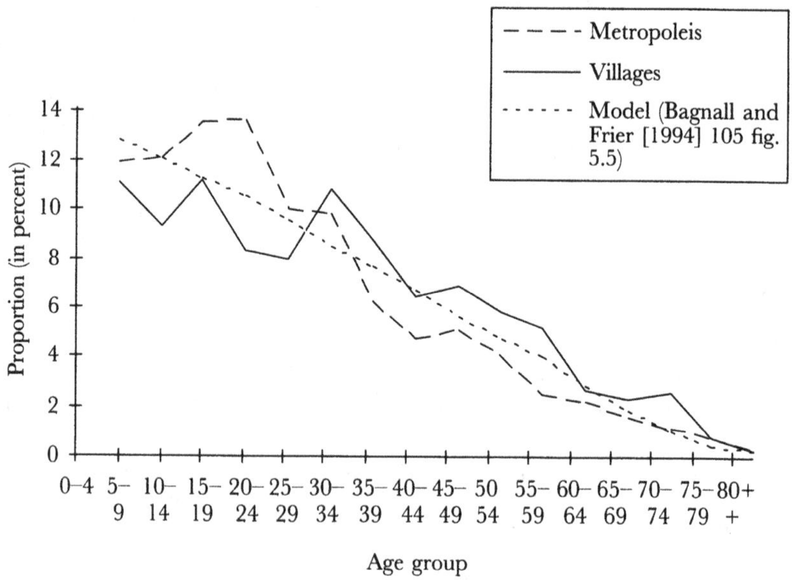

Figure 2.11 Age composition of the census population of Roman Egypt (seven-year moving averages)

[70] For this break-off age, see below, Figs. 2.12–13, 2.15.

sented in the urban record, their exclusion from the sample would erase the apparent deviation and 'flatten' the distribution. This, however, is clearly not the case: in this respect, the remaining 'core' population hardly differs from the aggregate urban total (Figs. 2.12–13). It should be noted that because of their small number, the removal of lodgers alone would not have any visible impact on the age distribution.[71] Moreover, there is no reason to suppose that manumitted domestic slaves regularly (or ever) left the cities. Hence, the corresponding exclusion of ex-slaves (who can only rarely be identified in the record) would offset the removal of slaves by rendering the latter segments of these curves steeper still: after all, freedmen were usually older than thirty, freedwomen over fifty.[72]

We lack other means of identifying temporary migrants in the census returns. The mean age of the members of 'solitary households' (single persons living without kin) is about forty. Hence, solitaries are 'probably most often the sole survivors of their families', and not unmarried young migrants. Households comprised of co-resident siblings are rare; although their typical age would fit young

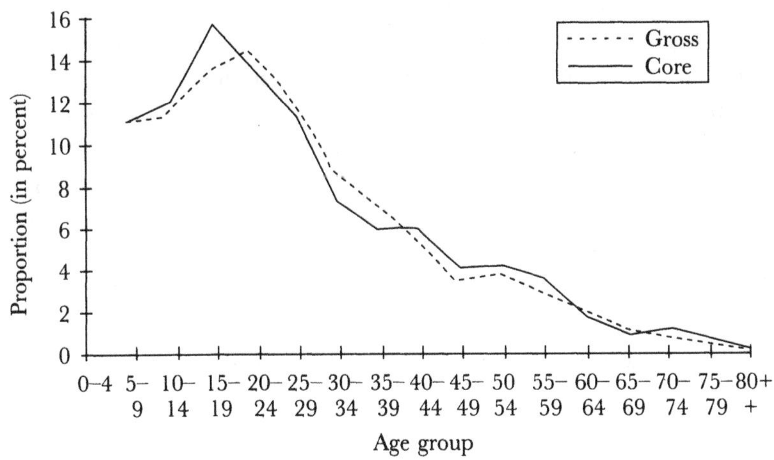

Figure 2.12 Female age composition of the metropolitan census population of Roman Egypt (seven-year moving averages)

[71] The mean age of urban lodgers aged 5+ of 27.9 is *higher* than that of the total urban population aged 5+ of 24.2.

[72] Cf. Bagnall and Frier (1994) 342–3 tab. D for urban patterns of manumission.

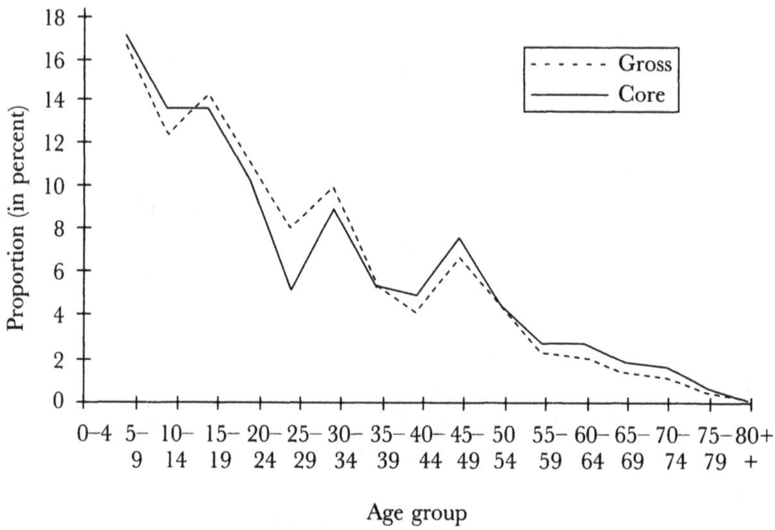

Figure 2.13 Male age composition of the metropolitan census population of Roman Egypt (seven-year moving averages)

migrants, Bagnall and Frier plausibly observe that this type 'doubtless usually resulted from the death of both parents' and were temporary in nature, lasting only until their members married.[73] The remaining categories include conjugal and extended families which cannot be associated with short-term teenage immigration.[74]

In view of this, there is nothing to suggest that the strong presence of teenagers and young adults in the urban record is caused by temporary migrants who were registered in the census. This is not to say that such individuals did not exist in significant numbers.

[73] Solitaries: Bagnall and Frier (1994) 60 (quote); co-resident siblings: 60–1 (quote: 61).

[74] Owing to the poor preservation of many documents, a fair share of all attested individuals cannot be linked to any particular type of household. Even so, it is impossible to speculate that most temporary migrants might belong to that group of individuals: in the absence of any logical association between the chances of preservation of individual papyrus texts and population structure, there is no obvious reason why the personal properties of the persons recorded in imperfectly preserved census returns should be significantly different from those of those persons who may be studied in context. There is likewise no reason to believe that the designation 'lodger' (*enoikos*) might be significantly more frequently missing from fragmentary texts than other specifications, such as age. The fact that entries on lodgers, who were listed near the bottom of census documents, are more likely to be missing altogether from incomplete specimens, is of no relevance here.

It is, however, far from obvious that they should be visible in the census documents. The exclusive focus of the Egyptian census on households (rather than individuals) may well have enabled temporary migrants to avoid registration. Comparative evidence indicates the possible scope of concealment. A demographic survey of households in Bangladesh conducted in 1961/2 established an urban sex ratio of 107.7 and a rural sex ratio of 106.1. The census of 1961, by contrast, which aimed to include every person, found the urban sex ratio to be as high as 153.2, compared to 105 in the countryside. Local observers explained this bewildering discrepancy with reference to the omission of messes, hostels and similar residential units from the survey.[75] Poor young temporary migrants may also have found shelter at their workplace or simply slept rough. In this case, registration centred on households proper missed at least one-sixth of the entire population. The structure of the Egyptian census facilitated comparable underreporting. In fact, a population count that took place every fourteen years was in any case an extremely rare event: the average teenager could expect to experience not more than two or three censuses in his or her lifetime. Under these circumstances, young men who fled their villages to evade taxation cannot have found it difficult to avoid registration in the cities. Arsinoe, which dominates the census returns and which was one of the largest—quite possibly the largest—Egyptian city outside Alexandria must have attracted many individuals of this kind.[76] There can be little doubt that certain segments of large urban populations, in the first instance temporary migrants to the urban centres of Middle Egypt, Arsinoe, Oxyrhynchus and Hermopolis Magna, were considerably less likely to be represented in the census returns than others. Unequivocal evidence of widespread concealment in the villages which highlights the deficiencies of the census procedure further corroborates this assumption (see below).

Among permanent urban residents, girls under the age of fifteen were also heavily underreported. The urban sex ratio is exceptionally high for the first five years of life (350; $n = 36$; $p < 0.0014$), and still markedly elevated from ages five to fourteen (152; $n = 78$;

[75] Muniruzzaman (1966a) 9 tab. 1.7, 10.

[76] As is well known, tax flight was a common occurrence in Roman Egypt: e.g., Braunert (1964). For the size of Arsinoe, see Bagnall (1993) 52; Davoli (1998) 149–50.

$p<0.0702$).[77] Since these high sex ratios do not persist into mature ages, they cannot be attributed to femicide. As has been argued more fully elsewhere, this apparent lack of girls should be seen as a function of the neglect of unmarried daughters. Concealment of such individuals is a common feature of underdeveloped societies, where they suddenly appear in the record once they are married.[78] As the Florentine Giovanni di Pagolo Morelli put it around 1400 in his *Ricordi*, 'there is no need here to make mention of the females, since they are very young; when they are old enough to marry, if they reach that age, then we shall mention them'.[79] In the ancient world, a comparable attitude is familiar from other hellenised settings. The lists of enfranchised immigrants on the walls of the Delphinion in Miletus (third and second centuries BCE) provide the most conspicuous example: the sex ratio of 360 for all co-resident children of fifty-seven two-parent families is made up of a sex ratio of 390 for minors and of 125 for marriagable children. This belated emergence of daughters is best explained with previous underreporting.[80] In the cities of Roman Egypt, many of the under-age females in residence are missing from the census returns.[81] This lack of girls in the census population—as opposed to the actual population—is the only reason why the male and female urban age distributions appear to differ between ages five and twenty (Fig. 2.14).

If, therefore, ages under fifteen are excluded, and the size of the age cohort from fifteen to nineteen is expressed as 100, the stan-

---

[77] The urban sex ratio from birth to age fourteen is 192; $n = 114$; $p < 0.0008$.

[78] The sex ratios in the Egyptian census returns are discussed by Scheidel (1996d) 39–40 and n. 41. In Bangladesh, for instance, it used to be 'generally regarded as a disgrace for a respectable family' to have unmarried daughters of marriageable age, leading to the understatement of age of such girls: Muniruzzaman (1966b) 12. The same has been suggested for India: Saxena, Verma and Sharma (1986) 131, and see Scheidel (1996d) 41–2 on the 1907 census of Egypt. Cf. also du Boulay (1974) 124, on Greece.

[79] Quoted by Herlihy and Klapisch-Zuber (1985) 135 n. 13.

[80] Thus Scheidel (1996d) 43 and n. 51; see the evidence in Rehm, ed. (1914) and Günther (1988), with discussions by Pomeroy (1983); Petropoulou (1985) 128–30, 177–99; Brulé (1990) and (1992) 68–9. For further references to implausibly high ancient sex ratios, see Scheidel (1996d) 44 n. 53–4.

[81] Bagnall (1997a) suggests that many newborn urban daughters were sold to villagers who raised them as slaves and later sold them back to city residents. This is not the place to judge the merits of this complex thesis which has no bearing on the present discussion. Since the urban 'core' population does not differ from the aggregate urban population (including lodgers and slaves) from age five, any such transfer would have had no effect on the adult age distribution.

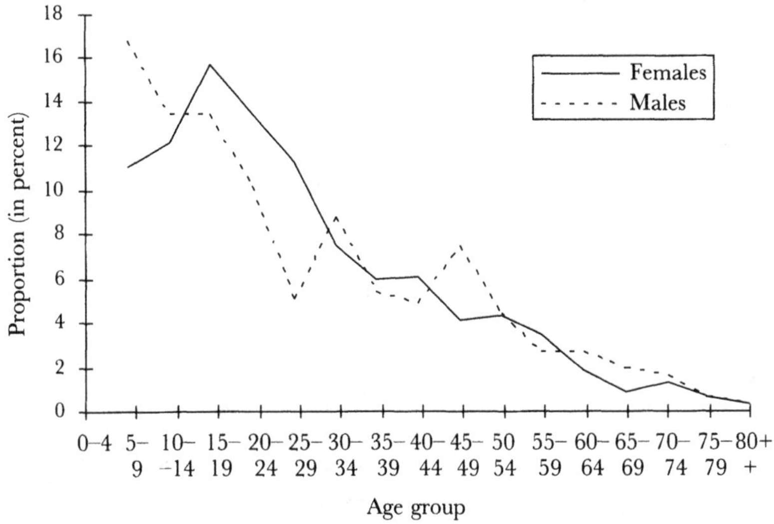

Figure 2.14 Age composition of the 'core' metropolitan census population of Roman Egypt (1) (seven-year moving averages)

dardised patterns for females and males broadly resemble each other (Fig. 2.15). As men became subject to the poll-tax at age fourteen and girls began to marry at about that age,[82] concealment becomes less likely from the mid-teens onwards, especially for women.

In terms of age-structure, both the female and the male urban 'core' populations deviate signally from the model life table selected by Bagnall and Frier even after age fifteen. Thus, these discrepancies cannot be explained away as reflecting irregularities of reporting at subadult ages (Figs. 2.16–17).

Owing to the poor quality of the subadult data, permanent immigration, which would increase the adult population relative to the juvenile age cohorts, is impossible to gauge. Permanent relocation of villagers to the cities may, however, have raised attrition rates in early adult life, provided that these immigrants were subject to higher mortality than those raised in and inured to an unhealthy, high-exposure urban environment. The fact that high attrition rates are attested for men and women alike is also consistent with the permanent immigration of couples or individuals of both sexes seeking to marry.

[82] See Bagnall and Frier (1994) 27 (taxation) and 112, 113 fig. 6.1 (female marriage).

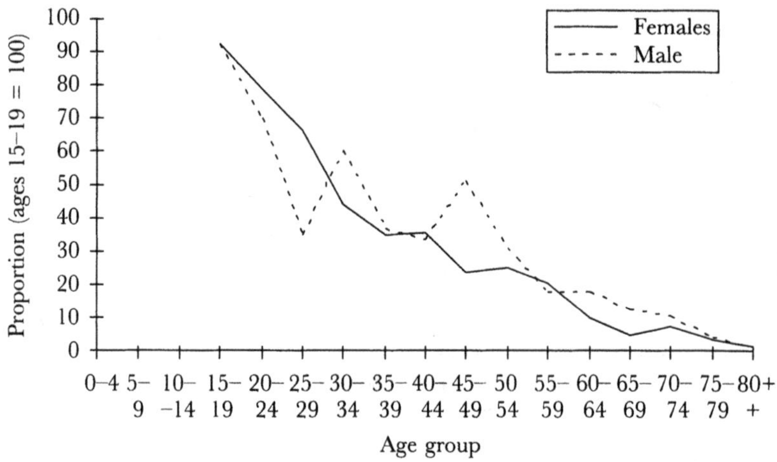

Figure 2.15 Age composition of the 'core' metropolitan census population of Roman Egypt (2) (seven-year moving averages)

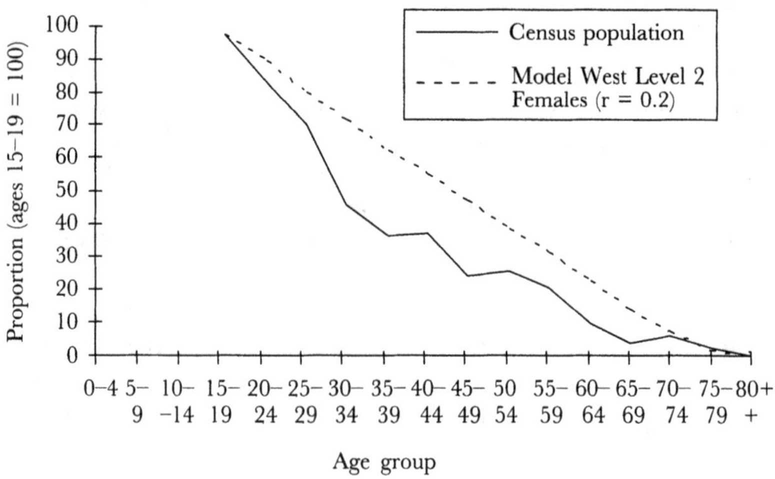

Figure 2.16 Female age composition of the 'core' metropolitan census population of Roman Egypt (seven-year moving averages)

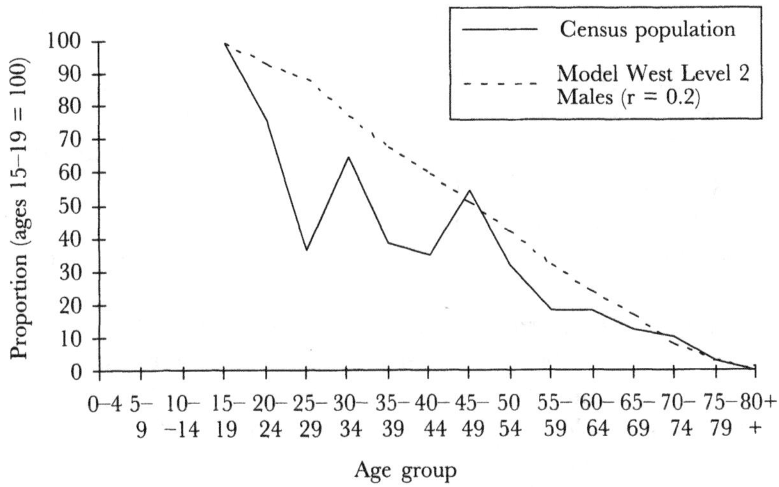

Figure 2.17 Male age composition of the 'core' metropolitan census population of Roman Egypt (seven-year moving averages)

Whatever the adult sex ratio, sex-selective migration cannot explain the observed patterns. The apparent slowdown of attrition in old age may partly be an artifact of age exaggeration: freedom from poll-tax beyond the early sixties may have encouraged some amount of shoving into higher ages, thus 'flattening' the age distribution at advanced ages. As will be seen below, the same effect is discernible in the tax lists.

A similar picture emerges from the census data preserved in *P.Oxy.* 984A which originate from a city in Upper Egypt, either Ptolemais or Lykopolis, and were probably compiled in 91/2 CE based on the census of 89/90 CE.[83] Because of their urban provenance, these data are best compared with the urban records from Middle Egypt.[84] Given the small size of the Upper Egyptian sample and its seemingly inferior quality, aggressive smoothing is necessary to elucidate the properties of the documented age pattern, and the resulting reconstruction can therefore only be tentative. When compared to Bagnall and Frier's model life table for Roman Egypt, the Upper

[83] Provenance: Bagnall in Bagnall, Frier and Rutherford (1997) 22–25, 56; date: ibid., 20–22.

[84] *Contra* Frier (1997) 101–03, who, pondering differences between *all* Middle Egyptian data and the exclusively urban Upper Egyptian data, fails to compare like with like.

Egyptian data, converted into three-quintile moving averages, fall into an inverted S-shaped curve similar to that for the Middle Egyptian cities, characterised by higher attrition rates between ages twenty and fifty than predicted by the model (Fig. 2.18).[85]

The records from Upper Egypt list very few slaves and no lodgers; moreover, four of the six attested slaves are not older than five and excluded from our sample. Thus, these texts contain no sign of temporary migration.[86] What, then, may have caused the non-standard age composition of either urban population sample? In theory, a high rate of natural growth might have skewed the urban age distribution in the observed fashion. The attested pattern is consistent with an annual rate of growth of one and a half per cent under the conditions of Model West Level 2 Females (Fig. 2.19). At this rate, however, a population doubles every forty-seven years. For that rea-

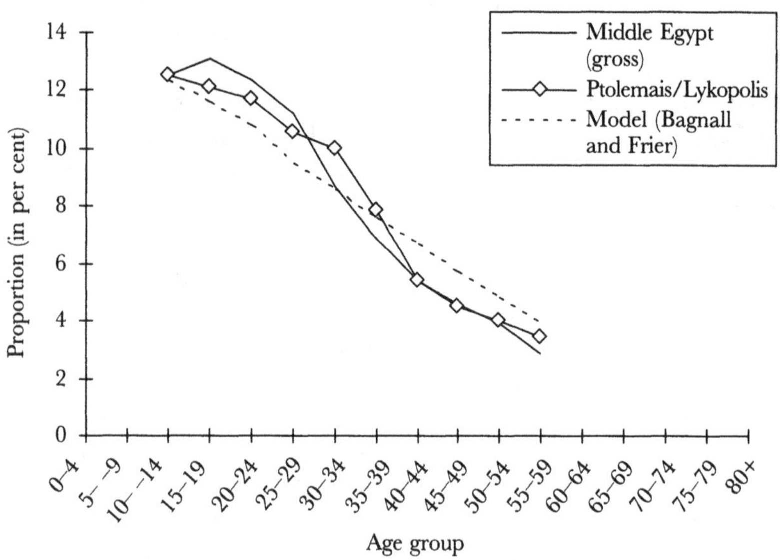

Figure 2.18 Age composition in two urban census populations of Roman Egypt (three-quintile moving averages of seven-year moving averages)

[85] The Upper Egyptian sample is based on the catalogue in Bagnall, Frier and Rutherford (1997) 57–88. In Fig. 2.18, all data are expressed as three-quintile moving averages of seven-year moving averages.

[86] Admittedly, this is an argument from silence. See Bagnall in Bagnall, Frier and Rutherford (1997) 26, on the lack of lodgers.

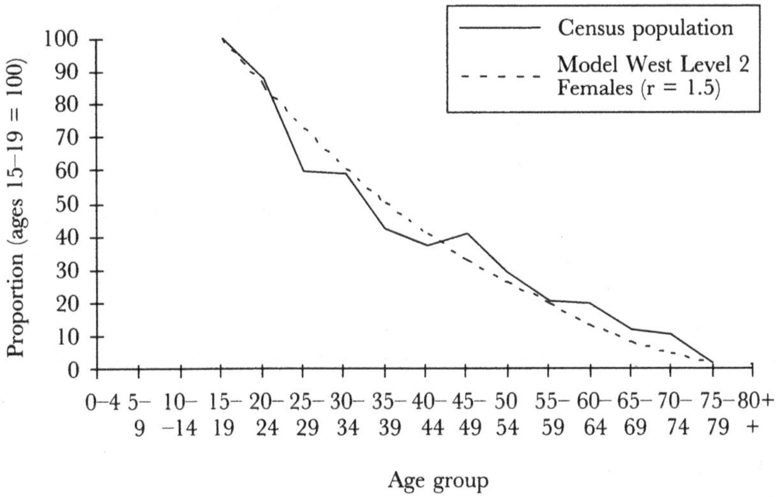

Figure 2.19 Age composition of the 'core' metropolitan census population of Roman Egypt fitted to a model life table (seven-year moving averages)

son alone, at any rate in the long term, this value seems impossibly high for any pre-modern population.[87] Since the cities of Roman Egypt cannot have doubled their size twice per century, an annual growth rate of one and a half per cent driven by immigration must also be ruled out.

Mortality is the only remaining factor. As we have seen in the previous section, under certain circumstances adult mortality rates may be considerably higher than predicted by standard model life tables. The metropolitan data from Middle Egypt suggest a probability of dying of sixty-three per cent between ages twenty and fifty.[88] While

[87] The most likely rate may be lower by as much as an order of magnitude: cf. Bagnall and Frier (1994) 87–8; but also below, Tab. 2.3.

[88] While this age pattern clearly deviates from the conditions simulated by standard model life tables (see above, p. 146), the evidence is insufficiently robust to establish precise age-specific rates of attrition and, hence, life expectancy. If taken at face value, the urban data are consistent with a mean life expectancy at age fifteen of the order of twenty-two to twenty-three years. This figure is about one-quarter lower than the most pessimistic estimate for a stationary population in Coale and Demeny (1983) 42 (Model West Level 1 Males). If we speculatively put mortality up to age fifteen at sixty per cent (again an extremely high rate, which, however, is corroborated by the attested mortality rates for Cairo from 1798 to 1801: see above, Chapter 1, p. 41), the average woman surviving to menopause would

rates this high are absent from Coale and Demeny's models, they tally well with the corresponding probability of dying of sixty per cent in the malarial population of mid-nineteenth-century Grosseto. They are also reminiscent of conditions in Crotonese, where mortality between ages twenty and forty was twice as high as expected.[89] The Egyptian pattern is furthermore compatible with a high incidence of tuberculosis, which raises death rates from ages five to forty. Both malaria and tuberculosis may have been prevalent in the cities of Middle Egypt, the former above all in Arsinoe (cf. above, Chapter 1.3.5). Permanent immigrants from less severe disease environments would have been particularly exposed to either infection. Unfortunately, osteological and biomolecular analyses of skeletal finds from these locations that could corroborate these ideas have not yet become available.

The attested age-composition in the Egyptian villages differs considerably from that in the cities (Fig. 2.20). Taken at face value, these data suggest that no men died between ages five and fifty. Indeed, there are more men aged forty to forty-nine than aged five to fourteen. None of this is at all possible. Bagnall and Frier accept that the existence of boys approaching the age of fourteen was frequently concealed in order to save them from imminent exaction of the poll-tax.[90] However, given that much of the adult age distribution is similarly distorted, underreporting clearly did not cease at that age. Either concealment continued on a large scale well into

have had to give birth to approximately seven children in order to keep the urban population from contracting. At the same time, owing to the very high rates of attrition among young adults implied by the census returns, the average woman could not have borne more than 5 to 5.5 children even if age-specific fertility had been between one-sixth and one-third higher than suggested by Bagnall and Frier (1994) 143 tab. 7.1. (It would appear imprudent to envisage even higher average fertility.) Reckoning with a mean rate of urbanisation of between twenty and twenty-five per cent, the resultant shortfall of around twenty-five per cent could have been counterbalanced by the transfer of about seven per cent of all rural births to the cities. In statistical terms, the attested urban age distribution is of course consistent with somewhat lower rates of adult mortality; hence, the required volume of immigration may well have been considerably smaller than this rough calculation suggests. In Tab. 2.3 below, I speculate that around five per cent of all rural births were required to offset urban excess mortality. In this context, greater precision is neither possible nor necessary. Suffice it to note that Wrigley (1978) 217–20, in a schematic model, considers it plausible that at a time when close to ten per cent of the English population resided in London, about four or five per cent of all English births outside London were necessary merely to counterbalance negative growth in the capital.

[89] See above, section 2.

[90] Bagnall and Frier (1994) 97–8.

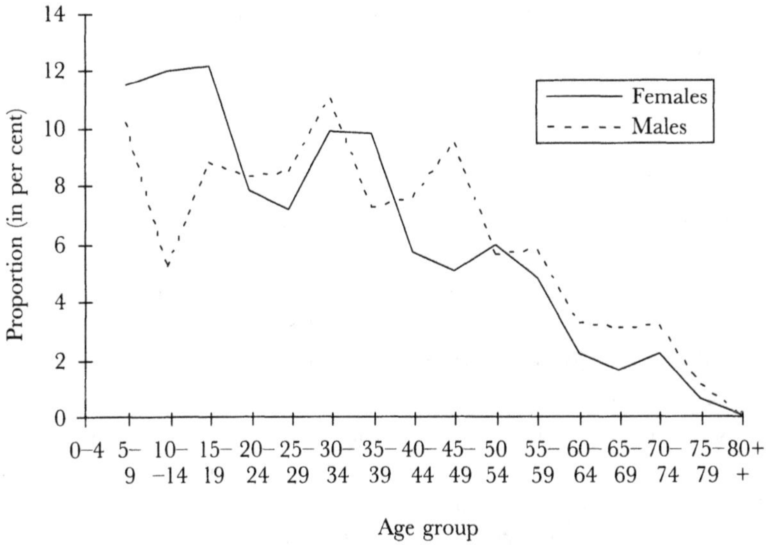

Figure 2.20 Age composition of the village census population of Roman Egypt (seven-year moving averages)

mature ages, or many village men lived in the cities where they went unregistered.[91] Both practices, which probably occurred side by side, are best understood as strategies of tax evasion. Comparative evidence from early Chinese and Japanese censuses corroborates this interpretation.[92]

---

[91] For the latter, cf. above, p. 149, and below, p. 162.

[92] Comparable levels of underregistration of male taxpayers mar the census documents from a number of villages in early medieval Japan (702–732 CE) studied by Farris (1985), with attested sex ratios of 77.1, 83.0, 88.9, 92.5 and 98.9 in five samples comprising 5,031 individuals. Farris 34 attributes this imbalance to attempted tax evasion. As a result, the records create the specious impression that male life expectancy exceeded female life expectancy (43). According to a paper by T.F. Liao given at the 25th Anniversary Meeting of the Social Science History Association in Pittsburgh (28 October 2000), original census documents from the T'ang period (seventh to ninth centuries CE) that have survived in the arid environment of Xinjiang south-west of Mongolia closely resemble the Roman Egyptian census returns (listing the name, age and position within the family of each member of a particular household) and record a comparable number of households and individuals (approximately 250 and 1,000, respectively). More importantly, these texts mimick the Egyptian village records in that in a sample of 588 persons whose sex and ages are known, reported women outnumber men from ages sixteen to forty; moreover, a trend curve fitted to the raw data for male ages improbably indicates virtually no mortality from ages thirty to sixty. In this period, in the same way as in Roman Egypt, adult men were subject to a poll tax that appears to have encouraged considerable concealment.

The serious deficiencies of the census records for male villagers are also reflected in the extant tax lists, all of which come from Arsinoite villages. These texts, compiled from census returns, record only males of tax-paying age. Bagnall and Frier claim that the age distribution of these individuals and that of all males in the (rural *and* urban) census returns between ages fifteen and fifty-nine 'are closely similar not only in their overall shape but also in their age-specific trends'.[93] This statement is misleading. First of all, Bagnall and Frier rely on a garbled version of the evidence in the tax lists.[94] Exploiting only published data, I use here a sample of 507 men aged fifteen to fifty-nine. More important, both their samples and our corrected dataset produce age curves that are clearly at variance with the predictions of high-mortality model life tables. These curves are similar to, but somewhat less distorted than, that for village men in the census returns (Fig. 2.21).[95]

The conspicuous dearth of ages fifteen to nineteen in the tax lists must be the result of concealment. Unlike in the village census returns, many of these men are documented from age twenty onwards: by then, the authorities seem to have caught up with them. The precipitous drop after age fifty can only be explained with reference to age shoving past age sixty to avoid further tax payments. The patterns of distortion come into focus when we eliminate ages under twenty.[96] Between ages twenty and forty-nine, the age pattern in the tax lists can be fitted to Model West Level 10 Males ($e_0(0)$ = 39.7) (Fig. 2.22). This model is clearly inappropriate for ancient populations. Comparable levels of life expectancy were not attained in Egypt until the second half of the twentieth century.

---

[93] Bagnall and Frier (1994) 102.

[94] Bagnall and Frier (1994) 102 n. 32 claim to have derived 462 male ages between fifteen and fifty-nine from a total of 527 male ages in the following documents: (1) *P.Harris* 72; *P.Mich.* inv. 890 and *P.Princ.* III 123; *P.Mich.* inv. 791; *P.Mich.* inv. 811: 129 ages; (2) *P.Mich.* inv. 619 recto: 33 ages; (3) *P.Brit.Lib.* 2253 and *P.Mich.* inv. 881 and *P.Mich.* inv. 877: 101 ages; (4) *P.Lond.* II 257–259: 264 ages. These data were supplied by A.E. Hanson. However, I find that *P.Lond.* II 257–258 contains 351 ages, and I have also used eighty-six ages in *P.Princ.* I 8 (not used by Bagnall and Frier because of some overlap with the unpublished texts in (3), which are excluded here), thirty-two ages in *P.Harris* 72, and forty-eight ages in *P.Princ.* III 123. This gives a total of 517 ages, of which 507 fall into the range from fifteen to fifty-nine. Consultation with B.W. Frier confirmed that their sample is somewhat defective.

[95] Fig. 2.21 is partly based on the raw data from the tax lists (n = 507): see above, n. 94. Cf. Bagnall and Frier (1994) 103 fig. 5.4.

[96] The tax lists contain 448 ages in the age bracket from twenty to fifty-nine.

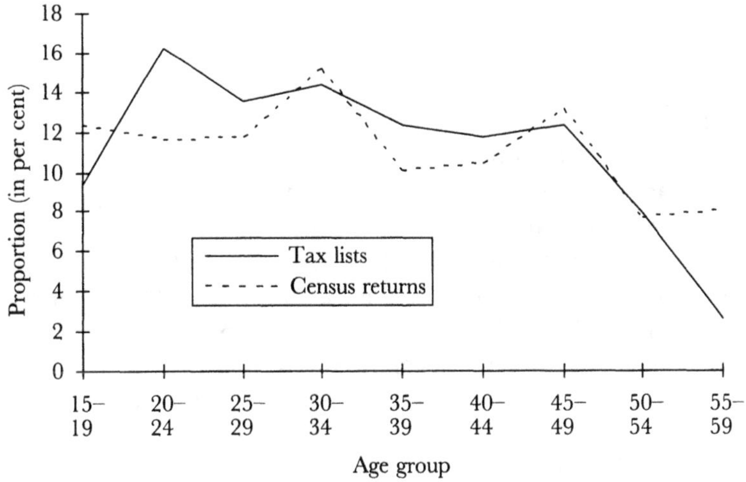

Figure 2.21 Male age structure in the village census returns and tax lists of Roman Egypt (census returns: seven-year moving averages; tax lists: raw data)

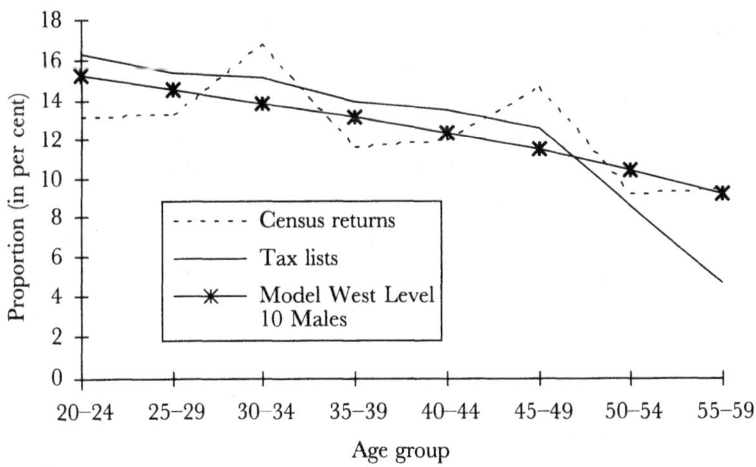

Figure 2.22 Male age structure in the village census returns and tax lists of Roman Egypt (seven-year moving averages)

As shown in Figure 2.23, the age data from the lists are incompatible with the model distribution proposed by Bagnall and Frier (Model West Level 4 Males, $r = 0.2$). The pattern generated by the village census returns for men deviates even more dramatically from that model, and cannot be made to fit any conceivable model life table. We are forced to conclude that the available age records for male villagers are irremediably flawed. This invalidates Bagnall and Frier's attempt to derive an 'average' male age distribution by conflating urban and rural data for men. The notion of a higher life expectancy for men than for women is merely a function of the distorted age pattern for rural men.[97] The marginally better quality of the data furnished by the tax lists is consonant with the lower incidence of age-rounding in these documents compared to the census returns.[98] The census returns and the tax lists for village men appear to be vitiated to different extents by the same reporting errors, and are thus unsuitable for demographic analysis.

The situation is completely different for village women. In this case, the proposed standard of Model West Level 2 Females ($r = 0.2$) fits the attested pattern remarkably well (Fig. 2.24). The closest match is with Model West Level 2 Females ($r = 0$), yielding a Weiss index of deviation value of zero.[99] A small amount of net growth may have been absorbed by the cities (see below, section 4), creating the impression of stagnation in the villages. Since there existed no obvious reason for the concealment of adult village women, this particular age distribution much more faithfully mirrors reality than that for their male counterparts. However, as I will argue below, the superior quality of these data has no bearing on their representative value.[100]

The female age distribution precludes the possibility that the 'steep' curve for urban males and the 'flat' curve for village males are caused by cyclical migration and cancel each other out, thereby producing a credible mean (cf. Figs. 2.15 and 2.18). Not only do the census returns fail to reflect temporary migration of this kind. Even more

---

[97] *Contra* Bagnall and Frier (1994) 100, who themselves express some doubts (107–9), conceding that 'we are permitted to speculate that male and female life expectancy did not differ widely' (108). In my view, this is not just 'speculation' but the most plausible interpretation.

[98] See Scheidel (1996a) 84–5.

[99] Cf. Weiss (1973) 65; Bagnall and Frier (1994) 85–6.

[100] See below, section 5, esp. n. 128.

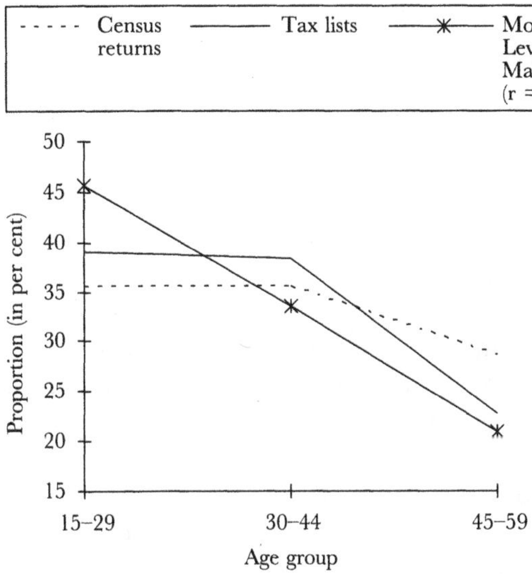

Figure 2.23 Male age structure in the village census returns and tax lists of Roman Egypt (seven-year moving averages consolidated into fifteen-year age brackets)

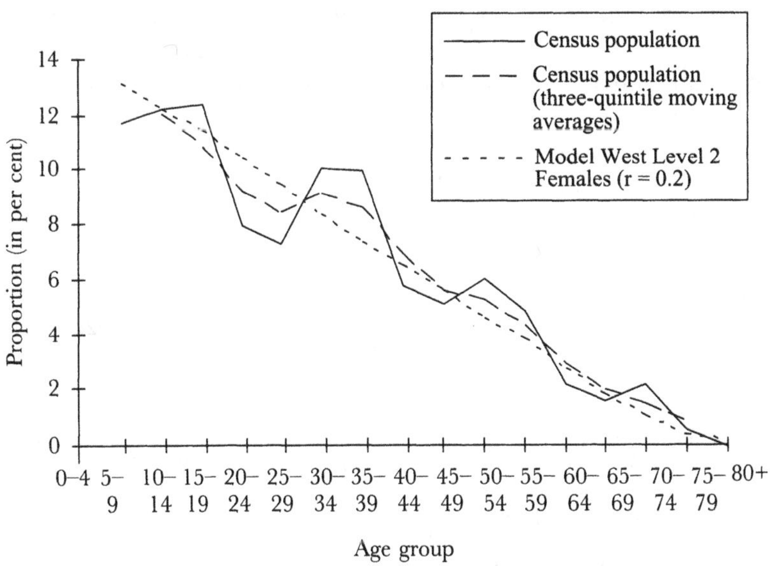

Figure 2.24 Female age composition of village census population of Roman Egypt fitted to a model life table (seven-year moving averages)

important, the similarly 'steep' curve for urban females is not counterbalanced by a correspondingly 'flattened' curve for village females (cf. ibid.). The missing male villagers either lived in their villages but eluded registration or had decamped to the cities where they likewise went unregistered.

I conclude that the discrepancy between the age distribution in the villages and the model is a function of the underregistration of rural males, whereas the deviation of the city pattern from the model may be explained with reference to urban excess mortality. Whereas the similarity of the male and female metropolitan patterns suggests that together they may provide a fairly representative mean for the urban populations covered by the census returns, the observed peculiarities of the records for rural males show that in much the same way as the geographically undifferentiated gender groups studied by Bagnall and Frier, the aggregate sample of all villagers does not represent a meaningful analytic category.

3.3. *The impact of the 'Antonine plague'*

From 166 into the 180s CE, the Roman empire was swept by a severe epidemic usually identified as smallpox.[101] While the death toll is unknown, the most plausible modern estimates reckon with the loss of seven to ten per cent of the total population of the empire, and of up to twice as many in large cities.[102] Papyrological evidence suggests that the epidemic affected at least Lower and Middle Egypt from about 166 into the late 170s CE, manifesting itself in 'sporadic, brief but devastating outbreaks in individual localities'.[103] Observing that similar numbers of census returns date from before and after the onset of this plague, Bagnall and Frier address the question of whether differences between these two subsets of data 'betray (. . .) signs of the plague's consequences'.[104] As can be seen in Figures 2.25–26, aggres-

[101] Gilliam (1961/86); Littman and Littman (1973); Salmon (1974) 133–9; Breitwieser (1995); Duncan-Jones (1996). For the identification with smallpox, see Littman and Littman (1973) 245; Sallares (1991) 248; cf. Duncan-Jones (1996) 116 n. 86.

[102] See Littman and Littman (1973) 252–5 for estimates of likely levels of mortality. McNeill (1977) 116 proffers an estimate of mortality of one-fourth to one-third in places affected; cf. Duncan-Jones (1996) 116 n. 88.

[103] Rathbone (1990) 119, who surveys the pertinent record (114–19) and suggests a drop in Egyptian population of twenty to thirty per cent (119). See now also Sharp (1999) 185–9.

[104] Bagnall and Frier (1994) 173–8, at 174.

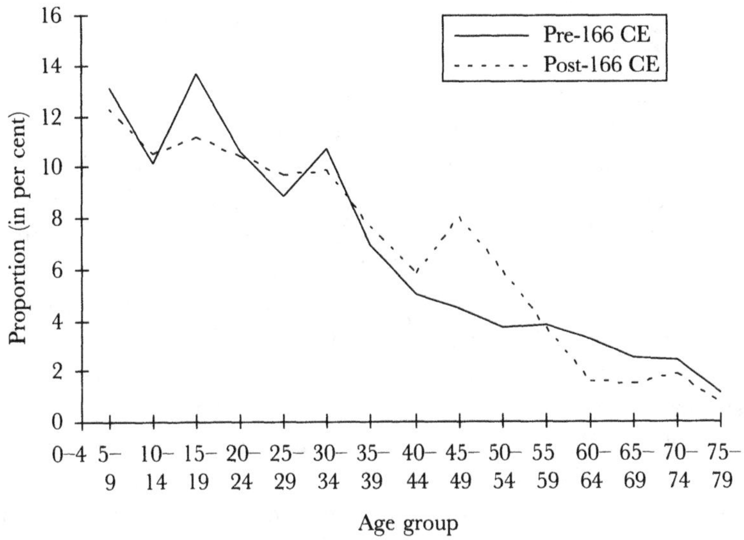

Figure 2.25 Age composition of the census population of Roman Egypt before and after 166 CE (seven-year moving averages)

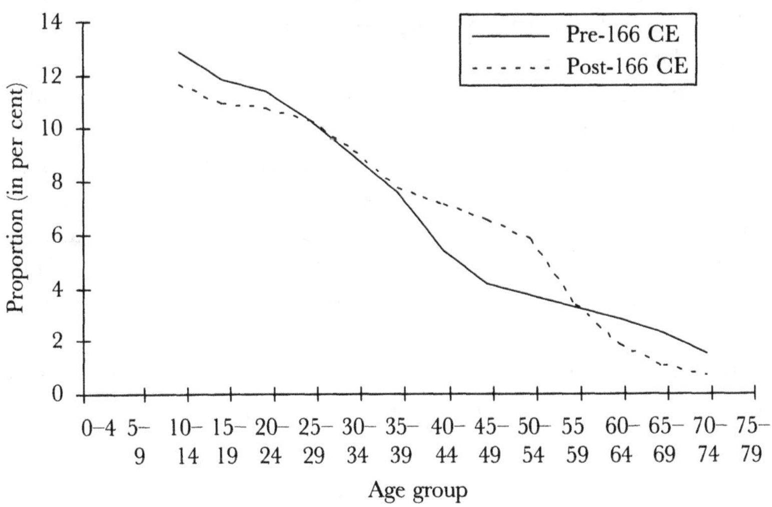

Figure 2.26 Age composition of the census population of Roman Egypt before and after 166 CE (three-quintile moving averages of seven-year moving averages)

sive smoothing of the evidence reveals a limited amount of variation.[105]

The pre-plague pattern seems to suggest somewhat higher attrition rates during much of juvenile and adult life, pointing to either lower life expectancy or higher fertility before 166 CE. Bagnall and Frier are ready to accept these discrepancies as evidence that 'the Egyptian population was not entirely stable over the long period covered by the census returns'.[106] Although this must inevitably be true, the observed fluctuations are of questionable significance. Because the grand total is composed of fairly equal shares of pre-plague and post-plague data, we lack an objective standard against which to measure either age distribution. If we somewhat arbitrarily assign predictive value to the earlier sample, the later age distribution can be shown to deviate significantly from that norm: 77.83 per cent of the pre-plague data from ages five to fifty-nine fall into the range from five to thirty-four, compared to 71.02 per cent of the remaining data ($p < 0.0119$). Due to smaller sample size, the significance of the difference from ages thirty-five to fifty-nine is weaker (19.73 against 26.15 per cent; $p < 0.0885$). Even so, it would appear that these discrepancies are not accidental.

However, two problems remain. It is uncertain whether the pre-plague data provide an objective standard. If that sample deviated somewhat from the actual mean pattern, in the first instance because of its modest size, the differences between the post-plague evidence and the 'norm' could be smaller than they now seem. In addition, the urban-rural split in the two subsamples differs. Based on the discussion in the previous section, we would expect a predominance of villagers to 'flatten' the curve up to age fifty. This effect may account for some of the observed deviation: the pre-plague data are split down the middle (49.45 per cent urban against 50.55 per cent rural), whereas the post-plague data are somewhat biassed in favour of villagers (44.2 versus 55.8 per cent). Together, these two factors help explain the discrepancies between the two subsamples without reference to the epidemic. Subtle theories of demographic change lack a basis in the available evidence.[107]

---

[105] Figs. 2.25–26 are based on the enlarged database in Appendix 2. The graphs in Bagnall and Frier (1994) 176 figs. 9.1–2 show the same patterns.

[106] Bagnall and Frier (1994) 177.

[107] *Contra* Bagnall and Frier (1994) 177, who argue that as a result of the plague, life expectancy was lower after 166 CE while the intrinsic growth rate was higher as the Egyptians tried to compensate for smallpox mortality. Under those circum-

Our scepticism is reinforced by a closer look at the data. The impact of smallpox should primarily be visible in the census returns from 173 and 187 CE, which are close to the event and dominate the record (two-thirds of the post-plague data come from these two censuses). This is not the case (Table 2.5). Children under five and adults over forty are most heavily affected by epidemic smallpox; its impact is weakest from ages five to twenty.[108]

Table 2.5 Proportional representation of age cohorts in different subsamples of the census returns of Roman Egypt (in per cent)

Age	Pre-166 CE (n = 370)	173 CE (n = 98)	187 CE (n = 125)	173/87 CE (n = 223)	Post-166 CE (n = 342)
0–9	24.9	25.5	**16.8**	20.6	22.8
10–14	8.1	10.2	12.0	11.2	9.1
15–24	20.5	20.4	24.8	22.7	19.0
25–59	38.1	**37.8**	**42.4**	**40.4**	43.9
60–79	8.4	6.1	4.0	4.9	5.3

Note: Underlined figures are expected to fall short of the pre-plague values, bold figures are expected to exceed them.

In the context of rampant smallpox, the following skewing is to be expected. In the data from 173 CE, six years after the first outbreak in Egypt, the age group from birth to nine years should have shrunk. This is not the case. By 187 CE, this cohort, then reflecting births between 177 and 187 CE, should have grown to compensate for previous losses. Again, the opposite is the case. By that time, the birth cohort from 163–172 CE would have moved into the range from fifteen to twenty-four, depressing that particular age bracket. Once more, the opposite effect can be observed. In both censuses, ages twenty-five to fifty-nine ought to be more common relative to lower and higher ones. This is only documented for 187 CE, when this distortion is expected to be weaker than in 173 CE. Finally, the ranks of the elderly should appear depleted in both years. This assumption can be reconciled with the data. Taken at face value, the evidence is best compatible with smallpox mortality between 177

stances, the post-epidemic age distribution curve ought to have become 'steeper' than it had been before; however, the opposite is the case (see above).

[108] See Sallares (1991) 465 n. 367.

and 187 CE. This is puzzling, given that the first outbreaks date to the late 160s and must have had a stronger impact than on subsequent occasions.

However, any interpretation of this material perforce remains guesswork. The data from individual censuses are few and random fluctuations inevitable. At the moment, we are unable to identify the consequences of smallpox mortality in the Egyptian census returns.

4. *Population change: migration and growth*

As I have noted above, Bagnall and Frier do not consider the different age distributions in cities and villages. Instead, they attempt to explore migrational patterns through the urban sex ratio.[109] In their view, the documented prevalence of men among metropolitan adults may in the first instance be explained with reference to male immigration from the villages. These men are mostly considered 'marginal' villagers, 'perhaps most often young men unable to find brides and form families, or unable to find work', and thought rarely to have returned to the countryside later in life. Because of this outflow, the village sex ratio for young adults hovered at or slightly below parity.[110]

This model is inadequate for a number of reasons. We may leave aside the question of whether urban sex ratios are intrinsically likely to be skewed in favour of men. Suffice it to note that comparative evidence points to predominantly female migration to pre-modern cities and that the population of Cairo at the time of Napoleon showed a strong female bias.[111] What is important here is that the

[109] Bagnall and Frier (1994) 160–9 (ch. 8: 'Migration').

[110] Ibid., 165, with reference to comparative evidence from late medieval Tuscany (cf. also 160–1).

[111] Bagnall and Frier (1994) 160 consider town-bound migration of young adult males part of a 'fairly typical pattern'. Bangladesh provides another example: see above, p. 149. Even so, high urban sex ratios are far from 'typical'. According to Sharlin (1978) 137, 'most urban censuses of the early modern period indicate significant surpluses of women over men' (which, however, 'cannot be relied on in any exact numerical way due to the likelihood of a selective undercount of transient males': ibid.; cf. above, p. 149). For low urban sex ratios in Italy and France, see Beloch (1937) 13–23 and Fauve-Chamoux (1994), respectively. De Vries (1984) 178 points out that 'urban sex ratios below 100 (. . .) distinguish European urban life from that of many other world civilizations', such as India and China. For this reason, it is important to note that all adult deaths reported in Cairo from 1798 to 1801 reflect a sex ratio of 74.1 (3,897 men and 5,261 women: Desgenettes (1813) 320). Of course, sex biases in migration may change over time: cf. Prominska (1972) 116–18, on Alexandria.

assumption of substantial male migration to the cities at ages fifteen to twenty-five and continuing albeit smaller transfers of older men is inconsistent with the attested urban age distribution at those ages. As shown in Figure 2.13, the male population of the metropoleis was subject to severe attrition rates from the late teens onwards when, according to Bagnall and Frier's hypothesis, it should have been bolstered up by townward migration. Moreover, the female age structure, which is supposed to have remained unaffected by comparable demographic transfers, exhibits exactly the same characteristics. Hence, there is nothing to suggest significantly divergent patterns of migration for men and women.

There are two ways of interpreting the sex-specific urban age composition. We might have to assume that there was little male immigration after age twenty and no female immigration at all, and that the indigenous population suffered from unusually high adult mortality levels. Alternatively, we may reckon with substantial immigration of male *and* female teenagers as well as weaker transfers at higher ages, resulting in exceptionally high adult mortality rates among these first-generation residents. Given that in the first scenario, the urban population could hardly have remained stable, let alone expanded (as it undoubtedly did during the early empire), the second interpretation appears to provide us with the only plausible model.

The high urban sex ratio, which could be taken to conflict with the latter scenario, need not be more than a statistical artifact. From ages fifteen to fifty-nine, the sex ratio is 118.7 for the cities of Middle Egypt (n = 199) and 133.3 in the sample from Ptolemais or Lykopolis (n = 70).[112] Owing to differences in sample size, these two rates are identical in terms of statistical significance. In both cases, there is a one-in-four chance that the attested deviation from perfect parity (50:50) is accidental ($p < 0.23$). Thus, the data are consistent with mature urban sex ratios at or slightly above parity, thus obviating the need for speculations about sex-biased migrational patterns.

If three-quarters of the Egyptian population lived in villages, the aggregate sex ratio for all weighted data for all ages stands at ninety-five. At four-fifths, it drops to ninety-two. Once again, whether these rates reflect any genuine deviation from parity remains doubtful.[113]

[112] Based on raw data from Appendix 2 and Frier (1997) 100 tab. 6.2.

[113] For a three-to-one rural-urban split, the difference between sex ratios of 95 and 100 is not significant ($p < 0.348$; n = 1,316), and only moderately significant for a four-to-one ratio ($p < 0.105$; n = 1,645). The latter scenario may be more plausible.

Moreover, the male age distribution in the villages enables us to explain the apparent shortfall in men as a function of widespread concealment. This suggests that at least several per cent of the total population, and a correspondingly higher proportion of adult villagers, may be missing from the census returns. Since the underreporting of village males was partly offset by the neglect of urban girls (see above, p. 149), the actual percentage may well be higher than indicated by the sex ratio proper. A low aggregate sex ratio (*if* it is more than a statistical fluke) is readily consistent with our argument that the attested male age distribution is fashioned by underreporting and therefore unsuitable for further demographic analysis. As a consequence, there is absolutely no reason for proposing a significantly elevated sex ratio for the total population of Roman Egypt.[114]

The graphs in Figure 2.27 further underline the futility of examining migration through age-specific sex ratios. First of all, the small number of data in any one fifteen-year age bracket *a priori* undermines the statistical significance of any particular finding. In purely impressionist terms, most of the observed variation can be attributed to reporting biases. Thus, the high juvenile sex ratio in the cities of Middle Egypt may reflect disdain for immature girls, while male predominance in old age is indicative of incremental age exaggeration, a common feature of elderly men in traditional societies.[115] At the same time, the sex ratio might also have been driven up by some indifference towards post-menopausal women. In the villages, the concealment of males only seems to have ceased at advanced ages.

By contrast, the sources from Upper Egypt are rather puzzling. While it might be tempting to interpret the sharp peak of the sex ratio among young adults as evidence of temporary male migration from and then back to the countryside, it must not be forgotten that the adult age structure in this one Upper Egyptian metropolis appears to be the same as in urban Middle Egypt (cf. above, Fig. 2.18). It is hardly possible to reconcile dramatic differences in the sex ratio—the Middle Egyptian pattern being inverted by the Upper Egyptian

---

[114] *Contra* Bagnall and Frier (1994) 104, deriving a hypothetical overall sex ratio of 118 from different model life tables for men and women (but cf. 108, for a probable sex ratio 'between 100 and 110'). As I have shown in section 3.2, the notion of higher male life expectancy is not supported by the data.

[115] For the neglect of girls, see above, p. 149; for age inflation among elderly men, see Bagnall and Frier (1994) 107 and n. 47; Scheidel (1996d) 45–6.

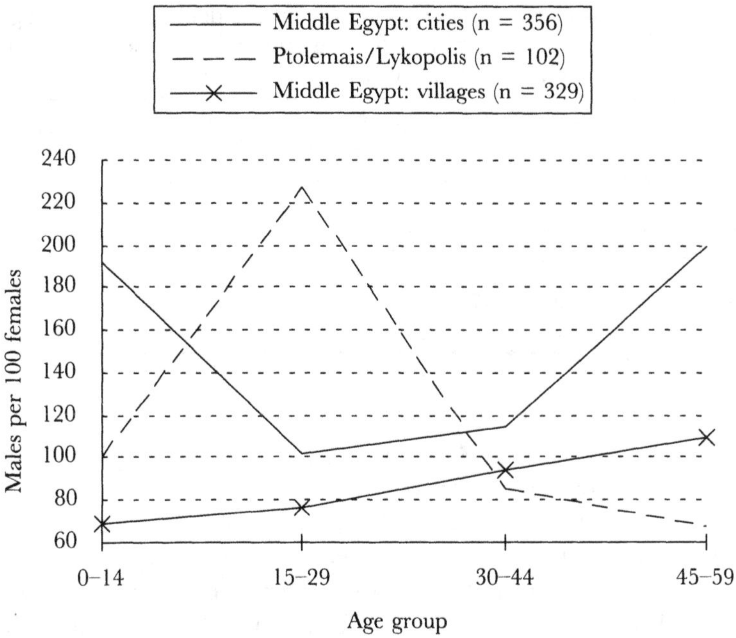

Figure 2.27 Age-specific sex ratios in two census populations of Roman Egypt (raw data)

distribution—with the complete lack of differences in the age composition. Something has to give: from the perspective of statistical significance, it seems advisable to discard the implied sex ratio in favour of the attested age structure. Moreover, the omission from *P.Oxy.* 984A of any census returns filed by women may well raise the attested urban sex ratio beyond the actual level.

The census returns of Roman Egypt do not permit us to trace patterns of migration. Hence, parametric modelling offers us the only opportunity to delineate, however imperfectly, the probable rythm of demographic change (Table 2.6).[116]

This schematic model is based on a few uncontroversial assumptions: that the population of Egypt was larger in 165 CE than it had been in 30 BCE; that both the cities and the villages grew during that period; and that the cities expanded at a faster pace than the villages,

[116] The uses of this type of modelling are well illustrated by Wrigley (1978). Jongman (1990) and Morley (1996) 33–54 have developed similar models for Roman Italy.

Table 2.6 A speculative simple model of annual demographic change in Roman Egypt from Augustus to the Antonines (population figures in cols. 2–4, 6–7 in 1,000; rates in cols. 5, 8–9 in per cent)

Date	Population		Rural births	Rural natural increase	Urban shortfall of births	Transfer Rural > Urban	Net gain	
	Urban	Rural					Urban	Rural
(1)	(2)	(3)	(4)	(5)	(6)	(7)	(8)	(9)
30 BCE	1,000	4,000	172	+0.3	7.5	10	0.25	0.05
165 CE	1,500	4,500	193.5	+0.3	11.25	12.5	< 0.1	~ 0

raising the overall rate of urbanisation. The individual figures are merely meant to capture likely orders of magnitude. While the model is relatively insensitive to changes in total population size, the urban-rural split is a more important variable. As has been argued elsewhere, a level of urbanisation of twenty-five per cent for the entire country including Alexandria (and of under twenty per cent outside the capital) in the second century CE is unusually high but perhaps not impossible.[117] It is even more difficult to estimate the respective figure at the onset of Roman rule. However, within the parameters of the model, it would make little difference if the share of the urban population had risen from twenty to twenty-five per cent, as suggested here, or from less than fifteen to twenty or from fifteen to twenty-five per cent instead.

Our model is furthermore predicated on the conventional assumption that in the cities, mortality was somewhat higher than in the villages.[118] Thus, immigration from the countryside both counterbalanced a small amount of natural decrease and supported net growth. In real terms, the urban population is thought to have grown at an average annual rate of around 0.15 per cent, increasing by one-half within two centuries.[119] Annual growth is expected to have slowed

---

[117] See below, Chapter 3, p. 247. Cf. Bairoch (1989) for a general discussion of pre-modern urbanisation.

[118] The figures chosen tally well with my tentative estimate of natural decrease in the largest cities: see above, n. 88. Cf. Wrigley (1978) and Wrigley and Schofield (1981) 166–70, for comparative material. See also below, section 5.

[119] This long-term rate seems readily consistent with the observation that 'during the most flourishing periods of the pre-industrial economies in Europe the fastest rates of urban expansion (concerning 3–4 decades) were about 0.4 per year': Bairoch (1989) 255.

down as the cities expanded: in the model, this effect is expressed as a gradual decrease from 0.25 per annum to a notional value close to zero. Because of continuing population transfers to the cities, the rural population expanded more slowly. By the time of the 'Antonine plague', the carrying capacity of Egypt may well have been pushed to its limits. In this scenario, the combination of very high levels of urbanisation and the absorption of rural natural growth by migration needed to sustain cities which could not grow much further would have forestalled continuing demographic expansion and exposed the Egyptian population to Malthusian positive checks.[120]

During the period covered by the census returns, the survivors of 10,000 or more rural births may have permanently moved to the cities every year. Immigration on this scale involved not more than approximately six per cent of all villagers and therefore remains invisible in the rural census returns. The fact that the removal of lodgers from the urban census samples does not raise the mean age of the adult population suggests that some immigrants failed to acquire their own households and, perhaps together with the urban-born poor, formed a permanent urban 'under-class' of lifelong lodgers.[121] Immigrants who managed to set up their own households in the cities cannot be identified on the basis of the census returns.[122] In practice, however, the uniquely endogamous marriage customs of the metropolitan census population, above all in the city of Arsinoe (which dominates the urban record), must have separated long-term residents from newcomers. Unfortunately, our sources do not permit us to trace any such fault lines within the urban population. With regard to the Fayum, we can only speculate that given the existence of incestuous unions in the villages, albeit at lower levels than in Arsinoe, recent immigrants were ready to blend into their new environment by embracing the prevailing metropolitan custom of brother-sister marriage.[123]

---

[120] Cf. below, Chapter 3, p. 247, and in general Frier (1999, 2000) and esp. (2001).

[121] This group was probably complemented by a transient under-class of temporary (male) migrants from the villages (cf. above, p. 149).

[122] The sources convey the impression that the legally privileged metropolitan population was meant to be fairly tightly closed off to outsiders. I have tried to show that for demographic reasons alone, this kind of separation was feasible only up to a point.

[123] For the statistics of brother-sister marriage in Roman Egypt, see Bagnall and Frier (1994) 127–33; Scheidel (1995), (1996a) 9–51, (1997a), and cf. also (1996b). In the second century CE, 37.0 and 20.6 per cent of all documented marriages

5. *Conclusions*

The census returns tell us both less and more about the demography of Roman Egypt than Bagnall and Frier maintain. On the one hand, this body of evidence is marred by a number of serious deficiencies that obscure much of the underlying demographic regime. Widespread neglect and underreporting of juveniles make it impossible to explore important issues such as sex selection and migration at subadult ages. In the villages, a substantial proportion of all men were concealed far beyond their teenage years, and in fact well into their forties. This practice, which also corrupts the extant tax lists, rules out any attempt to ascertain the age composition of the male rural population. This, in turn, prevents comparative demographic analysis along gender lines. In the villages, only the records for females appear largely free from systematic reporting biases. In the cities, by contrast, we find a similar adult age structure for both men and women. At the same time, the urban data differ significantly from those for rural women.

This observation reveals a previously unappreciated yet important feature of Egyptian demography. Thus, urban mortality rates at mature ages are not only much higher than among female villagers, but also much higher than predicted by those model life tables which have been thought to provide a reasonable approximation of Egyptian population structure. Bagnall and Frier opt for gender as the most important criterion in differentiating demographic patterns within the aggregate census population. As we have seen, however, the irreparable defects of the rural male data invalidate sex-specific analysis. What is more, the authors' focus on gender blocks out genuine differences between city and countryside. It is location, not gender (or period: cf. section 3.3), that should be considered the pivotal criterion of differentiation.

In his work on Egypt in late antiquity, Bagnall claims that its cities provided 'an environment even less healthy than the villages, with (like many other premodern cities) a lower life expectancy than

---

were between siblings in Arsinoe and in the surrounding villages, respectively (Scheidel (1997a) 362 tab. 1). The urban incidence of brother-sister marriage is so high compared to the possible maximum level (*c.* 25–50 per cent against < 40 per cent: ibid., 365) that if there was a significant amount of immigration, many of the newcomers must necessarily have adopted the same custom.

the countryside'.[124] Even so, in their subsequent joint study Bagnall and Frier neglect to address this important question with the help of the census returns.[125] This omission is all the more unfortunate given that evidence of disproportionately high urban death rates is of relevance far beyond the study of some province of the Roman empire. While variation in mortality along gender lines is primarily associated with social and cultural norms and practices, such as preferential allocation of resources to one sex and different labour regimes, elevated urban mortality is most likely to be a function of density-dependent disease. Thus, whereas higher life expectancy for men (if it were documented) might shed light on the valuation of the sexes in Roman Egypt, lower life expectancy for city residents of either sex helps reinforce the concept of large pre-modern cities as 'population sinks'.[126] The bulk of the urban census returns originates from Arsinoe, perhaps the second-largest Egyptian city after the provincial capital itself, with a population of forty thousand or over. Most of the remaining documents in this category were filed in Oxyrhynchus and Hermopolis Magna, cities of several tens of thousand inhabitants each. District *metropoleis* of this kind may have been

---

[124] Bagnall (1993) 50, with express reference (50 n. 38) to the—then forthcoming—study of Bagnall and Frier (1994).

[125] According to Bagnall and Frier (1994) 49, 'major demographic distinctions divide metropoleis from villages (. . .). For example, village families are larger and internally more complex than those in metropoleis; houses in villages are much likelier to be owner-occupied; and metropolitan households contain significantly higher numbers of both slaves and non-kin lodgers. Metropolitan women may also marry a few years later than village women, and they are much more likely to enter brother-sister marriages; and, perhaps most significant, the attested village sex ratio differs appreciably from that in metropoleis.' These and other discrepancies between city and countryside are explored in considerable detail, e.g., age-rounding (46), household structure (66–7), family size (67–9), house ownership (69–70), slaveholding (70–1), occupations (72–3), sex ratio (93, 95), age of marriage (117–18), sibling marriage (128–9), and migration (160–9). It is only in the chapters on age structure that the data are not disaggregated according to location. But cf. their isolated and unexplained remark, which is not borne out by anything in their own text, that villages 'may even have had a slightly higher life expectancy than nome metropoleis' (87); and see the previous footnote.

[126] De Vries (1984) 175–98, in a balanced discussion of the model of urban excess mortality and its critics, cautiously favours this concept. Bairoch (1989) 261–2 reiterates the notion of urban excess mortality, estimating that in pre-industrial Europe in general, urban infant and adult mortality may have been sixty and twenty per cent higher than in the countryside, respectively. Scheidel (2001) 28 n. 106 cites further literature. For ancient medical allusions to the health hazards of urbanism, see Nutton (2000) 66–7.

thirty or forty times as large as the average Egyptian village and could easily have generated a more aggressive disease environment than rural settlements.[127] Under these circumstances, and allowing for particularly high attrition rates among adult immigrants, it is possible that the non-standard age distribution suggested by the urban census returns reflects conditions in an high-exposure environment characterised by severe mortality (even) at mature ages. This interpretation of the urban census data receives support from the epigraphic evidence for seasonal mortality patterns discussed in the previous chapter. Extraordinary levels of seasonal mortality variation (even) among young and middle-aged adults such as those attested by the epitaphs of the Nile valley and the Fayum—many of which come from an urban background or other locales with high population densities, such as monasteries—are fully consistent with very high mortality rates overall. From this perspective, census returns and epitaphs simply record two different aspects of the same phenomenon.

This re-assessment of the Egyptian census data casts further doubt on the universal applicability of model life tables. Attempts to reconcile heterogenous population samples with standard models only divert our attention from local differentiation. No fewer than seventy per cent of the data in known census returns fall into patterns that are not consistent with the predictions of standard model life tables; this proportion rises to seventy-five per cent if the evidence from Upper Egypt is included. It is true that the largest segment of the Egyptian population that appears to be reliably documented by the census returns, i.e., female villagers, conforms to the predictions of a plausible Coale and Demeny model (Model West Level 2 Females; $e(0) = 22.5$). Given that at least four-fifths of the Egyptian population outside Alexandria must have lived in the countryside, and speculating that in terms of mortality, men did not differ significantly from women, we might be tempted to conclude that this sample alone suffices to give us a rough but fairly representative impression of mortality in Roman Egypt in general. However, owing to the relatively small number of pertinent references, and notwithstanding the apparent fit in terms of the overall *shape* of the age distribution, these

[127] For the cities of Middle Egypt, see briefly Rathbone (1990) 120–1, and forthcoming work by L. E. Tacoma. Cf. also above, n. 88. Rathbone 124–37 discusses the size of Egyptian villages.

data are fully compatible with a whole range of models with both lower and higher rates of life expectancy.[128] This fact alone seriously weakens the predictive value of this subsample. To make matters worse, the age data for village women are marred by a comparatively high incidence of rounding and numerical preference.[129]

Moreover, we must also allow for the possibility of demographic variation in the countryside. In the same way as the urban data, the majority of the census records for villagers come from the Fayum, which has traditionally been the most malarial region of Egypt south of the lower reaches of the Nile Delta. The observed anomalies in the urban age composition may be explained with reference to malaria or tuberculosis, a combination of both or a mixture of these and other endemic diseases (cf. above, section 2). Even though the female village data do not display a comparable pattern, we have good reason to expect some amount of malaria infection in substantial parts of the Fayum.[130] In this case, mean life expectancy in the Fayum in general—and hence in our sample population of female villagers—may well have been somewhat lower than in the country as a whole. The relatively small number of age records from outside the Fayum regrettably forestalls meaningful comparison between that region and

---

[128] When we divide the sample of 141.1 female villagers aged fifteen to sixty-nine into two roughly equal halves, we find 51.45 per cent to be younger than thirty-five (based on seven-year moving averages). In terms of statistical significance, this proportion is readily consistent with Model West Females Levels 1 ($p < 0.4$), 2 ($p < 0.484$), 3 ($p < 0.873$), 4 ($p < 0.897$), 5 ($p < 0.689$) and 6 ($p < 0.516$), with values of $e(0)$ from 20 to 32.5 years. According to the chi-square test for eleven five-year age brackets within the same range, there are more than seven and more than five chances in ten that the underlying age pattern would also match Levels 1 and 6, respectively (but cf. above, n. 69, for the limited utility of this test). Note that the (larger) metropolitan sample is incompatible with any of these models (see above, pp. 144–5), and that it would therefore likewise be incompatible with the rural female age distribution were it considered a normative standard.

[129] The value of Myers' Index of Deviation, a standard test of age-preference, is 20.4 per cent for adult village women, against 10.4 per cent for adult village men and an average of 9.2 per cent for all adults in Egyptian census returns: Scheidel (1996a) 64 tab. 2.6, with 66–70, 85 tab. 2.19. Most of this distortion results from age-heaping on multiples of five. In addition, avoidance of the final digit 'seven', presumably motivated by superstitious concerns, is strikingly common among village women: ibid., 65. By contrast, the urban age data utilised in section 3.2 are remarkably precise by pre-modern standards.

[130] See above, Chapter 1, section 3.5. This undermines the claim by Bagnall and Frier (1994) 6 that 'there is no particular reason to believe that these Middle Egyptian nomes were on the whole significantly different from the rest of the country in demographic characteristics'.

other parts of the country. It is, however, interesting to note that in the 1920s, at a time when the average life expectancy at birth of Egyptians was still below thirty years, the Crude Death Rate reported for the Fayum was much higher than in any other Egyptian district outside the crowded capital and the (malaria-ridden) oases.[131]

In view of all this, we cannot reasonably claim to be able to estimate the most likely *average* life expectancy or age structure of the population of Roman Egypt. The Egyptian census returns do not advance our knowledge of these important issues beyond the position taken on *a priori* grounds by Hopkins in 1966, namely, that mean life expectancy at birth in the Roman world probably fell in a range from twenty to thirty years.[132] Whilst the evidence for village women may superficially point to a value close to the lower end of that range, this impression is lacking in statistical significance. The data for male villagers in the census returns as well as in the tax lists are unsuitable for demographic analysis but for that very reason throw important light on the limits of bureaucratic control over the rural population. At the same time, the urban records evince a demographic pattern that cannot be reconciled with the predictions of reasonable standard models. I have argued that mortality was the principal factor in shaping the metropolitan age composition in the observed fashion. If this interpretation is correct, the census returns of Roman Egypt provide the earliest quantitative evidence of urban excess mortality in world history. In any event, the close match established by Bagnall and Frier between the age distributions generated by all female and all male age data on the one hand and two superficially plausible model life tables on the other thus turns out to be coincidental. As a consequence, extrapolations from these particular model life tables, such as the calculation of a mean Total Fertility Rate of 5.979, remain unsupported by the evidence.[133]

---

[131] *Annuaire statistique 1926–1927* (Cairo 1928), 61 gives CDRs of 31.5 (Fayum), 25.5 (Lower Egypt), 25.1 (Upper Egypt), 34.5 (Cairo) and 40.6 (Frontier districts). All these figures are clearly marred by extensive underreporting (cf. below, Chapter 3, p. 214). Thus, the higher death rates in Cairo may partly be due to higher standards of registration. By contrast, there is no obvious reason why deaths in the then backward Fayum region should have been more assiduously reported than in other rural areas.

[132] Hopkins (1966) 264. For this range, see above, n. 9.

[133] *Contra* Bagnall and Frier (1994) 138–9. The findings in n. 128 suggest that the TFR cannot strictly speaking be fixed at any particular point within the probable range from about 4 to 6.5. Even so, a relatively high rate seems plausible *a priori*.

This is an important epistemological point. I do not mean to suggest that Bagnall and Frier's reconstruction of Egyptian age structure and levels of life expectancy is somehow intrinsically implausible, or that they fail to offer a reasonable proposal of what the demographic regime of Roman Egypt *may* have looked like.[134] However, in as far as in their scrutiny of the surviving census returns they aim to move the study of ancient mortality away from sheer probabilistic modelling and to anchor it (at least in a complementary fashion) in the quantitative analysis of ancient source material, their project must be judged largely unsuccessful. Whilst the urban data are of considerable interest in their own right, they contribute little if anything to the reconstruction of life and death among the much larger rural majority of the population. Unfortunately, owing to the deficiencies of the male age data from the villages (corroborated by the tax lists), it would not be appropriate to consolidate all rural sources into a single total. At the same time, the sample of rural female age data on its own is too small for us to derive from it a sufficiently robust age distribution that could be used, albeit in a somewhat speculative manner, to correct reporting errors in the dataset for male villagers. However, given that levels of life expectancy in the rural census population cannot be fixed with greater precision than merely within the conventional range of between twenty and thirty years or so that entirely depends on models and comparative evidence, the census returns cannot replace *or even supplement* model life tables in our search for mortality and life expectancy in, mostly, the Arsinoite and Oxyrhynchite nomes of Middle Egypt.

Even more importantly, even if these vital functions were known, they would tell us little about the scope of local and regional variation. Perhaps depending on their size or location, cities appear to have been even less healthy than villages. The exceptional scale of seasonal mortality variation (Chapter 1, section 2.3) and comparative evidence of malaria infestation in the Fayum indicate that in terms of attrition and survival, this region gravitated towards the lower end of the spectrum for the entire province. The Nile Delta,

---

[134] Thus, for instance, our schematic model in Tab. 2.3 is based, for the rural population, on the projections of Model West Females Level 3, which resembles Bagnall and Frier's model for the total Egyptian population: ibid., 105 fig. 5.5. Cf., e.g., Zhao (1997) for (implied) levels of *e*(0) of about twenty-seven to thirty years in a (privileged) Chinese clan from 1 to 1000 CE which are corroborated by much larger population samples from 1000 to 1749.

home to more than half of the Egyptian population, is barely visible in the census record. Mystifying differences between the seasonal mortality patterns of Upper and Lower Egypt point to otherwise indetectable interregional diversity. Hence, the notion of an average age structure proves an elusive concept even when applied to the population of a single province of the Roman empire.[135]

* * *

This brings us back to the central argument of this book. In their own words, Bagnall and Frier 'are convinced that the returns provide solid support for the emerging picture of life expectancy in the early Roman Empire'. But unlike beauty, solidity is not just in the eye of the beholder. I have stressed the problems of determining average Egyptian life expectancy even as a purely mathematical mean. Leaving this issue aside, any further extrapolation raises additional questions. It may well be 'likely that overall Egyptian life expectancy at birth was in the lower twenties'. After all, one would favour a comparable estimate on the basis of comparative evidence alone.[136] It is considerably more doubtful to what extent this estimate supports broad generalisations about the demography of the Roman world. Owing to its unmatched levels of population density and singular ecological conditions created by its inundation schedule, Egypt is a special case *a priori*.[137] High population density sustains endemic infections and facilitates the introduction of novel diseases. Local levels of seasonal mortality fluctuation comparable to those found in the mega-city of Rome tend to confirm this picture. So do ancient as well as more recent accounts of Egypt as a hotbed of infectious disorders. The notorious prevalence of leprosy in that country which is now being studied by Sallares and which set it apart from the remainder of the Roman empire is only one exam-

---

[135] For seasonal mortality in the Fayum and in Lower Egypt, see above, Chapter 1, sections 2.3 and 2.4.

[136] Quotes from Bagnall and Frier (1994) 110 and 109. For comparative evidence from early twentieth-century Egypt, see below, Chapter 3, p. 214.

[137] Average population density in Egypt may have been in excess of 200 persons per km^2 (and closer to 300 per km^2 of arable), compared to 30/km^2 in Italy and around 15/km^2 in the empire as a whole: see below, Chapter 3, p. 247, for Egypt, and Frier (2000) 812, 814.

ple; the early presence of bubonic plague is another. We have considered the possibility that in terms of health and longevity, the Fayum may have been one of least favoured parts of Egypt. An analogous case can be made with regard to Egypt's position within the empire. Most of the sparse quantifiable sources for ancient demography come from either Egypt or Rome. Neither area can justifiably lay claim to representing an environment that is 'typical' and therefore representative of the Roman empire as a whole. Not only does evidence of conspicuous mortality variation in other traditional settings, such as early modern England, cast doubt on the very idea of 'typical' death rates or age distributions. If anything, at least in ecological terms, the populations of the Nile valley and the Seven Hills of Rome might be considered two of the *least* typical concentrations of humans anywhere in the empire.

Throughout this book, I have argued that Roman population history can only be studied within the context of its wider ecological framework. Reviews of particular samples of ancient data that neglect their ecological background invariably fail to advance from description to explanation. In keeping with the emerging consensus among historical demographers concerned with more recent periods, I have identified disease as the crucial variable in Roman mortality variation.[138] A few years ago, I concluded a previous book by emphasising the scope of diversity in Roman demography.[139] Given the intense fragmentation of the disease environment of an area as vast and disparate as the Roman empire, my present study of the demographic impact of disease further reinforces this impression. The hyper-uniformitarian retrojections embodied in model life tables have been helpful in gaining insight into various processes from the workings of Athenian democracy to the transmission of property in the Roman family that would not otherwise have been possible.[140] At the same time, these interpretive crutches have also made it easier to forget that such ancient demographic evidence as there is inevitably reflects local conditions and may be unsuitable for generalising extrapolations.

[138] The persistent deficiencies of paleodemographic analysis make it difficult to relate the nutritional status of Roman cemetery populations to life expectancy. However, disease is a more important factor determining life expectancy than access to resources: see Johansson (1994a). Quantifiable evidence for the Roman elite suggests that wealth and power did not significantly raise mean life expectancy: Scheidel (1999a).

[139] Scheidel (1996a) 165.

[140] See above, n. 12.

By the same token, generic models that may conceivably provide a rough approximation of overall averages cannot necessarily be applied to any particular geographical or social context or matched with local samples of data. Instead, it is the interdisciplinary study of disease that holds the key to an improved understanding of the demographic landscapes of the Roman world.

CHAPTER THREE

POPULATION SIZE AND DEMOGRAPHIC CHANGE

1. *The size of Roman populations*

Consideration of gross population size has traditionally been given pride of place by ancient historians with demographic interests.[1] The relative abundance of pertinent references in Greek and Roman literature may help to explain this preoccupation. But appearances are deceptive: in general, the reporting of numbers in ancient texts can be shown to be very heavily controlled by literary conventions. While some figures may well be based on actual counts, many references are no more than symbolic values, at best indicative of a certain order of magnitude and deployed to lend emphasis or colour to an author's exposition.[2] Regardless of these obstacles, however, population size matters, and is of more than merely antiquarian interest. In fact, it can be critical for our perception of the levels of development of ancient societies. Thus, our views on the true extent of political participation and military mobilisation in classical Athens or its dependence on food imports from overseas depend on our estimates of its gross population. To an even higher degree, the fortunes of classical Sparta were determined by changes in manpower.[3] Among Roman historians, the debate has largely revolved around the problem of the size of the citizenry in the late Republican period, which is the crucial determinant of any estimate of the total population of the Italian peninsula in antiquity.

---

[1] This section draws heavily on my more extensive discussion of recent scholarship on Roman population size in Scheidel (2001) 49–72, esp. 49–59.

[2] A number of studies of prices and other amounts of money in Roman literature clearly prove this point: see Duncan-Jones (1982) 238–56; Scheidel (1996c); Duncan-Jones (1997). Analogous surveys of military tallies are still missing. For rhetorical stylisation in other types of accounts, see Dreizehnter (1978); Fehling (1990); Rubincam (1991).

[3] For Athens, see, e.g., Hansen (1985, 1988, 1994), on the political system and warfare; Garnsey (1988) 183–95, on the food supply, with a survey of recent controversies in my addendum (ibid., 195–200). For Sparta, see Hodkinson (1989).

Assessments of the number of Roman citizens depend entirely on a series of recorded census results, many of which may be based on documentary evidence of actual population counts but were transmitted via literary texts or more rarely in inscriptions. With regard to the late Republic, the debate has long oscillated between two competing and mutually incompatible positions. The attested census totals jump from about 900,000 in 69 BCE to close to four million in 28 BCE and comparable figures in the following decades.[4] In the Republic, only men of fighting age were enumerated in the census. However, given that under Augustus, most Roman citizens must still have resided in Italy and indeed largely in its peninsular half, the reported totals of four to five million imply a gross population of Roman Italy—including women, children, aliens and slaves—that would be difficult to reconcile with comparative evidence from the early modern period. Not only is the resultant grand total very high to begin with, but we also need to allow for a certain amount of census underreporting as well as further population growth during the early Principate. Beloch sought to solve this problem by assuming that the Augustan census figures referred to the entire citizen population instead of adult men only. This conjecture was until recently almost universally accepted as the most plausible interpretation.[5] Over the past few years, however, the legitimacy of this reading has repeatedly been called into question.[6] Depending on our interpretation of the early imperial census figures, the Roman citizenry at the turn of the millennium *either* numbered four or five million *or* was approximately three times as large. There is no obvious middle route between these dramatically divergent estimates.[7]

Unfortunately, neither scenario is particularly compelling. The supposed Augustan change in reporting practice is not directly attested and may be unlikely *a priori*; Beloch's population tally seems low relative to the large number of cities in Roman Italy—in excess of 400—and implies an exceptionally high degree of urbanisation even when the capital itself is excluded from the sample: the proportion

---

[4] Livius, *Periochae* 98 (900,000) and Phlegon *FGrHist* 257 F 12 (910,000) for 69 BCE; *Res Gestae Divi Augusti* 8 (4,063,000 for 28 BCE, 4,233,000 for 8 BCE and 4,937,000 in 14 CE); Tacitus, *Annales* 11.25 (5,984,072 for 47 CE).

[5] Beloch (1886) 370–8. See also (e.g.) Brunt (1971); Hopkins (1978) 33, 68; Parkin (1992) 5; Morley (1996) 46–50; Scheidel (1996a) 93.

[6] Lo Cascio (1994a, b, 1996, 2000).

[7] See Scheidel (2001) 53 n. 212.

of urban residents has been put at about one-third including Rome and one-fifth without it.[8] To make matters worse, the 'low' estimate also implies staggering levels of military mobilisation.[9] Moreover, it requires us to assume that the free Italian population outside the city of Rome shrank slightly during the first century BCE and demographic growth was limited to the servile element: under these circumstances, fully one-half of the non-metropolitan urban population ought to have consisted of slaves.[10] On the other hand, the 'high' estimate is very high indeed, raising the population of peninsular Italy outside Rome to a level equivalent to that close to the end of the nineteenth century.[11] Thus, while the 'high' estimate renders Roman Italy exceptional in terms of overall population density, the 'low' estimate makes it look exceptional in almost any other respect from the level of urbanisation to the share of slaves in the total population.

Modern assessments of the size of the population of Roman Egypt are plagued by similar uncertainties. Two mutually incompatible population totals arrived at under unknown circumstances are of little help to the demographic historian (see below). As a consequence, ancient literary and modern comparative evidence has been marshalled in support of significantly divergent estimates from four or five to more than eight million inhabitants during the Principate.[12] These calculations create a familiar dilemma: while the 'low' estimate of four or five million appears to be too cautious given the number and size of the Egyptian cities of that period, a 'high' total in excess of eight million implies a degree of popolousness equivalent to that close to the end of the nineteenth century but reduces the share of the non-agricultural population to more plausible levels, from around one-third to maybe one-fifth or less.[13]

Population density and the proportion of urban residents or the non-agricultural workforce are functions of economic performance

---

[8] Hopkins (1978) 68–9; for criticism, see Lo Cascio (2000).

[9] Lo Cascio (2001), and cf. already Hopkins (1978) 31–7; Scheidel (1996a) 93–7.

[10] Thus Hopkins (1978) 68–9; cf. in general Scheidel (2001) 55–6.

[11] Scheidel (1996a) 168.

[12] E.g., Beloch (1886) 258 (five million); Rathbone (1990) 108 (five million); Issawi (1981) 377, 379 (six to seven million); Bagnall and Frier (1994) 56, 103 (four to five million); van Minnen (1997) 40 (7.5 million); Lo Cascio (1999) 160 (eight to nine million).

[13] E.g., Rathbone (1990) 123 (at least twenty-five per cent); Bagnall (1993) 312 (thirty per cent); Bagnall and Frier (1994) 55–6 (thirty-seven per cent). See below, p. 247.

and productivity. Population totals of the Roman period that significantly exceed corresponding tallies in subsequent periods and in fact well into the nineteenth century imply a degree of efficiency in land use that appears remarkably and perhaps suspiciously high by pre-modern standards. Conversely, more modest estimates which inevitably increase the share of the urban population raise questions about the association of urbanisation with economic development in the form of rising agrarian productivity and intensive (i.e., per capita) economic growth.[14] These are the principal reasons why any evaluation of Roman economic performance and development critically depends on our understanding of the demographic background. It is my aim to provide a more solid foundation for the study of 'development' in Roman Egypt. In this, the distinctive properties of the Egyptian disease environment and their changes over time once again prove to be of pivotal importance.

2. *The case of Roman Egypt: from ancient texts to modern evidence*

Ancient sources offer two figures for the size of the population of Greco-Roman Egypt. Diodorus, with reference to the middle of the first century BCE, puts the number of inhabitants at three million, down from seven million in some unspecified past, whereas Josephus, in a speech meant to highlight Roman power, makes King Agrippa II allude to a total of seven and a half million, excluding the residents of Alexandria, in the time of Nero. As the population of Alexandria is usually assumed to be close to half a million, this latter statement implies a grand total of some eight million for the country as a whole.[15] The dubious background of either figure has been explored in exemplary fashion by Dominic Rathbone and need not detain us here.[16] There is no viable alternative to his conclusion

[14] For this crucial issue of Roman history, see Saller (forthcoming); Scheidel (forthcoming c).

[15] Diodorus 1.31.6–9; Josephus Flavius, *Bellum Judaicum* 2.385. Diodorus' figure is sometimes emended to seven million. For Alexandria, see Delia (1988); Bagnall and Frier (1994) 54. Diodorus 17.52.6 assigns more than 300,000 free inhabitants to that city, a figure that conveniently equals one-tenth of his population total for Egypt. For Josephus' total, see below, n. 286.

[16] Rathbone (1990) 103–7, who compares Diodorus' figures to similarly round and symbolic numbers in other accounts of pre-Roman Egyptian manpower, undermines Josephus' claim to have estimated Egyptian population size from poll tax

that 'they were rhetorical currency, necessary in their persuasive context', and even though the discussion of these texts will probably go on for the foreseeable future,[17] I see little point in resuming a stale debate that cannot be expected to yield firm conclusions.[18]

Instead, my focus will be on comparative evidence from early modern Egypt.[19] The fact that unlike most other former parts of the Roman empire, Egypt did not undergo fundamental socio-economic change and progress until well into the nineteenth century facilitates relatively straightforward comparisons with conditions in the Roman period. Thus, it has been a common practice among students of Graeco-Roman Egypt to use vital statistics from the nineteenth century, including population size, as a benchmark for their assessments of the situation in antiquity. Even so, although ancient and early modern Egypt can be shown to have been similar in many respects, some significant differences tell against any oversimplifying equation of ancient and more recent conditions.

I will try to show that while basic demographic functions do not seem to have changed much over the course of several millennia, the distinct disease environment of late eighteenth and early nineteenth century Egypt would have put its inhabitants at a disadvantage compared to their ancient forebears, and that, as a consequence, the relatively low population totals of that period cannot *a priori* be taken to represent upper limits for the Roman period (sections 3 and 4). In terms of the production of and trade in foodstuffs, the carrying capacity of Roman Egypt need not have been markedly inferior to that of much of the country for much of the nineteenth century (section 5).[20] Estimating population size from carrying capacity is a hazardous business,[21] and my quantitative models for ancient and early modern Egypt will, at best, sketch out the limits of the plausible

---

records, and reminds us of wildly inflated population tallies supposedly calculated in the same manner by early Arabic authorities.

[17] See Lo Cascio (1999), who argues in favour of Josephus' figure.

[18] For a critical survey of modern attempts to determine the size of ancient populations, see Scheidel (2001) 49–72; and compare Henige (1998) for parallels in the historiography of other regions and periods.

[19] Here and in the following, I will refer to the nineteenth century as the 'early modern' period of Egypt. The standard chronological categorisation of 'medieval' and 'modern' makes little sense in the Egyptian context.

[20] See Bowman and Rogan, eds. (1999) for a series of papers on Egyptian agriculture from antiquity to the present. The study of Roman Egypt would greatly benefit from further collaborative projects of that kind.

[21] As shown by Cohen (1995).

(section 5.6). Yet even allowing for considerable margins of error, these rough models suggest that the population of Roman Egypt probably peaked at a level that fell between the two contemporary claims of three and eight million, and was probably situated in the upper half of this range (section 6).

3. *Disease and dislocation: constraints on population growth in nineteenth-century Egypt*

3.1. *Disease*

Well into the nineteenth century, Egypt was ravaged by deadly diseases which were unknown or relatively uncommon in the early Roman period, such as plague, cholera and smallpox.[22] While a wide range of other infectious diseases, such as gastro-intestinal disorders, malaria and tuberculosis, which resulted in continually high death rates, had already been common in antiquity,[23] recurrent epidemic outbreaks set the early modern disease environment apart from ancient conditions. Comparative evidence from better documented populations shows that isolated mortality crises, if they are sufficiently severe or frequent, have a significant impact on demographic development by stalling net population growth or even causing temporary contractions.[24] The incidence of epidemic mortality peaks is an important factor of demographic development. The presence of certain endemic infectious diseases, such as smallpox, tuberculosis, malaria or most recently AIDS, also helps shape the overall pattern of mortality and, thus, fertility.[25] In the case of early modern Egypt, both epidemic and endemic infections arguably played a major role in determining the rate of population growth.

---

[22] There is no evidence for smallpox in Roman Egypt prior to the 'Antonine plague' of 166 CE. It is true that to judge from Rufus of Ephesus (in Oribasius, *Collectiones Medicae* 44.14, *CMG* 6.2.1), bubonic plague need not have been uncommon in Egypt, Libya and Syria under the early empire: see above, Chapter 1, n. 288. However, the scale of such outbreaks remains unknown; no catastrophic epidemics are attested. See in general Casanova (1984) 164–81. For further discussion, see above, Chapter 1, section 3.8.

[23] See above, Chapter 1, section 3.

[24] See below, n. 124, on early modern England.

[25] On smallpox, see above, Chapter 2, p. 134, and below, esp. n. 83. On malaria, see above, Chapter 2, p. 132. AIDS: Cohen (1995) 340–51.

> Avec une température à peu près constamment égale, un ciel toujours serein, l'Egypte ne peut avoir qu'un petit nombre de maladies, mais elles sont la plupart terribles. La peste ravage l'Egypte à des époques plus ou moins éloignées. La petite vériole, si longtemps funeste à nos contrées, continue ses ravages en Orient. Elle est terrible en Egypte et s'y présente d'une manière bien plus effrayante qu'en Europe. Les enfants en bas âge échappent rarement à sa malignité.[26]

3.1.1. *Plague*

According to a conventional guess, one-quarter to one-third of the population of Egypt perished in the Black Death.[27] In the catastrophic if belated outbreak of 1429/30, for instance, more than 100,000 people may have died in Cairo alone.[28] Following the pandemic of 1347, plague frequently flared up throughout the Near East.[29] Dols lists twenty major epidemics in Egypt in the period from 1347 to 1517, at average intervals of eight to nine years.[30] Comparable cycles are known from Syria and Europe.

Plague was *comparatively* rare in the Middle East during the sixteenth and seventeenth centuries, but it never left for good and eventually intensified over the course of the eighteenth century. In Egypt, plague outbreaks were reported in 133 years out of a total of 378 years from 1517 to 1894. Thirty-three major epidemics occurred between 1571 and 1835, again at a mean interval of about eight years.[31] Early European travellers to Egypt bore witness to the regularity of plague outbreaks in that country, a scourge to which the indigenous population was helplessly exposed.[32]

---

[26] M. de Chabrol in 1822, cited by Panzac (1982) 92.

[27] Dols (1977) 218. He deals at length with the demographic effects of the pandemic in Egypt and Syria (143–235); see also Dols (1981). For the first plague pandemic, which struck Egypt in 541/2, 639/40 and 686 CE, cf. Biraben and Le Goff (1969); and Dols (1977) 13–35 (on the Middle East). Egypt was never entirely free of plague throughout the Middle Ages: Kuhnke (1971) 101. On plague in history in general, see Biraben (1975).

[28] Dols (1977) 212.

[29] Dols (1979) 184–9 provides a useful year-by-year overview of plague outbreaks from the fourteenth to the nineteenth centuries in different parts of Europe, Africa and Asia.

[30] Dols (1979) 168–9 and n. 11. During that period, plague outbreaks were reported for 58 years in Egypt and Syria: Dols (1977) 223.

[31] Dols (1979) 175–6. See also Raymond (1972) 204–7, on the years 1601–1791. On early plague, cf. briefly Winter (1992) 234–6.

[32] Father Antonius Gonzales, who went to Egypt in 1665/66, observed that in Cairo, plague broke out every four or five years: *Hierusalemsche Reyse* (Antwerp 1673), bk. 4, ch. 28, p. 140. See also *Sandys Travels* (London 1673), p. 76; Pococke (1743)

Extremely severe epidemics occurred less frequently. In the seventeenth and eighteenth centuries, nine catastrophic outbreaks took place within a period of 184 years, at an average interval of twenty-three years.[33] Thus, plague would abate to allow a new generation who had not been strongly exposed to an epidemic to grow up, and would then strike again with force. Major epidemics of this kind usually followed food crises or famines caused by insufficient inundations of the Nile. Although casualty figures are rare and represent hardly more than contemporary guesses, there can be little doubt that the most severe outbreaks resulted in serious mortality crises. 300,000 people are said to have died from 1623 to 1626. Another great epidemic occurred in 1696 after a famine in 1694, but no figures are available. Following two years of food crisis, the plague struck again in 1718. On that occasion, at the peak of the outbreak 5,000 to 6,000 inhabitants of Cairo are alleged to have died every day, and a total of 300,000 lost their lives in the entire country. Numbers aside, this epidemic was considered the worst in a century. A similar catastrophe occurred in 1758 and 1759, when an estimated 400,000 people died in Lower Egypt alone. Again, up to 5,000 people were said to have died in Cairo on each of the worst days, and, perhaps more plausibly, 17,000 of the 40,000 to 50,000 inhabitants of Alexandria reportedly succumbed to the plague.[34]

In urban centres, a death toll of about forty per cent is not without parallel. 4,000 to 5,000 people out of 10,000 died of the plague in Colchester in 1665/66, and on a similar occasion, thirty-five per cent of the people of Penrith in Cumberland were killed.[35] In 1656, the plague destroyed half of the 300,000 inhabitants of Naples. In

---

196; Volney (1788) vol. 1, 253–8 (every four or five years); Antes (1801) 32–61. In the late sixteenth century, plague was reportedly treated by bloodletting: Alpin (1980) 165. The quality of medical intervention would not significantly improve in the following centuries, and many observers testify to the fatalistic attitude of the population in the face of plague.

[33] Raymond (1972) 208.

[34] Raymond (1972) 209 (1623–26), 205 (1696), 205–6, 209 (1718), 206, 209 (1758–9). For reported daily death tolls in Cairo in 1419 and 1429/30, cf. Dols (1977) 178–9, 208–9. With respect to the latter occasion, Dols concludes that a daily mortality rate of *c.* 5,000 'would not be unreasonable' (212), but this assumption rests on a forced reading of the evidence and some calculations of dubious validity.

[35] Colchester: Dobson (1997) 485; Penrith: Appleby (1980) 162. In the years from 1603 to 1666, the plague killed at least 190,000 inhabitants of London: Appleby (1980) 162. Two-thirds of a million people may have died in England between 1570 and 1670: Slack (1985) 174.

Venice, about one-quarter and one-third of the population were killed in two outbreaks in 1575/77 and 1630/1, respectively.[36] The isolated outbreak of 1720/22 carried off 50,000 of 100,000 people quarantined in Marseille.[37] In the plague epidemic of 1784/85, between one-sixth and one-third of the population of Tunisia seems to have been killed, and the plague from 1818 to 1820 claimed the lives of about one-quarter of the inhabitants of the city of Tunis.[38] In an outbreak in Baghdad in the spring of 1831, up to 1,000 or 2,000 people were said to have been killed every day.[39]

With a view to comparative evidence, Raymond considers it plausible that the worst outbreaks could have carried off as many as 100,000 or even 150,000 out of the 300,000 residents of Cairo. As a consequence, the population of Cairo in the seventeenth and eighteenth centuries must have stagnated or perhaps even shrunk.[40] The impact of plague on the countryside is much more difficult to ascertain. It seems that apart from numerous smaller localised outbreaks, the major epidemics would sweep through the country and add substantially to the urban death toll, albeit presumably at proportionally lower levels.[41]

A pair of serious epidemics struck at the unusually short interval of seven years in 1784 and 1791. In the first case, 1,500 people were said to have died in Cairo on a single day, and similar estimates, ranging from 1,000 to 2,000 per day, are offered for 1791, when the ruler of Egypt, Ismail Bey, was among the victims.[42] While these two outbreaks may have been less devastating than the ones described above, their proximity in time produced an epidemiologic double blow which, in conjunction with hunger, epizootic and political disorder, weakened Egypt on the eve of French intervention.

---

[36] Benedictow (1987) 424 and n. 107 (Naples), 424 and n. 102 (Venice). See also Corsini (n.d.) 128 on the plague of 1656 (Salerno).

[37] Benedictow (1987) 410 tab. 3 A. Forty-four per cent of 208,000 people in those parts of the Provence affected by this outbreak died (ibid.). For a more extreme case, see ibid. 403: in 1721, of 2,060 people who remained in Marvéjols, a small town in Languedoc, when the plague struck, 1,596 died, 400 survived the disease, and only sixty escaped unharmed.

[38] Valensi (1969) 1547 and n. 9 (1784/5), 1558 and n. 2 (1818–20).

[39] Groves (1832).

[40] Raymond (1972) 209–10.

[41] The issue of rural versus urban plague mortality is discussed by Benedictow (1987, 1993); see below, p. 193.

[42] Raymond (1972) 207.

These problems were in no way limited to Egypt; in fact, that country merely shared in the demographic stagnation and contraction of much of the Islamic world in the eighteenth and early nineteenth centuries in general, a development in which epidemics played a major part.[43] Aleppo is a case in point: a recent study counts four epidemics in the sixteenth and five in the seventeenth centuries, but eight in the eighteenth and four in the first quarter of the nineteenth centuries, a disturbing intensification that is in line with the Egyptian and Middle Eastern experience.[44]

Plague became fully endemic in Egypt from the 1780s onward (see below, Figs. 3.2–3). McCarthy reckons with plague epidemics in twenty-one of the forty-four years from 1801 to 1844, whereas Panzac classifies as many as as thirty of the fifty years from 1799 to 1848 as years of plague.[45] 'Plague was so constant in early nineteenth-century Egypt that it can generally be considered as a usual source of death, just like tuberculosis and dysentery.'[46]

These annual local outbreaks sometimes grew into larger epidemics, such as in 1801, when both the Delta and Upper Egypt were severely affected.[47] Outbreaks from 1813 to 1825 were mainly confined to the Delta, with peaks in 1813 and 1816.[48] The impact of the 1801 plague on the population of Cairo was captured by the earliest Western statistic, drawn up by members of the French expeditionary forces (Fig. 3.1).[49] These observers considered plague to be a major attrition factor for the urban population.[50]

The string of local outbreaks that lasted for much of the first half of the nineteenth century was punctuated in 1835 by the most violent epidemic in memory, considered worse than the outbreak of

[43] See, e.g., Valensi (1969) 1560; and in general Panzac (1985) 339–80.

[44] Marcus (1989) 256–8; see also 339: 'The plague epidemics alone, of which twelve struck the city between 1700 and 1830, each carried off as much as 10–15 percent of the population in the course of a year or so. How this order of mortality affected fertility and migration, and how soon the community replenished the heavy human losses, are among the many unanswerable questions about the population dynamics of the period.'

[45] McCarthy (1976) 12; Panzac (1987) 18.

[46] McCarthy (1976) 12. On plague in nineteenth-century Egypt, see ibid. 12–15; Panzac (1982) 94–8. For a contemporary account, cf. Clot-Bey (1840) 348–50.

[47] Sandwith (1905) 157 cites a French source to the effect that in 1800, 100,000 people may have died of plague in Upper Egypt. According to Wilson (1803) 256, 60,000 inhabitants of Upper Egypt succumbed to the plague in 1802.

[48] Kuhnke (1971) 111–15; Panzac (1987) 18.

[49] Source: Panzac (1982) 96 tab. 9. On this outbreak, see ibid. 95–8.

[50] Renati (1800) 187.

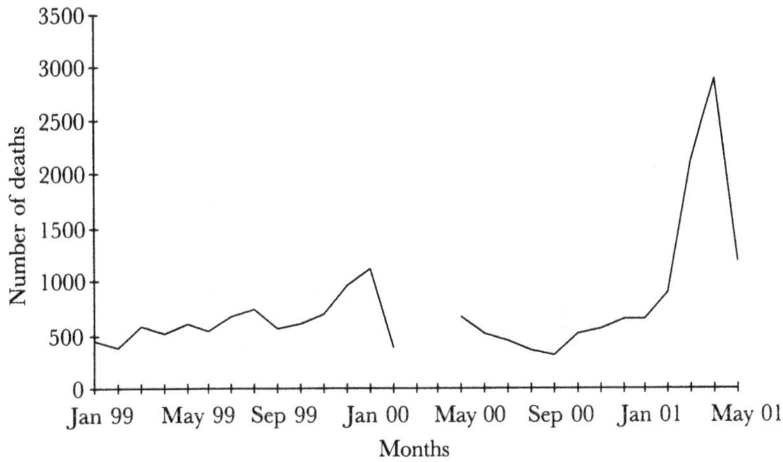

Figure 3.1 The earliest European statistics of Egyptian plague mortality: monthly incidence of deaths, Cairo, 1799 to 1801

1783/84.[51] While the ferocity of this event cannot be in doubt, reliable figures are hard to come by. According to one source, 30,000 people died in 1834, well before the epidemic peaked in March and April 1835.[52] The best account gives a total death toll of 150,000 for the entire country, of which 75,000 occurred in Cairo and 18,000 in Alexandria.[53] This report, however, suffers from various shortcomings: first of all, the numbers for the two major cities are the only ones that would have been based on some kind of official count while the figures for the remainder of the country cannot have been much more than guesswork. Moreover, the count ended with 30 June 1835, when the plague was unlikely to have run its course in the Delta. If taken at face value, this estimate also ascribes an unrealistically high proportion of all deaths to the two urban centres: 93,000 deaths equal about one-quarter of the combined populations of Cairo and Alexandria, while 57,000 deaths outside these two places amount to not more than something like 1.2 to 1.3 per cent of the rural population. This assumption is at variance both with

[51] See Kuhnke (1971) 116–47 and Panzac (1985) 348–52 for recent discussions.
[52] Jagailloux (1986) 227.
[53] McCarthy (1976) 12; Panzac (1985) 349. Cf. Kuhnke (1971) 132. The daily death toll reportedly peaked on 19 April with 1,350 fatalities: Panzac (1985) 349. Panzac estimates that thirty-five per cent of the population of Alexandria was wiped out (350 tab. 33).

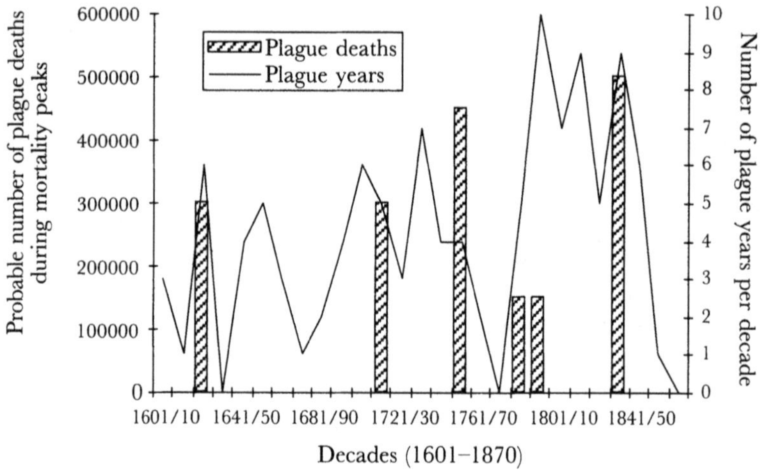

Figure 3.2 Incidence of plague and mortality peaks in Egypt, 1601 to 1870

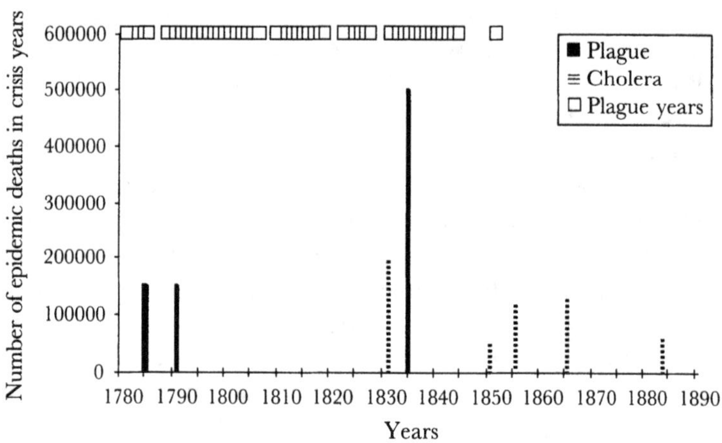

Figure 3.3 Mortality crises and the endemicity of plague in Egypt, 1780 to 1890

contemporary accounts of the ensuing devastation of the countryside and with comparative evidence of the much less severe but also much better documented plague of 1899, when fifty-five per cent of all deaths occurred in Upper Egypt. For all we can tell, in the 1830s the authorities were not in any position to establish an accurate death count for much of the country.[54] It is true that plague often prefers larger settlements and does not necessarily evenly spread across the countryside;[55] hence, the urban death toll per capita was probably higher than the national average. At the same time, there is a considerable amount of previously neglected evidence supporting the conclusion that 'morbidity rates of plague epidemics in southern Europe in the seventeenth and eighteenth centuries were as high in the countryside as in the cities'.[56] Even if a mere five per cent of the rural population had died, the total death toll would have doubled to 300,000. Panzac reckons with 100,000 urban and 200–300,000 rural deaths.[57] McCarthy considers 500,000 a reasonable estimate for the whole country.[58] In this scenario, the metropolitan death rate would still have been three times that of the villages; roughly one Egyptian in ten would have succumbed to the disease. In the following, this estimate will be used for computational purposes; in this context, 100,000 more or fewer would not make any palpable difference.[59]

Following this disaster, some measures were taken to curb plague,[60] but when the disease largely disappeared after 1844, it was probably

---

[54] The various deficiencies of their counts are discussed by McCarthy (1976) 13–14.

[55] Cf., e.g., Dobson (1997) 484 (on England).

[56] Benedictow (1987) 419. He shows that Biraben's thesis that plague was a predominantly urban phenomenon is ill-founded (413), and offers a case study of plague in Cilento, a rural region in the Kingdom of Naples in 1595 (413–6). On that occasion, the epidemic spread widely through the individual parishes and killed 3,179, or one-third, of 9,235 people on record (414 tab. 4). For corroborative evidence from India and China, see ibid. 419–21. Appleby (1980) 162 notes that English villages could be as severely affected as cities.

[57] Panzac (1985) 351. This equals eight to ten per cent of what he holds to be the total population of Egypt at that time.

[58] McCarthy (1976) 15, who concludes that it 'could have been considerably higher, but not lower'. Marsot (1984) 157 also reckons with 500,000 dead.

[59] If 500,000 seems high, one ought to consider the aggregate impact of minor outbreaks which are not otherwise taken into account, as well as the tens of thousands of excess deaths resulting from conscription and war-related diseases in the 1830s (see below, section 3.2). Thus, a death toll of half a million is a resonable and perhaps even modest estimate for excess mortality in the 1830s excepting the cholera outbreak of 1831 which will be discussed in the next section.

[60] See Panzac (1985) 463–75. Cf. Pruner (1847) 389–91, on the plague outbreak of 1840/1.

not because of human intervention, even though later improvements in public health may have helped to keep it at bay. In terms of mortality, the short-lived return of the plague in 1899 was negligible compared to previous epidemics. The ultimate cause of the disappearance of plague remains obscure, not just for Egypt but for the entire Middle East.[61]

3.1.2. *Cholera*

Shortly before the great plague of 1835, Egypt was visited by an entirely new disease, cholera.[62] Modern cholera first appeared in India in the late eighteenth century, and spread in a first pandemic in 1817 which spared Egypt. The country was, however, less fortunate during the second pandemic of 1831. On this occasion, in a way typical of a new infectious disease, cholera spread through the entire country from the Delta to the Thebaid.[63] Again, numerical evidence is poor, not just because of deficient reporting but also because it was problematic to identify the disease, which resembled other dysenteric disorders, as a clinical cause of death. To all appearances, the epidemic claimed a very large number of lives.[64] McCarthy puts the total death toll at 180,000, 10,000 of whom died in Cairo which serves as a basis for extrapolation.[65] Panzac states that 32,000 died in Cairo and 4,000 in Alexandria.[66] Other sources give 36,000 deaths in Cairo (with 2,500 per day at the peak), and 150,000 in the whole country. Some figures are even higher: in 1834, Clot Bey estimated that 30,000 people died in Cairo and 400,000 in Egypt, while Lane speaks of 80,000 deaths in Cairo and 200,000 in the whole country.[67] The disease lingered until 1837 but did not cause high mortality.

---

[61] See briefly Jagailloux (1986) 226. Much the same is true for Europe: Flinn (1979) 138–43; Appleby (1980); Slack (1981).

[62] On the spread of cholera from India, see Cook (1996); on cholera in Egypt, see Kuhnke (1971) 64–78; Panzac (1985) 411–45.

[63] McCarthy (1976) 7–8.

[64] Cf. Cook (1996) 21–2 for comparative evidence: from 1847 to 1849, more than one million people died from cholera worldwide, 53,000 of them in England. An epidemic in 1854 killed another 23,000 people in England and Wales, despite public health measures. From 1910 to 1952, over ten million people in India died of cholera: Lancaster (1990) 69–70.

[65] McCarthy (1976) 8. Panzac 1985: 440 considers 150,000 a plausible total for Egypt (cf. also Kuhnke (1971) 64, 74). Again, the difference does not matter here.

[66] Panzac (1985) 440.

[67] Jagailloux (1986) 231 and nn. 11–12. Clot Bey's mortality estimates tend to be inflated: see below, on smallpox.

Subsequent outbreaks appear to have been somewhat less violent. In 1848, some 20,000 people may have died, and perhaps twice as many in 1850.[68] McCarthy reconstructs a death toll of 116,000 and 122,000 for the last two major epidemics in 1855 and 1865, respectively. Both figures are based on extrapolation from official counts but seem reasonable. In 1883, after the disruption caused by the British invasion, another outbreak was said to have killed 50,000 to 60,000, despite countermeasures including the setting up of sanitary cordons. Later outbreaks were of comparatively minor importance.[69]

3.1.3. *The demographic impact of epidemic disease*

These figures, which may not be more than indicative of the right order of magnitude, ought to be viewed in relation to total population size. Thus, cholera and plague in the 1830s killed off about one-eighth of Egypt's inhabitants.[70] By contrast, 60,000 cholera deaths from 1848–50 amounted to hardly more than one per cent of the population, and the two cholera epidemics of 1855 and 1865 to about two per cent each, or about half the regular annual death toll. From this, it becomes apparent that the period of severe excess mortality ended with the 1830s. It is worth considering the aggregate impact of epidemics on mortality during the fifty-two-year period from 1784 to 1835. Assuming that the four epidemics of 1783/4, 1791, 1831 and 1834/5 together killed about one million people, and that each year of local plague outbreaks raised the average death rate by five per cent,[71] we arrive at something like 1.3 million excess deaths over fifty-two years, or an average of 25,000 per annum.[72] In a population of, say, five million (see below), this translates to an annual mean of five deaths per 1,000 population, or, roughly, to a ten per cent rise of the annual death rate from, say, forty to forty-five or from forty-five to fifty per 1,000. In other words, these mortality crises alone could have offset an annual natural growth rate

[68] Jagailloux (1986) 231; McCarthy (1976) 8–9.

[69] McCarthy (1976) 8–12, on 1850 to 1883. For a tabulation of various estimates of Egyptian cholera mortality from 1831 to 1918, see Jagailloux (1986) 234.

[70] 680,000 out of 5,350,000. For population size, see below, sections 4.1–2. I here use the mean of my two scenarios. The mean of McCarthy's and Panzac's estimates yields similar rates.

[71] According to Panzac (1985) 352 tab. 34, plague was responsible for 3.9 per cent of all deaths in Alexandria from 1836 to 1844.

[72] In India, the plague killed an estimated 12.6 million people from 1898 to 1948: Pollitzer (1954) 26–7.

of 0.5 per cent. These calculations are no doubt highly schematic and are of not more than illustrative value.[73] Even so, whichever way we might tinker with individual variables, there can be little doubt that by putting a brake on population growth, epidemic mortality played a significant role in the demography of Egypt in the late eighteenth and early nineteenth centuries.

3.1.4. *Smallpox*

If the so-called 'Antonine plague' in 166 CE was indeed smallpox, as is now commonly assumed,[74] and if it was then a 'new' disease, as seems likely, endemic smallpox as a major killer of infants and small children must have been unknown in early Roman Egypt. Indeed, apart from this catastrophe, there is otherwise no trace of smallpox in ancient Egypt from the time of Ramses V down to the sixth century CE.[75] By the end of the Middle Ages, however, smallpox had become a common feature of the Egyptian disease community. In the 1580s, Prosper Alpinus referred to annually recurring smallpox among children, and later observers concurred.[76]

Comparative evidence shows that smallpox has considerable effects on mortality and is capable of curbing demographic growth. Perrenoud, in his study of the demography of early modern Geneva, for instance, accords great significance to the impact of smallpox.[77] In Europe, the decline of smallpox in the eighteenth century, engineered through vaccination, has been considered an important precondition of nineteenth-century population growth.[78]

[73] The notion that all epidemic deaths are excess deaths is questionable: some of these victims would have died anyway in the same year, only of other causes. However, in the case of major epidemics, this consideration is bound to be of minor importance.

[74] See Littman and Littman (1973) 245; Sallares (1991) 248; cf. Duncan-Jones (1996) 116 n. 86.

[75] See Hopkins (1983) 14–16, 164. He claims it was common in Alexandria in the 620s CE (166–7). Smallpox can be identified in human skeletal remains: Ortner and Putschar (1981) 227–9. See above, Chapter 1, pp. 95–6.

[76] Alpin (1980) 87–8, 97. For the eighteenth century, see Volney (1788) vol. 1, 245–52.

[77] Perrenoud (1979) 454–77. From 1580 to 1799, he observes 42 outbreaks which caused more than 10 per cent of all annual deaths, and another 22 which accounted for 5 to 10 per cent of annual mortality (455–7). He also notes that the most violent outbreaks coincided with outbreaks of plague (457), a finding that is relevant for plague-prone Egypt.

[78] Mercer (1985), (1990) 46–73; Brunton (1992) 425.

By analogy, smallpox has been seen as a means of curbing population growth in Egypt as well.[79] As usual, reliable quantitative data are unavailable and we are left with general appraisals of the severity of this disease. The only figure given by a contemporary source from the early ninteenth century, when smallpox still ran unchecked, is Clot Bey's claim that around 1827, smallpox was killing 50,000 to 60,000 children per year. We have no way of knowing how he arrived at this figure. At that time, the causes of death of children were hardly subject to medical scrutiny. Although some scholars have elected to treat this estimate as plausible,[80] their confidence seems unwarranted. If we assume that these 50–60,000 annual deaths occurred during the first five years of life, and if we put the population at five million, the Crude Birth Rate (CBR) at fifty per 1,000 and mortality up to age five at fifty per cent,[81] forty to fifty per cent of deaths under the age of five (and, as a consequence, twenty to twenty-five per cent of *all* deaths) would have been directly caused by smallpox, which seems rather improbable.[82] Speculating that, perhaps, one-fifth of deaths in early childhood were due to smallpox, we arrive at 25,000 deaths per year, or roughly one-tenth of all deaths. In England in the early eighteenth century, perhaps ten to fifteen per cent of all deaths were caused by smallpox, although estimates as high as twenty per cent have also been put forward.[83] From all this, there can be little doubt that Clot Bey's figure is too high. This is even more true of his related estimate that the smallpox death toll stood at 20,000 per million, implying some 100,000 deaths per year.[84]

---

[79] Panzac (1982) 93–4, (1987) 17–8. On smallpox in Egypt, see Jagailloux (1986) 233–6.

[80] Panzac (1985) 278, (1987) 17–18. Cf. Kuhnke (1990) 112 (but also (1971) 208).

[81] For these figures, see below, p. 214.

[82] It is intriguing to note that Panzac, although he purports to accept Clot Bey's figure, sets the total death toll from smallpox in the first half of the nineteenth century at 600,000, or 12,000 per year ((1982) 98). This discrepancy apparently stems from the fact that he reckons with 12,000 deaths per year-of-age-cohort from birth to age five (an annual total of 60,000), yet in his further calculation only includes infant mortality, conveniently forgetting about the remaining four-fifths of supposed smallpox mortality, which, if included, would raise his total to three million.

[83] Brunton (1992) 404 (with references). Mercer (1990) 73 refers to rates from eight to twenty per cent in different parts of Europe.

[84] This variant is presumably due to the contemporary misconception that the population of Egypt numbered no more than three million (cf. below, p. 203). The absurdity of this latter estimate is appreciated by Jagailloux (1986) 69 n. 23, who however attempts to salvage it by assuming that it only refers to years of epidemic

The eradication of smallpox was a drawn-out affair, beginning in 1819 with a decree issued by Muhammad Ali to convince his people of the benefits of vaccination.[85] Under the influence of Clot Bey, the drive for vaccination gained momentum from 1827 onward. At first, vaccination was regularly practised by the army, and gradually introduced among the population as a whole, which initially greeted it with some resistance but was slowly persuaded of its benefits. In the absence of medical personnel (see below, section 4.3), vaccinations were mostly performed by local barbers. Between 1837 and 1840, 61,000 vaccinations were administered, most of them presumably in Cairo. Progress was indeed most rapid in the capital, where half of all newborns had been immunised by 1848. Clot Bey reckons with a total of 80,000 vaccinations from 1827 to 1850.[86] By the end of Muhammad Ali's reign, perhaps fifteen to twenty-five per cent of all newborns had been vaccinated. This rate is similar to rates of inoculation in eighteenth-century Europe which may have been sufficient to reduce overall mortality.[87]

In 1851, a decree regulating the health administration of the provinces ordered the sheikhs to present all children for vaccination.[88] In 1862, Schnepp was able to say that smallpox was less severe than in the past; by that time, vaccination was practised in all parts of the country.[89] For whatever reason, Egypt was spared the smallpox epidemics that hit the Levant in the mid-nineteenth century. In 1870/72, seventy-four per cent of all newborns in Alexandria and eighty-five per cent in Cairo were said to have been vaccinated. At the same time, in 1871, as few as 0.7 and 0.4 per cent of all deaths in Alexandria and Cairo, respectively, were attributed to smallpox.[90] By 1883, seventy-two per cent of the children in the major cities had been vaccinated, but only twenty-seven per cent

---

outbreaks, which, to judge from European data, may have occurred every six years or so. He ends up with an annual mean of 20,000 deaths, as good a guess as any.

[85] Jagailloux (1986) 69; Panzac (1987) 19. On the history of vaccination in Egypt, see Kuhnke (1990) 111–21. Jagailloux (1986) 69–72 discusses measures under Muhammad Ali.

[86] Jagailloux (1986) 71; Panzac (1987) 20. Cf. Clot-Bey (1840) 358, on the impact of the vaccination of children.

[87] Jagailloux (1986) 272.

[88] Jagailloux (1986) 71.

[89] Schnepp (1862) 550–1.

[90] Panzac (1985) 375 tab. 47.

nationwide.[91] In 1890, smallpox vaccination was made mandatory.[92] Vaccination improved considerably from then on, aided by the establishing of an 'Institute for Vaccination' and the linking of vaccination to entry into the birth register. By 1901, the number of smallpox vaccinations equalled ninety-four per cent of all reported births. By then, smallpox mortality had dropped to 0.05 cases per 1,000 population.[93]

From this, it will be clear that the eradication of smallpox was primarily an achievement of the second half of the nineteenth century, and thus coincided with the disappearance of plague after 1844 and the abating of cholera after 1865. Benefits from reduced mortality would have increased throughout the second half of the century.

3.1.5. *Epizootic*

We might note in passing that in 1841/42, a catastrophic epizootic, reputed to be *cholera morbus*, struck the country. 400,000 to 665,000 livestock were said to have been killed. Nearly all cattle in Lower and Middle Egypt died, while the disease swept all the way to Aswan and also affected sheep.[94] This crisis, too, must have added to the burden that already rested on the population, and may have had some impact on the rates of death and survival.

3.2. *Corvée and conscription*

Apart from disease, the population of Egypt under Muhammad Ali also suffered from other disruptions. His ambitious irrigation and reclamation projects put a heavy strain on the farming population.[95] These large-scale operations changed the traditional pattern of corvée: where peasants had formerly maintained the irrigation works of their own villages, they were now dragooned to work far from their homes, with little or no compensation and under unhealthy living conditions.[96] Hundreds of thousands of peasants seem to have been employed

---

[91] Jagailloux (1986) 233. It should be noted that the latter figure is based on a deficient population count, and that the proportion was therefore lower still.

[92] Omran (1973a) 11.

[93] Jagailloux (1986) 233, 235.

[94] Rivlin (1961) 156; Jagailloux (1986) 244. Rivlin reckons with 150,000 to 200,000 dead cattle.

[95] On the burden of corvée, see, e.g., Marsot (1984) 150–1; Toledano (1990) 188–95; Cuno (1992) 121–3.

[96] Richards (1982) 22–3.

on the Mahmudiyya Canal, having been rounded up by soldiers and brought to work with cords around their necks. Estimates of casualties on this project alone range from 12,000 to 100,000 over a three-year period.[97] Even the low estimate would have raised the annual CDR for men by at least three per 1,000 during that period.

Military service came to be similarly burdensome. Owing to Muhammad Ali's policy of expansion in the eastern Mediterranean, the strength of Egypt's armed forces multiplied under his reign at considerable cost to the population. This military build-up was achieved through the drafting of ordinary peasants: shunning mercenaries, Egypt's army and navy was mainly made up of brutally conscripted native Egyptians.[98] The size of the armed forces rose from 16,000 in 1821 to 62,000 in 1829. In the 1830s, when the Pasha occupied Syria and advanced into southeastern Asia Minor, the expansion stretched Egyptian manpower to its limits: in 1832, around 125,000 men served in army and navy. This number rose to 157,000 by 1838 and peaked in 1840, when French sources put the total strength at 207,000, of whom 130,000 were regular infantry and cavalry.[99] If this is true, one in eight adult males had been drafted, and even allowing for some exaggeration, a very sizable proportion of all able-bodied males—hardly under one-tenth—were kept away from agriculture. Given the heavy toll the epidemics of 1831 and 1835 had taken on the population, this kind of displacement must have been particularly oppressive. Large numbers of soldiers would die of war-related diseases, and in the villages, the absence of so many men would depress the birth rate. Not surprisingly, conscription was intensely unpopular among peasants who frequently resorted to flight (and self-mutilation) to escape the draft. As early as 1831, one-quarter of the cultivable land of Upper Egypt was said to lie barren because of manpower shortage.[100]

When in 1841 the intercession of European powers forced Muhammad Ali to abandon his designs, he committed himself to cutting his army to 18,000 men. However, instead of fully demobilising the large majority of his soldiers, formally discharged soldiers were often put

[97] Richards (1982) 23.

[98] On the burden of conscription, see, e.g., Toledano (1990) 181; Cuno (1992) 123. Fahmy (1997) is the most recent account of Muhammad Ali's army.

[99] Rivlin (1961) 209; McCarthy (1976) 37 n. 77.

[100] Rivlin (1961) 204–5. See 201–212 on the effects of conscription on farming. Self-mutilation: e.g., Yates (1843) 138–9.

to work on irrigation projects.[101] In 1848, his successor Ibrahim still kept an army and navy of some 80,000 men. Matters finally changed with the accession of Abbas, who slimmed the army to 22,000 men and put an end to forced conscription.[102] Canal dredging was scaled down in the 1850s and some projects were even cancelled.[103]

Thus, from the 1840s onward, ordinary Egyptians were less likely to face dislocation and social disruption than before. As we have seen, this development coincided with an amelioration of the disease environment, thereby facilitating steady population growth.[104]

4. *The population of nineteenth-century Egypt*

4.1. *Contemporary sources and modern discussions*

For most of the nineteenth century, the size of the population Egypt cannot be established from contemporary counts and estimates. Many of the weaknesses of the available source material have been exposed by McCarthy, and there is no need to repeat his discussion. The earliest figures are the results of the extrapolations of a French scholar, Jomard, of the population of Cairo and the whole country in 1800. His estimates for Cairo of between 253,000 and 263,000 people can be shown to rest of flimsy foundations. McCarthy replaces them with a (similarly dubious) total of 211,000, based on the assumption that on average, every house was inhabited by eight persons.[105]

Jomard's grand total for the entire country of 2,488,950 individuals excluding nomads (which another source put at 130,000) is much farther of the mark. It is based on Jomard's investigation of a single province, Minya, which he thought yielded a mean rate of population density. McCarthy shows that this assumption must be wrong;[106]

[101] Rivlin (1961) 209. Population estimates for Alexandria point to continuing dislocation in the 1840s: Panzac (1978) 196–7 reckons with about 100,000 inhabitants in the 1830s, 164,359 according to the census of 1846, but only 104,189 in 1850 and 180,000 in 1865.

[102] Rivlin (1961) 211.

[103] Toledano (1990) 190. Cf. however, Owen (1981a) 143, for large-scale corvée in later years.

[104] Cf. Toledano (1990) 187: 'conscription and war (. . .) during the reign of Mehmet Ali Pasa (. . .) is estimated to have contributed significantly to the low rate of population growth in the first half of the nineteenth century'.

[105] McCarthy (1976) 1–3.

[106] McCarthy (1976) 3–6. It is hard to understand how as late as 1981, Crecelius (1981) 366 could refer to the French guess as a 'reliable estimate'.

instead, he uses his own estimate of the population of Cairo which, he holds, equalled 5.5 per cent of the total Egyptian population, a value taken from the census of 1846. (According to Jomard's estimate, Cairo's share in 1800 was an implausible 10.6 per cent.). In this way, McCarthy arrives at a total of 3,835,633 inhabitants in 1800.[107]

This model does not necessarily bear much weight. The grand total has been extrapolated from the figure for Cairo which is itself the result of an extrapolation based on the French count of 26,000 urban houses. It seems likely, however, that many of these city houses were crowded with lodgers and retainers. The census of 1897 reports an average of 11.1 persons per household in Cairo, as opposed to 10.5 in Alexandria and 6.8 in the countryside.[108] Thus, if McCarthy were right to reckon with eight persons per house, the average *house* in Cairo would have comprised fewer people than the average *household*, an implication that is hard to accept. Yet even with not more than nine people per house, Cairo's population rises to 234,000, and if five per cent of the total population lived in the capital (instead of 5.5 per cent), there may have been as many as 4,680,000 Egyptians. This simple calculation shows that a margin of error of a mere ten per cent in either extrapolation (from the number of houses to the population of Cairo and from the population of Cairo to that of Egypt) creates a discrepancy of some 850,000 people.[109] The variables on which McCarthy's estimate are based support a substantially higher total for Egypt, i.e., a figure in excess of 4.5 million instead of under four million. (In theory, a lower estimate of say, three million, is equally possible but far less likely because of the high rates of growth during the following decades it would require: see below.) We are forced to admit that these estimates only provide us with a very rough idea of the limits of the possible order of magnitude. As my best guess, I would reckon with ten people per house in Cairo and with a five to 5.5 per cent share of the capital in the population of Egypt, and thus with a grand total of 4.73 to 5.2 million Egyptians. A rough estimate of five million is readily consistent with this model.[110]

---

[107] McCarthy (1976) 6. Raymond (1981) 687 assumes that Egypt's population exceeded four million at the end of the eighteenth century.

[108] Panzac (1987) 15. The census of 1882 gave 8.1 for Cairo and 8.9 Alexandria, presumably due to some underenumeration.

[109] Whether the French house count is correct is anyone's guess.

[110] See below, section 4.2.2.

A census held in 1821 reported 2,536,400 people in Egypt. Whereas this count is in line with the discarded French estimate of 1800, it is impossible to reconcile with the next census in 1846, implying as it does an increase of the population by three-quarters within a quarter of a century which, to make matters worse, was characterised by catastrophic mortality crises. Both an annual net rate of growth of 2.3 per cent and, factoring in epidemic mortality, an intrinsic growth rate of the order of three per cent are impossibly high (see below). If the count for 1846 had itself involved some underenumeration, as it probably did (see below), the required growth rates would have been higher still. The only possible conclusion is that the 1821 figure is defective beyond redemption.[111]

French sources refer to a total of 618,000 tax-paying households in 1827, and report that in 1833, Muhammad Ali made a reference to 870,000 men aged seventeen and over who were liable to pay the poll tax.[112] Unfortunately, these two figures seem mutually incompatible. In 1882, an average of 7.0 people were registered per household, and 6.9 in 1897.[113] This ratio implies a total population of 4,264,000 to 4,326,000 people in 1827, presumably excluding nomads. These figures, however, are lower than McCarthy's 4.6 million for that year, an estimate which, as we will see, is itself likely to be too low. The figure of 870,000 men aged seventeen and over is even more problematic. Under the conditions of Model Life Table West Mortality Level 4 Males ($r = 0.5$), this figure suggests a total population of 2.9 million, or about two-thirds of the previously implied total.[114] If anything, Muhammad Ali's statement indicates that tax evasion must have been rife. If the actual population was close to five million, something like forty per cent of all adult males went uncounted, and even a somewhat lower estimate for the total population could not push this rate under one-third. Once again, this discrepancy should warn us against taking official numbers at face value.

The census of 1846, including nomads, recorded 4,476,440 people. Strangely enough, this count was dismissed by contemporary European observers as exaggerated. These critics proffer rival estimates ranging from 1.5 (!) to three million. A particularly imaginative

---

[111] Cf. below, p. 212.
[112] Panzac (1987) 14.
[113] Panzac (1987) 15.
[114] Panzac (1987), who does not check the implications of the second figure, remains unaware of this incongruity.

source reckoned that not more than 800,000 out of 2,235,500 people were 'peasants'.[115] As McCarthy correctly observes, 'examination of these figures reveals them all as impossible'.[116] The lowest and the highest guesses vary by 100 per cent. The only of these estimates that is not just an ostensibly arbitrary round figure, Barnett's estimate of 2,158,580, of which 1,708,580 (or seventy-nine per cent) were 'agrarian', implies a rate of growth of 3.3423 per cent per year from 1846 to the (corrected) figure of about eight million in 1882. Sustained growth at that pace is not only incompatible with comparative evidence but would also have required the birth rate to be twice as high as the death rate, which is inconceivable for nineteenth-century Egypt.[117]

There is no compelling reason to believe that the census of 1846 was particularly accurate or that it did not, as imperfect censuses usually do (and indeed still did in 1882), underenumerate the existing population. However, McCarthy takes little account of this likely source of bias. Rather, he decides to use the figure given by the census, 4,476,440, as a reasonable approximation. His only reason for doing so seems to be that this conjecture yields a credible growth rate for the period from 1846 to 1882 of 1.7143 per cent per year (excluding the impact of the major cholera epidemics). But this rate is higher than the probable rates in the periods from 1882 to 1897 and from 1897 to 1907, and thus rather suspicious. McCarthy's claim that 'the virtue of Mohammed Ali's census is that its figures are probable' raises crucial methodological questions. Strictly speaking, for this figure to reflect reality, the census would have had to be absolutely accurate. Given that subsequent population counts were far from perfect, this idea would be hard to maintain and is, indeed, not explicitly advocated by McCarthy. Otherwise, he would have to assume that the authorities deliberately inflated the census figures so

---

[115] For these sources, see Rivlin (1961) 278–9. Rivlin (1961) was perhaps the last modern scholar to take these criticisms seriously: she accepts reported but worthless low counts for 1800 and 1821 and dismisses the high rate of growth between 1821 and 1846 implied by these data: her conclusion, however, that for this reason the 1846 figure must be too high is only one of two alternative solutions; and as we have seen, the other explanation—that the previous estimates are far too low—must be correct. Rivlin's misplaced faith in these low population estimates extends to unrealistically low estimates of agricultural output in the same period (see below, n. 213).

[116] McCarthy (1976) 18. It is disconcerting to note that as late as 1862, a French observer would put the indigenous population of Egypt at a mere four million (Schnepp (1862b) 531).

[117] McCarthy (1976) 18–9. See below, section 4.3.

that the result of a defective count, if only by coincidence, came to resemble the actual number. In this, however, McCarthy would follow the misguided criticism of the European observers which he so cogently demolishes. In fact, we have no reason to suspect that Muhammad Ali tampered with reported population figures. His reference to the number of adult men in 1833 tells against any such notion: at a time when his imperialist ambitions were still alive, Ali did *not* succumb to the temptation to impress Westerners and the Sublime Porte by inflating the number of potential soldiers under his command but contented himself with what must have been a massive underestimate. The same is true for the census of 1821.

Modern scholars agree that the total of the census of 1882 is too low because it implies unreasonably high rates of growth between 1882 and 1897. Thus, the population would have had to grow from 6,817,000 to 9,734,000, or at 2.39 per cent p.a. over fifteen years.[118] By comparison, the growth rate from 1897 to 1907 was only 1.5 per cent. Since the 1882 count was held under rather chaotic circumstances in the wake of the British takeover, its shortcomings do not come as a surprise. The actual total must have amounted to about eight million.[119]

In Table 3.1, I set out the estimates of population size at different moments in time proposed in the fundamental studies by McCarthy and Panzac. Table 3.2 shows the mean annual rates of growth required to produce these figures. Table 3.3 presents Baer's set of figures, retrapolated from the census of 1897, which are similar to Panzac's results.

Table 3.1 Contemporary assessments and modern estimates of the population of Egypt[120]

Year	McCarthy	Panzac	Census	Mean McCarthy/ Panzac
1800	3,853,633	4,500,000		4,200,000
1810	4,115,165			
1821	4,423,396	(4,894,000)	2,536,400	
1830	4,692,681	5,000,000		4,850,000

[118] McCarthy (1976) 25.

[119] McCarthy (1976) 25 reckons with 7.84 million, Panzac (1987) 15 with eight million. The actual total may even have been higher than that: see below, p. 212.

[120] McCarthy (1976) 33–4; Panzac (1987) 15 tab. 2. Figures in parentheses have been calculated by me.

Table 3.1 *(cont.)*

Year	McCarthy	Panzac	Census	Mean McCarthy/ Panzac
1840	4,303,510	5,000,000		4,650,000
1846	4,476,439		4,476,439	
1848	4,631,237	5,400,000		5,000,000
1850	4,752,088			
1860	5,506,253	(6,231,000)		5,850,000
1870	6,393,594	(7,020,000)		6,700,000
1882	7,840,271	8,000,000	6,817,262	7,900,000
1890	8,776,852			
1897	9,734,405	9,734,405	9,734,405	9,734,405
1907	11,287,359	11,287,359	11,287,359	11,287,359

Table 3.2 Intercensal growth rates of the population of Egypt[121]

	Attested	McCarthy	Panzac
1800/40		0.6587	
1800/30			0.4
1830/40			0
1840/48			1.0
1846/82	1.3227	1.7143	
1848/82			1.2
1882/97	2.4830	1.5142	1.3
1897/07	1.5246	1.5246	

Table 3.3 Baer's estimates of the population of Egypt[122]

Year	Number	Growth rate
1821	4,230,000	1.0 (1821–46)
1846	5,290,000	1.4 (1846–82)
1882	7,930,000	1.5 (1882–97)

[121] McCarthy (1976) 16, 20, 25; Panzac (1987) 15 tab. 2. McCarthy's rates exclude the death toll of major epidemics, which is subtracted separately; hence the higher growth rates.

[122] Baer (1969) 135–6.

There are two ways of estimating population size prior to 1897. McCarthy combines one of the earlier figures (in this case, the census of 1846) with plausible intercensal rates of growth, whereas Baer and Panzac disregard any reported data and simply retrapolate from 1897. In many respects, both approaches yield similar results. According to McCarthy and Panzac, the population reached six million around 1860 or 1865, seven million around 1870 or 1875, and eight million in 1880 or a few years later. One major discrepancy remains: in Panzac's view, the five million mark was passed in 1830, but not until the early 1850s according to McCarthy.[123] As we have seen before, McCarthy's lower estimate is based on his inexplicable faith in the 1846 figure and is therefore less attractive than the higher alternative. Both authors broadly agree on the mean rate of growth from 1800 to 1830: Panzac reckons with 0.3 to 0.4 per cent per year (but uses 0.4 for his calculations) and McCarthy with *c.*0.66 per cent. For the 1830s, Panzac assumes that excess mortality from epidemics and other causes was sufficient to wipe out any net growth but does not predict an actual contraction of the population ($r = 0$). In this, he appears to underestimate the scale of plague mortality in 1835. McCarthy, on the other hand, by balancing a mean growth rate of *c.*0.66 per cent against the loss of 680,000 lives through cholera and plague ends up with a contraction by 8.3 per cent between 1830 to 1840. This assessment is to be preferred to Panzac's estimate.[124]

At the same time, Panzac proposes more reasonable growth rates for the remainder of the nineteenth century than McCarthy. If the annual rate of growth from 1882 to 1897 was similar to that from 1897 to 1907, the population in 1882 must have been approximately eight million. Reckoning with 1.2 per cent annual growth from 1848 to 1882, the population in 1848 would have been about 5.4 million, implying that about one-fifth of the population escaped registration in 1846.[125] During the 1840s, growth must have been somewhat lower than later on, perhaps in the order of one per cent; thus, the

---

[123] Cuno (1992) 122 also believes that the population may have reached five million by 1830.

[124] See above, sections 3.1.1–2. For comparative evidence of demographic contraction caused by epidemics, see Wrigley and Schofield (1981) 208–9 tab. 7.8, 210: the population of England reached 5.281 million in 1656, fell by eight per cent to 4.865 million in the mid-1680s, and took until 1717 to return to the 1656 level. No net growth occurred within a sixty-year period.

[125] Panzac (1987) 12–13.

population in 1840 can be put at about five million. However, since Panzac's estimate for demographic development in the 1830s is too optimistic (see above), the population would have had to be larger than five million in 1830, and was therefore probably close to five million in 1800.

McCarthy's acceptance of the 1846 figure, by contrast, forces him to reckon with higher growth from 1846 to 1882. In fact, the proposed rate for that period of *c.* 1.7 per cent is higher than that for 1882 to 1907, which is rather unlikely. However, if the rate of growth from 1846 to 1882 is scaled down to bring it in line with later evidence, we must conclude that the 1846 census figure was too low (see above). I am inclined to follow Panzac in assuming that the mean rate of growth increased during the nineteenth century as health improved and the economy expanded. As a consequence, the population of Egypt in the 1840s probably did not fall short of five million.

4.2. *Population size and population growth: a reconsideration*

Having considered existing discussions, I shall devise two scenarios of my own in a further attempt to delineate the limits of the plausible. Both reconstructions are based on retrapolation from 1907 and do not take account of earlier reports. The first model rests on the assumption that the 'base population'—in 1800 and before—was *relatively* small and, therefore, annual growth was *relatively* high. In the second scenario, a somewhat larger base population is thought to have grown at somewhat lower rates. I must stress that in this context, labels such as 'high' and 'low' only describe differences within the model but need not refer to variables that are in and of themselves particularly high or low.

4.2.1. *'Low' population, 'high' growth*

My starting point is the first census held in the twentieth century, which recorded 11,287,359 people in 1907. It is interesting that even this count was the target of contemporary criticism for supposedly underenumerating the existing population. One critic charged that up to one-quarter of the populations of Cairo and Alexandria had gone uncounted.[126] And indeed, it would be unwise not to allow for

[126] Eid (1907) 55–61, cited by Owen (1969) 237 n. 1.

a certain amount of underregistration in this and other modern censuses. Controlling for this bias, we may raise the total to 11.5 million (although the implied undercount of 1.85 per cent will seem unrealistically low), of whom close to 300,000 were foreigners which must be excluded from any retrapolation that aims to assess the indigenous population. Hence, we start with a total of 11.2 million Egyptians. Growth rates will be staggered to reflect the gradual increase in annual growth throughout the nineteenth century.

At a mean annual rate of growth of 1.5 per cent from 1897 to 1907, the native population in 1897 numbered 9.7 million, compared to 9,734,405 in the census (including foreigners). Again, this figure seems rather low when set against the census. From 1882 to 1897, the population may have grown by 1.4 per cent a year, starting with 7.9 million natives in 1882. Putting growth from 1850 to 1882 at 1.3 per cent, a figure that already accommodates the impact of 250,000 to 300,000 cholera deaths up to 1865, we arrive at 5.2 million people in 1850. If we define these cholera deaths as excess mortality, the actual growth rate would have been more like 1.45 per cent. Growth from 1840 to 1850 can be put at 1.2 per cent, no doubt overly optimistically. This gives us 4.6 million in 1840. If natural growth is put at one per cent from 1830 to 1840, and 700,000 people are subtracted to account for major epidemics and other extra deaths, the population in 1830 must have been about 4.8 million. If the underlying rate of growth was lower, as it likely was, e.g., 0.5 per cent, the population in 1830 would have amounted to 5.1 million. If the population numbered 4.8 million in 1830 and growth from 1800 to 1830 is put at 0.5 per cent, there were 4.25 million Egyptians in 1805, at the beginning of Muhammad Ali's reign. At 0.75 per cent growth, it would have risen from 4.25 in 1805 to 5.1 million in 1830. Both rates of growth seem plausible; hence, 4.25 million, perhaps plus minus ten per cent, might seem a reasonable guess for 1805. It so happens that this figure is close to the mean of McCarthy's and Panzac's estimates. Allowing for 0.5 per cent growth under the unfavourable circumstances of the preceding decades, and for a total of, say, 400,000 plague deaths, the population of 1783 must have been of the same order of magnitude. My best guess for this scenario is that with a reasonable rate of growth of 0.5 per cent, the population of Egypt in the seventeenth and eighteenth centuries would oscillate between 4 and 4.25 million or so, periodically curbed by plague and generally held down by endemic smallpox.[127]

In my view, this scenario offers nothing more than a lower limit of what is plausible. We must always bear in mind that there is no reasonably reliable information on population size prior to the end of the nineteenth century, and that it would therefore be methodologically unsound to discriminate against alternative scenarios of higher population and lower growth on the basis of existing but unfounded preconceived notions of 'early' (i.e., small) population size. It is, for instance, perfectly possible that average rates of growth in the nineteenth century were generally lower than we usually assume. The net difference between CBR and CDR need not yet have risen to the levels reported for the early twentieth century, and the depressing picture of disease in nineteenth century Egypt sketched out above suggests that this could very well be true.

As a general rule, the lower the rate of growth, the larger the base population must have been. In view of rates of 1.5 per cent and over frequently proposed for the nineteenth century, it is rather disturbing that the mean rate of growth from 1897 to 1937 was approximately 1.25 per cent. Net growth really took off only from the 1940s onward. Although one might argue that by the early twentieth century, the population had outstripped local agricultural resources (see below, section 5.5) and population growth had temporarily slowed down, we know that it was above all the poor who were the driving force behind growth. It also seems plausible that on average, health in the first third of the twentieth century may have been marginally better than in the preceding sixty years or so. All this should make us reluctant to posit a net rate of growth in excess of 1.25 per cent for any extended period of the nineteenth century.[128]

---

[127] An ambitious reconstruction of the population of Egypt from the Roman period to the end of the Middle Ages has been attempted by Russell (1966). There is no need here to discuss his arguments in detail; suffice it to say that they are inevitably based on evidence whose reliability is impossible to check and which usually pertains to tax-payers or taxed land. Because of the latter, variations may therefore reflect changes in administrative practice or acumen as much as changes in population size. Russell deserves credit for eschewing inflated estimates but tends to go too far in the opposite direction; cf. Dols (1977) 149, 198, who criticises some of his figures as being too low.

[128] Comparative evidence of premodern rates of growth should also give us pause for thought. According to Wrigley and Schofield (1981) 186 tab. 6.11, in times of elevated mortality (such as from 1630 to 1700), decadal mean annual rates of growth fluctuated between -0.06 and 0.52 per cent (excepting migration). It is true that English fertility was lower than in Egypt, but so was mortality.

If the population was ten million in 1900, steady growth began in the 1840s, and mean annual growth from 1840 to 1900 was 1.25 per cent, the base population for 1840 of 4.6 million suggested by the scenario presented above seems remarkably small. After all, at a mean rate of growth of 1.25 per cent, the population would have risen from 4.6 million in 1840 to 9.7 million in 1900, and we must bear in mind that this calculation does not account for the hundreds of thousands of excess deaths caused by cholera epidemics. The mean intrinsic rate of growth between years of epidemic outbreaks must therefore have been higher than 1.25 per cent, and thus in conflict with the basic assumption of this model. We are forced to conclude, therefore, that the actual net growth rate in that period may well have been lower, and that the population in 1840 is unlikely to have been smaller than five million.

4.2.2. *'High' population, 'low' growth*

These considerations tell in favour of an alternative model of lower growth rates and, consequently, a larger base population. Starting with 11.5 million Egyptians in 1907 (still an undercount of under five per cent), the total for 1897, at 1.4 per cent growth from 1897 to 1907, is ten million. 1.3 per cent growth from 1882 to 1897 lead to 8.25 million in 1882. At 1.2 per cent growth minus 300,000 cholera deaths from 1850 to 1882, we arrive at 5.9 million in 1850, and 6.75 million in 1865 (when the major cholera outbreaks stopped). At 1.0 per cent growth from 1840 to 1850, the population in 1840 was 5.35 million. At 0.5 per cent minus 700,000 extra deaths from 1830 to 1840, we may reckon with 5.75 million in 1830. At 0.75 per cent growth from 1805 to 1830, the total for 1805 is 4.8 million. At 0.5 per cent growth minus 400,000 extra deaths from 1784 to 1805, 4.7 million inhabited Egypt in 1784. This, in turn, points to a total of around 4.25 million immediately after the plague of 1759. In Table 3.4, I juxtapose the figures generated by these scenarios.

With all due caution, for the reasons discussed above, I am inclined to consider the second set of figures to be considerably more likely to reflect reality than the other (Fig. 3.4). Moreover, it is certainly possible to propose even lower rates of growth for the nineteenth century, suggesting an eighteenth-century base population of around five million, which was kept from growing only by recurrent plague and endemic smallpox. With respect to Roman Egypt, these schematic calculations strongly suggest that at its apex, *ceteris paribus*, the population of Roman Egypt may very well have been in excess of five million, and would hardly have fallen short of this mark.

4.3. *Demographic structure in Egypt in the nineteenth and early twentieth centuries*

In section 3.1.3, I suggested that plague alone may have raised the mean Crude Death Rate (CDR) between 1784 and 1844 by up to five per thousand. Smallpox, with its impact on infant and child mortality, may have had a similar effect (see above, section 3.1.4). Needless to say, in all of this we will never progress beyond vague

Table 3.4 Scenarios of population growth in Egypt

	Scenario I (3.2.1)	Scenario II (3.2.2)	Mean
1600–1780	3.75–4.25	4.25–4.75	4–4.5
1784	4.4	4.7	4.65
1805	4.4	4.8	4.6
1830	4.8–5.1	5.75	5.35
1840	4.6	5.35	5.0
1850	5.2	5.9	5.55
1865	6.15	6.75	6.45
1882	7.9	8.25	8.1
1897	9.7	10.0	9.85
1907	11.2	11.5	11.35

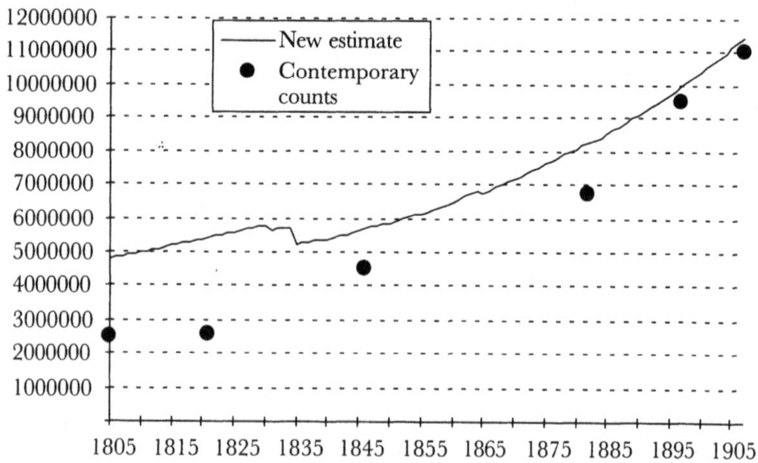

Figure 3.4 The probable size of the population of Egypt (excluding foreigners), 1805 to 1907

estimates. Panzac, in a speculative balance sheet, reckons with 12.5 million births and 11.6 million deaths from 1800 to 1850, implying mean annual growth by 0.5 per cent from 4.5 to 5.4 million.[129] He schematically reckons with ten million 'ordinary' deaths, to which he adds 700,000 from plague, 600,000 from smallpox, 150,000 from cholera, and 150,000 from famine and war.[130] Crude as it is, his guess is as helpful as anything we can hope for. At any rate, his figures, though to some extent arbitrary, seem unlikely to be wildly inaccurate. He and others put the Crude Birth Rate (CBR) at around fifty per 1,000, and in the light of comparative evidence it is hard to imagine that it could have been much lower.[131] Fertility must have been very high; women would marry early, between ages twelve and fifteen, female celibacy was rare, and remarriage was common.

Such figures are simply meant as an illustration of the situation aptly summarised by Panzac: 'The old demographic pattern still persisted under the rule of Muhammad 'Ali: a very high endemic mortality, mainly among children, aggravated time and again by famine and deadly epidemics of smallpox and plague.'[132] After the 1840s, cholera occasionally slowed down demographic growth, yet apparently without dramatic effects.[133] If the rather sudden departure of plague and the gradual eradication of smallpox had lowered the mean CDR from, say, fifty or forty-five to forty-five or forty, a CBR of around fifty-five would have resulted in mean annual growth by 1.0 to 1.5 per cent, a range which does not seem unreasonable and makes sense within the context of the models presented in section 4.2.

Reported birth and death rates from nineteenth-century Egypt are generally worthless.[134] However, data from the early twentieth century rule out a substantially lower CDR (and thus, CBR). The mean *reported* CDR for the cities of Egypt (which is more reliably documented than for the villages but far from perfect) from 1906 to 1917

---

[129] Panzac (1982) 98–99.

[130] For the basis of most of these figures, see above, section 3.

[131] E.g., Jagailloux (1986) 273.

[132] Panzac (1987) 19.

[133] Toledano (1990) 20–21. As a result of perennial irrigation, schistosomiasis became much more common than it had been before: Rivlin (1961) 248; Toledano (1990) 20.

[134] As McCarthy (1976) 19–24 cogently demonstrates. Registration problems persisted well into the twentieth century: in the late 1950s, districts covered by 'health bureaux' reported an average infant mortality rate of 14.9 per cent, compared to 8.6 per cent in other areas (Valaoras (1972) 22).

was as high as 36.2 per 1,000.[135] Allowing for some underreporting of perinatal and neonatal deaths and taking account of net growth, the CBR must have been at least fifty per 1,000. An attempt to reconstruct the actual rates of birth and death from imperfect data yields even higher figures: from 1910 to 1934 (excluding the influenza epidemic of 1918), the mean CBR was about fifty-seven per 1,000, while the CDR stood at forty-five per 1,000, resulting in an annual rate of net growth of about 1.2 per cent. Infant mortality is put at thirty per cent.[136]

Corrected figures for infant mortality in Egypt in the late 1920s suggest mortality of twenty-six to twenty-eight per cent under age one; life expectancy at birth would be thirty to thirty-three years.[137] Around 1900, infant mortality was higher, about thirty per cent or over.[138] In 1922, 35.1 per cent of all reported deaths in Cairo were infant deaths; deaths from age one to five accounted for another twenty-eight per cent.[139] In the poor quarters of Cairo in 1913/14, reported infant mortality was thirty to forty per cent, compared to twenty to twenty-two per cent among the wealthy.[140] Only from the late 1940s did infant mortality and CDR decline sharply. As a result, life expectancy at birth rose from thirty to thirty-five years in the early 1930s to fifty-five years in 1976.[141]

Progress of this kind was unknown to the nineteenth century. While the CDR dropped far enough to permit steady net growth, the figures cited in the previous paragraphs leave no doubt that this was the result of a precarious balance of very high mortality against even higher fertility. Panzac plausibly maintains that throughout the second half of the nineteenth and the first third of the twentieth centuries, death rates remained fairly stable. 'Gastrointestinal infections, pulmonary diseases and poverty were the causes of high infant mor-

---

[135] Jagailloux (1986) 277. In 1918, the influenza pandemic drove the CDR up to 51.5 per 1,000.

[136] Panzac (1985) 369 (based on a study by Fergany). It deserves attention that these rates, if correct, resemble those generated by Model West Levels 2 and 3 Females under the given rate of growth. Thus, the demography of early twentieth-century Egypt may have been much more 'ancient' than one might expect.

[137] *Estimation* (1982) 12 tab. 2. This estimate of life expectancy seems to be at variance with the variables presented above. Cf. also De Chamberet (1909) 162 for extremely high child mortality in Cairo in 1906.

[138] Omran (1973b) 46 fig. 4. See also the data listed in Jagailloux (1986) 274.

[139] Panzac (1982) 86. This rate is consistent with Model West Level 6 Females, at r = 1.5.

[140] Jagailloux (1986) 275.

[141] *Estimation* (1982) 1, 12 tab. 2.

tality; none of these were new to Egypt, and they in fact constituted the demographic patterns of the country.'[142]

The modest but important reduction of the CDR from the mid-nineteenth century owed little to medical intervention. The disappearance of plague remains mysterious; quarantine measures helped to keep epidemics at bay, but proved sucessful only from the end of the nineteenth century onward. Smallpox vaccination appears to have been the only important medical contribution to public health. Otherwise, demographic growth should be attributed to the whim of micro-organisms and to economic expansion rather than to public health measures.[143] What is known about public health in the nineteenth century supports this interpretation. Progress was slow: although a Western-style medical school was established in 1827 and provincial health services and hospitals set up in the 1804s, these facilities catered only to the elite and did not touch the lives of the rural masses.[144] Before the British takeover of 1882, questions of sanitation were neglected in the villages and in most of the towns.[145] In 1856, there was one medical doctor for every 50,000 Egyptians.[146] The number of doctors rose from an average of fifty-four in the 1830s to 273 in the 1880s and 1,411 in the 1920s. The number of hospital beds per Egyptian rose from one per 225,000 in 1826 to one per 90,000 in 1846, one per 55,000 in 1887 and one per 33,000 in 1916.[147] Not surprisingly, a comprehensive survey of the Egyptian health services in the nineteenth century comes to the conclusion that they did not cover basic needs and were mediocre and inefficient.[148] Smallpox eradication aside, they had no palpable impact on the lives of the common people.[149]

---

[142] Panzac (1987) 25.

[143] Omran (1973a) 11.

[144] Toledano (1990) 20–21. On the medical school, see also Jagailloux (1986) 49–53. Public health measures under Muhammad Ali are discussed by Jagailloux (1986) 45–75.

[145] Jagailloux (1986) 82. Even measures in Cairo were limited in scope (83–6). On public health from 1850 to 1882, see ibid. 77–108.

[146] This is based on the finding by Clot Bey that 145 doctors were then in charge of the inhabitants of 3,717 villages inhabited by four million people (Jagailloux (1986) 87). Given that the population was larger than assumed (see above, p. 212), the actual ratio was even more extreme.

[147] Doctors: Jagailloux (1986) 164; hospital beds: ibid. 144. Even these meagre resources were unevenly distributed, favouring the large cities: ibid. 148–151.

[148] Jagailloux (1986) 161–220, at 220. On improvements after 1900, see briefly Omran (1973a) 14–15.

[149] Jagailloux (1986) 221–78.

4.4. *The demography of ancient and early modern Egypt*

In demographic terms, many ordinary Egyptians of the early twentieth century do not seem to have been significantly better off than their ancestors in the Roman period. Even then, reported levels of infant mortality were still comparable to the range of rates predicted by the model life tables that have been thought to be consistent with the census returns from Roman Egypt (but cf. above, Chapter 2). By implication, conditions in the second half of the nineteenth century were even closer to the ancient pattern. In fact, we might venture the guess that conditions in the late eighteenth and early nineteenth centuries may actually have been somewhat less favourable than under the Romans. Plague does not seem to have been of particularly great importance in early Roman Egypt, and in all probability, smallpox and cholera were unknown.[150] Ancient peasants were not subject to wide-ranging conscription and not normally hauled away from their villages for stints of forced labour in the northern Delta.

Neither the conditions in Roman Egypt nor in early modern Egypt are sufficiently well known to support an accurate comparative assessment. All the same, the patchy evidence suggests two general conclusions. First, the pattern of mortality and fertility in Egypt during much of the nineteenth century is unlikely to have been significantly more benevolent than in the Roman period. This rules out the conceivable argument that because of intervening improvements in life expectancy, the Roman population of Egypt could not not have exceeded the population of that country at almost any time during the nineteenth century. Second, the interaction of intensifying plague with the new disease of cholera, endemic smallpox, and social disruption, culminating at several junctures from the 1780s to the 1830s,[151] suggests that the size of the population of Egypt—which can only be estimated with great uncertainty—was smaller than it would have been in the absence of these unusual attrition factors. This, in turn, makes it seem possible that the population of Roman Egypt, at its best, and again *ceteris paribus*, could have been larger

[150] To judge from the sketchy evidence (Casanova (1984)), during the first two centuries of Roman rule (i.e., from 30 BCE to the Antonine epidemic), Egypt does not seem to have been affected by major disasters. This is also the view of van Minnen (1997) 14. For bubonic plague in ancient Egypt, see above, Chapter 1.3.8.

[151] For a summary of the severe economic crisis and near-anarchy during the final two decades of the eighteenth century, see Raymond (1981) 703–5.

than the depressed population of Egypt in the eighteenth and the first half of the nineteenth centuries. This notion will be further explored against the background of agricultural production in nineteenth-century Egypt, and re-evaluated in more general terms in the concluding section of this chapter.

5. *The agricultural basis of ancient and modern Egypt*

5.1. *Tradition and progress in Egyptian agriculture*

From ancient times, most of Egypt's agriculture depended on the inundation that started in late June and receded by late October; crops were grown and harvested in the winter and the spring. This winter system of cultivation involved a series of basins made by long dikes at right angles to the river, which were allowed to fill with water as the river reached its height in September and October. After the water had deposited its sediment and thoroughly penetrated the dry earth, it was drained off into nearby canals or back into the Nile, now flowing at a lower level. Summer crops required a different method of irrigation. As they were generally not harvested until after the Nile had started to rise, they were grown on slightly higher ground and had to be protected by embankments from the flood waters, which would have ruined the standing plants. They also needed an artificial system of watering to keep them irrigated through the summer months, when the Nile was often ten to twelve feet below the level of the ground on either side. This system usually consisted of a network of small canals fed by waterwheels turned by oxen (*saqiyas*), or buckets on the arm of a long pole which could be swung down into the river and then up to the canal mouths. Both appliances were expensive in manpower and, in the case of *saqiyas*, animal-power. In the first place, summer cultivation was confined to areas with ready access to summer water, *viz.*, along the Nile or one of the few Delta canals dug deep enough to allow them to take off water from the river when it was at its lowest. Elsewhere, the introduction of summer cultivation was dependent on an extension of the area supplied with summer water, a project only the government had the resources to undertake.[152]

[152] Owen (1969) 8, 10.

For all we can tell, the irrigation system had been properly maintained until the 1780s, when it was disrupted first by internal political conflict and then by the French invasion. The network of dikes and canals progressively fell into disrepair. In conjunction with rampant epidemic disease, this neglect precipitated agricultural decline and the abandonment of land. In 1808, 160 villages in the Delta were plausibly reported to be uninhabited.[153]

Muhammad Ali's takeover lead to a revival of Egyptian farming.[154] In a first phase of expansion, up to about 1821, work centred on the repair and extension of existing canals and dikes.[155] To a large extent, these projects merely recovered lost ground. From the 1820s, the expansion of the cultivation of long-staple cotton for export required far-flung extensions of the canal system in Lower Egypt. Old canals were deepened and new ones dug to provide water for the irrigation of this new summer crop.

By the end of his reign in 1848, Egypt's integration into the world economy had gathered pace: cash crops expanded and the volume and value of agricultural exports kept rising.[156] However, these early advancements must not be overrated. It is true that a considerable amount of idle land was brought into cultivation but much of this merely restored the status quo ante. The success of the first few decades of the expanding of summer irrigation is unclear, and some scholars have offered a cautious assessment of Ali's achievements with respect to irrigation.[157] Major progress was yet to come. With insignificant exceptions, the 'basin system remained the only system of irrigation in Middle and Upper Egypt and was used in Lower Egypt for the irrigation of winter crops'.[158] The period of his reign witnessed no technological improvements of tools and other equipment. Farming implements were simple, cheap and easy to repair.[159] Incipient industrialisation, centred on the processing of cotton into textiles, peaked in the mid-1830s and declined from then on. Once

---

153 Rivlin (1961) 238; Owen (1969) 11; Cuno (1992) 30–2.

154 On agricultural changes under his reign, see Marsot (1984) 137–61; Cuno (1992) 112–17; on irrigation projects, Rivlin (1961) 213–49.

155 Rivlin (1961) 245; Cuno (1992) 112. On economic policy from 1805–1819, cf. Owen (1969) 17–27.

156 Owen (1969) 81; Toledano (1990) 11.

157 Rivlin (1961) 248–9; Cuno (1992) 116.

158 Rivlin (1961) 246.

159 Rivlin (1961) 167–9; Owen (1969) 12. Rabie (1981) 63 stresses continuity in tool design from ancient times. Even in the second half of the nineteenth century, western machinery was mostly confined to the royal estates: Owen (1981b) 534.

these early factories had been disbanded, Egypt was turned into a mere supplier of raw materials.[160]

Modern estimates that are based on a comparison of data from the early and from the middle of the nineteenth century tend to exaggerate the rate of growth in that period, because much of the early evidence is of distinctly inferior quality (see below). Artificial irrigation really took off under the reign of Ismail (1863–79) who had 8,400 miles of canal dug, the longest among which was the Ibrahimiyya Canal in Middle Egypt which brought perennial irrigation to that part of the country for the first time in history.[161] By and large, the expansion of irrigated land for cotton production had no effect on food production: cotton could not be eaten and the export of this cash crop was not balanced by imports of foodstuffs. It is not clear whether or to what extent peasants profited from rising cotton prices in the 1850s and 1860s. Revenues from cotton were slim for peasants; gold earned was mainly put to economically unproductive uses. The surge of food prices in the 1860s seems to have had a much greater beneficial impact on the rural population at large.[162] Only gradually did the emergence of a market economy open up a gulf in terms of wealth between Lower and Upper Egypt and between cities and countryside.[163]

From this, there is no compelling to reason to assume that Egypt, by the middle of the nineteenth century or even a bit later, had become capable of supporting a larger population than ancient Egypt would ever have been able to.[164] In the following, this question will be addressed in greater detail, looking in turn at the extent of arable, the productivity of the land, and the volume of trade in basic foodstuffs. Ancient evidence, such as it is, will be juxtaposed with the data from the nineteenth century.

---

[160] Marsot (1984) 162–95.

[161] Owen (1981a) 135; Richards (1982) 30. By comparison, 686 miles were dug under Ali, bringing the total to 1,200 miles: Rivlin (1961) 248.

[162] Owen (1969) 107, 109–10; Toledano (1990) 255 n. 18.

[163] Baer (1982) 243–5. Before the nineteenth century, Upper Egypt had not been significantly less wealthy than the Delta.

[164] I agree with van Minnen (1997) 40 n. 165 that 'Egypt's growing integration into a global economy dominated by capitalism and industry' (Rathbone (1990) 107) or 'the introduction of perennial irrigation and Egypt's partial integration into European industrial economies' (Bagnall and Frier (1994) 53–4) are of little relevance for an assessment of Egypt's carrying capacity during much of the nineteenth century and, thus, for the application of modern data to the Roman period. Cf. Alleaume (1999) on industrialisation in nineteenth-century Egyptian farming.

5.2. *The cultivated area*

The total amount of arable land in ancient Egypt at any given time is unknown. The only ancient text that purports to record pertinent figures, an inscription in a temple at Edfu from the reign of Ptolemy V, inspires little confidence in their validity.[165] In this source, the total area of Egypt is put at 27,000,000 *sṯ3t*, i.e., arouras, a figure that happens to equal three times three times three million. One-third of this total, 9,000,000 arouras (or three times three million), is classified as arable. This latter figure is split into two subtotals, 2,400,000 (or four times 600,000, or 2 × 3 × 4 × 100,000) and 6,600,000 (or eleven times 600,000, or 2 × 3 × (4 + 3 + 4) × 100,000). Parallels for the first two values, nine and twenty-seven million, suggest that they are not more than symbolic figures indicative of a very large amount.[166] For the same reason, it seems unlikely that the total of nine million is the sum of the two subtotals: rather, the two subtotals may have been chosen to fit a predetermined total. The smaller of these subtotals is conventionally taken to refer to Upper Egypt, the larger to Lower Egypt, although the text does not actually say so in so many words. As a consequence, we are asked to believe that in the second century BCE, the total area under cultivation was 24,800 km^2, 18,200 of which lay in the Delta. As we will see in a moment, these values are improbably high.

Medieval data suggest a very considerable extent of variation over time, from 1.5 million to 2.4 million feddans in the eighth to twelfth centuries to 3.6 million in the first half of the fourteenth century.[167] Rather than interpreting this rise as evidence of massive population increase,[168] it might be preferable to explain this apparent difference in terms of the different background of these sets of data and the possibility that the early data suffer from an indeterminable amount of undercount. What is perhaps of some interest here is that the medieval maximum of 3.6 million feddans, at 4,200 m^2 per feddan, amounts to some 15,120 km^2, or, at 4,417 m^2 per feddan, to 15,901 km^2,[169] both reasonable figures when compared to early modern evidence.

---

165 Discussed in detail by Schlott (1969) 160–9, who, however, treats this text with unwarranted reverence.

166 Scheidel (1996c) 224, 229.

167 Russell (1966) 74 tab. 1, 77 tab. 3. All his counts are based on a set of preconceived notions that remain impervious to verification.

168 Thus Russell (1966) 75–6.

169 Higher conversion rates, which would yield 19,270 to 21,344 km^2 (see below, n. 170), seem unlikely.

Table 3.5 charts the increase of cultivated land during the nineteenth century. This tabulation is beset by two problems, the fact that prior to the 1860s, the precise metric equivalent of the feddan is not certain,[170] and by the very real possibility that the two counts from the first half of the century are defective. Thus, it remains uncertain whether the cultivated area actually increased by 600,000 feddans between 1844 and 1852.[171]

Table 3.5 Cultivated area in Egypt (in 1,000 feddans and 1,000 km^2)[172]

Year	feddans	km^2
1813	3,054	12,827 or 13,488
1844	3,569	14,995 (?)
1852	4,160	17,475 (?)
1877	4,742	19,920
1879	4,810	20,206
1880	4,719	19,824
1881/85	4,780	20,080
1886/90	4,900	20,584
1891/95	4,912	20,634

It ought to be stressed that these figures, especially the early ones, are to be taken simply as an indication of the likely order of magnitude. Alternative counts are known,[173] and even in the second half of the century, subtotals for land under particular crops do not always add up to the grand totals recorded here.[174] By and large, however, the general trend is clear. The total amount of agricultural land seems to have increased quite considerably during the first three

[170] See Owen (1969) 381: before 1813, a feddan could have been 5,353 or 5,929 m^2; from 1813 to 1823, 4,416.5 m^2; in 1840, *perhaps* 4,083.3 m^2, and only since 1861 has it been firmly established as 4,200.8 m^2, or 1.038 acres.

[171] This rate is taken at face value by Richards (1982) 21. Both figures come from cadastral surveys. It seems reasonable to suspect that the latter was executed with greater care than the former.

[172] From O'Brien (1968) 172 tab. 3; the annual data have been converted into means from 1881 onward.

[173] Cf., e.g., Cuno (1992) 114 tab. 6.2 (cultivated land in 1,000 feddans): 3,055 (1813/14), 3,856 (1830s), 3,672 (1843), 3,590 (1844). O'Brien (1968) 173 thinks that the 1844 figure refers to taxed land only, whereas Cuno (1992) 114 tab. 6.2 takes it to pertain to all cultivated land. Cf. also the figures cited by van Minnen (1997) 29 n. 118. It seems inconceivable, however, that the total amount of arable could have doubled between 1813 and 1840, as indicated by Garbrecht, ed. (1986) 13.

[174] Compare the aggregate totals for the years 1879 and 1889 in O'Brien (1968) 165 tab. 1, with the grand totals in my Tab. 3.5.

quarters of the nineteenth century, even though the actual rate of increase is obscure. We can be fairly certain that it was smaller than indicated by these numbers but it is impossible to tell by how much.

Throughout the last third of the century, the total amount of agricultural land hovered around 20,000 km^2. This is not to say that expansion had by then ground to a halt. Egyptian farmland is classified in two different ways, as cultivated and cropped area. The latter category reflects the fact that some of the land produces more than one crop per year. Further progress was made mainly through the conversion of growing portions of inundated land into perennially irrigated land. As a result, the cropped area grew at a much faster rate than the cultivated area. According to figures of dubious reliability, the area under summer cultivation (i.e., perennial irrigation) grew from 250,000 feddans in 1798 to 600,000 in the early 1830s.[175] However, according to the count of 1844, not more than 508,000 feddans were then under artificial irrigation, or one-seventh of all cultivated land. Usable figures for cropped and cultivated land start as late as in 1894. By that time, the ratio of cropped to cultivated land had risen to 132 to 100, which means that one-third of all land was cropped twice a year.[176]

The available statistics indicate that in the course of the nineteenth century, wheat and maize expanded at the expense of barley and beans (Table 3.6). This impression is in keeping with the attested importance of wheat for export and the replacement of lesser grains by wheat.

Table 3.6 Area devoted to major crops in Egypt (in 1,000 feddans)[177]

Year	Wheat	Maize	Barley	Beans	Rice	Cotton
1844	914	799	872	840		
1886–7	1,241	1,125	520	756	150	865
1893–4	1,296	1,475	460	689	181	966
1899/1904	1,270	1,727	537	647	164	1,305
1909/13	1,269	1,838	373	524	246	1,670

175 Richards (1982) 21. Owen (1969) 7–8 estimates that before 1805, one-eighth of Lower Egypt was irrigated for summer crops such as sugar-cane, rice, and short-staple cotton. Cf. also Maury (1987).

176 O'Brien (1968) 171–2. He rightly dismisses an isolated figure for 1877 which gives 4,762,000 feddans of cropped versus 4,742,000 feddans of cultivated land, an impossibly low ratio of 104 to 100 (174).

177 1844: Rivlin (1961) 258 tab. 12; 1886 to 1913: Owen (1969) 247 tab. 44.

The total area devoted to the production of cereals expanded only modestly during this period (Table 3.7). Rising output was mainly due to higher yields (see below, section 5.3). It must however be noted that even after 1900, the figures for crops other than cotton were not perfectly accurate; on one occasion, for instance, the returns for wheat, beans and barley have been found to be exaggerated.[178]

Table 3.7 Total area devoted to the production of basic foodstuffs in Egypt (in 1,000 feddans)[179]

1844	3,425
1886–7	3,642
1893–4	3,920
1899/1904	4,181
1909/13	4,004

One final point on the question of the surface of arable land. Historians of ancient Egypt often assume that the total cultivated area in the Roman period was of the order of 25,000 km^2.[180] This view conflicts with comparative evidence. The total cultivated area rose from 20,100 km^2 in 1879 to 23,100 km^2 in 1900, 28,500 km^2 in 1957 and 31,000 km^2 in 1982.[181] A continuously cultivated area of 25,000 km^2 was not attained until the early 1950s,[182] and, given the expansion of farming in the Nile Delta that had taken place by then, a corresponding value is hardly conceivable for premodern times. Once again, precision is impossible, but we have no reason to believe that the respective total for Roman Egypt could have been significantly in excess of 20,000 km^2.[183]

[178] Owen (1969) 247.

[179] Source: Tab. 3.6, cols. 1–4.

[180] E.g., Bowman (1990) 13; Rathbone (1990) 107–8 (cf. 139 n. 14); Bagnall (1993) 20 and n. 25 reckons with 23,000 km^2 as a rough model for late Roman Egypt. This idea can be traced back to Barois (1889), who reports 24,105 km^2 for Egypt in 1882. Butzer (1976) 92 even gives 27,659 km^2 for 1882; Schnebel (1925) 148 cites 26,670 km^2 for 1904.

[181] Béthemont (1987) 95.

[182] See O'Brien (1968) 188 tab. 10. In 1949/50, 24,982 km^2 were under cultivation: Kees (1955) 1; Schlott (1969) 161 and n. 1. By 1990, arable had expanded to 28,300 km^2: Yates and Strzepek (1998) 264 tab. 1.

[183] Durliat (1990) 259 cautiously reckons with 16,000 km^2 of arable from the sixth to the early ninteenth century centuries. Bagnall (1985) 304 calls 18,500 km^2 'not an unrealistic figure'. This does not preclude disproportionally higher development in particular areas in antiquity, such as the Fayum: see below, p. 244. Van Minnen (1997) 30 considers 20,000 km^2 a 'reasonable, conservative hypothesis'; I agree.

5.3. *The productivity of the land*

With respect to wheat (and also barley), historians of Roman Egypt conventionally reckon with an average of a tenfold return on one artaba of seed per aroura.[184] Once again, the margin of error is far from negligible but much of the available evidence is roughly consistent with this assumption.[185] It is also in line with evidence of yields from the nineteenth century, at a time when chemical fertilisers had not yet come to play a role in Egyptian farming.[186] As usual, the nineteenth-century data are to be taken with a grain of salt but provide some general orientation.[187]

Table 3.8 Average yields on state domains in Egypt (in ardebs per feddan)[188]

	Wheat	Barley	Beans
1844*	2.772	3.557	2.673
1844 (estimate)	3	4	3
1872*	2.21	2.02	1.84
1881/1885	3.364	2.21	2.256
1886/1890	3.818	3.33	2.656
1891/1895	4.70	3.894	3.118
1896/1900	5.16	3.696	3.8
1901/1905	5.798	3.758	3.628

[184] E.g., Crawford (1971) 127; Rathbone (1990) 108; (1991) 242–4, esp. 243 and n. 45 (with references). See van Minnen (1997) 24–7 for further discussion: he reckons with a mean of 12 artabas per aroura during the first two centuries of Roman rule but with lower yields in the following centuries (26–7).

[185] The land in the Fayum studied by Rathbone (1991) was characterised by an average yield of 11.5 artabas per aroura, a result which he considers 'quite respectable' given that this land lay in a marginal corner of the Fayum where irrigation could be problematic (243). Lo Cascio (1999) 164–5 stresses the difficulties of establishing an average value.

[186] However, even in the mid-twentieth century Kees (1955) 37 n. 5 refers to an average wheat yield of not more than 235 litres per 1,000 m^2 and to a maximum of 377 litres per 1,000 m^2.

[187] Cf. Owen (1969) 250–2. Like the feddan, the ardeb was subject to changes over time: in 1798, it equalled 184 litres, but by 1870 had risen to 197.75 litres, equivalent to 133.6 kg of wheat or 151.3 kg of barley: Owen (1969) 381–2.

[188] From O'Brien (1968) 169 tab. 2; Owen (1969) 250 tab. 45. The figures for 1844 come from Rivlin (1961) 258 tab. 12, 261 tab. 15, 262 tab. 16, the figures for 1872 from O'Brien (1968) 167. 1844 and 1872 refer to all land rather than merely state domains.

Table 3.8 *(cont.)*

	Wheat	Barley	Beans
converted into litres per 1,000 m²			
1844	131	168	126
1844 (estimate)	141	189	141
1872	104	95	87
1881/1885	159	104	106
1886/1890	180	157	125
1891/1895	222	184	147
1896/1900	243	174	179
1901/1905	273	177	171
estimate/antiquity	140		

5.4. *Crops and the volume of agricultural production*

Sources for the Hellenistic Fayum point to a diet mainly comprised of wheat, barley and *olyra* (emmer), plus lentils and beans. In this respect, Graeco-Roman Egypt resembled early modern Egypt, when millet and sorghum had replaced *olyra*.[189] Tetraploid emmer and barley were staple crops up to the Ptolemies, when durum wheat became more important.[190] Crop rotation can be traced in some detail: both two-field and three-field systems were in use, either alternating a year of grain and a year of something else, or two years of cereals and one year of grass or leguminous crops.[191] Multiple cropping is first attested in the third-century BCE Fayum; the cultivation of summer wheat on irrigated land is one example.[192] Multiple cropping was also practised later, in the Roman period, but it is impossible to tell how common it was.[193]

Farming techniques and dietary habits were quite similar during much of the nineteenth century. In the Delta, the main winter crops were wheat, barley, beans and clover, grown in a biennial rotation (wheat and barley one year, beans and clover the next). Barley and clover were used as animal fodder, while a mixture of wheat and

[189] Crawford (1971) 114–5; 1979: 142. Egyptian *olyra* was emmer, not oats: Sallares (1991) 495–6 n. 227; Lewis (1994).

[190] Crawford (1979) 140; Bagnall (1993) 24.

[191] Schnebel (1925) 220–8 lists the evidence. See in brief Crawford (1971) 116.

[192] Crawford (1979) 140–1.

[193] Schnebel (1925) 145–60, esp. 154.

barley flour formed the staple diet of the human population. Summer crops included sesame, cotton and rice. Summer crops required considerably more care and attention than the majority of winter crops. Maize, for instance, could be grown without any preliminary ploughing and with only a very occasional hoeing during growth.[194] The main winter crops in Upper Egypt were wheat, maize, barley, lentils, beans and flax. Wheat and barley was used largely for the payment of taxes in kind. Maize provided the main part of the peasants' diet in those areas where it was common. Summer crops were rare compared to the Delta.[195] The basin lands were cropped only once a year, wheat and barley alternating with beans and *birsim*.[196]

Richards has questioned the assumption that maize was very important as a staple item of the peasants' diet.[197] Beans were a staple throughout Egypt, and millet in particular was the staple cereal of Upper Egypt. The situation in the Delta was more complex: although maize had probably already been introduced in the seventeenth century, its need for water may have limited its distribution prior to the nineteenth century. Richards discusses this problem and concludes that the evidence is mixed, with some sources asserting that peasants ate maize early in the ninteenth century, whereas most sources claim that their main food crop was sorghum or millet.[198] 'On the whole, then, the consumption pattern was beans and millet bread in Upper Egypt and beans and wheat-millet, wheat-sorghum, wheat-barley, or wheat-maize bread in the Delta, with the consumption of maize spreading in the latter region.'[199] Vegetables would supplement this diet. Hence, excluding maize, whose importance for peasant subsistence should not be overrated, the situation was pretty much the same as in antiquity.[200]

---

[194] Owen (1969) 9, 11.

[195] Owen (1969) 9.

[196] Owen (1969) 12; Richards (1982) 15.

[197] Richards (1982) 15–17.

[198] It deserves attention that even in the 1880s, *sorghum vulgare* was known to be the most important cereal in Upper Egypt and Nubia, as opposed to the (by then more advanced) Delta: Woenig (1886) 171–2. Sandwith (1905) 287 refers to a poor resident of the Fayum who in 1903 stated that he mostly lived on a diet of millet.

[199] Richards (1982) 19.

[200] On beans in Egypt, see below, p. 237. It is surprising, though, that millet keeps a low profile in ancient sources from Egypt. *Panicum miliaceum* and *P. italicum*, main staples for poor peasants in Roman Italy and other parts of the ancient Mediterranean (see Spurr (1986) 89–102), are not unambiguously attested in Roman Egypt. Some kind of sorghum was however grown then: Hartmann (1923) 53.

At first, the expansion of cotton from 1820 onward had little impact on diet and the production of foodstuffs.[201] It was the cash value of cotton as an export good that made it overshadow traditional subsistence agriculture in which crops, tools and techniques had changed little from ancient times. Thus, in the years up to the 1860s, when cotton often provided up to half of the country's export revenues, it was cultivated over only one-tenth of the Delta in any one season.[202] Part of this was land that had previously been available for basin cultivation, and, indeed, was still used for the production of cereals in years when cotton was not planted there. Initially, the promotion of cotton by the authorities met with resistance among the peasants since it required greater labour input and entailed closer supervision: 'formerly beaten at harvest time (a practice which continued), the peasants were now also beaten throughout the eight month cotton-growing season'.[203] Wheat and other cereals continued to possess advantages for the poor peasant: they were easier to cultivate, provided quicker returns and occupied the ground for a shorter period of time. These attractions would limit the size of the area given over to cotton even at a time when cotton provided a higher income than other crops, during the 1840s and 1850s.[204] Only with the cotton boom triggered by the American Civil War did cotton production really begin to affect the whole of Egypt's economic life and the strategic decisions of ordinary peasants.

This evidence makes it clear that the impact of Egypt's integration into a global market economy must not be overrated. The rise in output, both in total and per capita, measured in monetary terms, can only be explained with reference to the expansion of cotton production, which increased fifty times between 1821 and the 1870s alone. 'Egypt's agricultural revolution rested overwhelmingly upon the introduction and expansion of a single cash crop'.[205] It can be shown, by way of a thought experiment, that had Egyptian farmers not been given the opportunity to grow cotton for sale to the West and had the land that was under cotton in the 1870s been allocated

---

[201] On the history of the expansion of cotton in Egypt, see Rivlin (1961) *passim*; Owen (1969) *passim*; Richards (1982) 19–22.
[202] Owen (1969) 354.
[203] Richards (1982) 21–2. It seems probable that with artificial irrigation, peasants worked more days per year than before (39).
[204] Owen (1969) 81.
[205] O'Brien (1968) 184–5.

to foodstuffs, the agarian economy would have grown far more modestly and largely in keeping with the growth of the population.[206] As a consequence, there is no reason to suppose that up to the 1870s or so, Egypt had reached a level of development that set it fundamentally apart from previous periods.

From the 1870s to the late 1890s, the cultivated area barely expanded, although multiple cropping became more common.[207] By the first decade of the twentieth century, the majority of cultivators in Lower Egypt had changed from a triennial to a biennial cotton rotation; the more intensive use of this land had been further increased by the growth of an additional crop of summer or *Nili* maize made possible by the extra supplies of water. At the same time, yields of all major crops were significantly increased, if only at the cost of serious soil exhaustion.[208] This, of course, was a harbinger of the change of Egypt's status from net exporter to net importer of foodstuffs as agricultural output could not keep pace with population growth. Chemical fertilisers, the only way to tackle this problem, were only slowly adopted. In 1910 it was estimated that five per cent of the total cultivated area was being artificially manured.[209] A comparison with the 1960s indicates that by the end of the nineteenth century, Egypt's agriculture had already become quite well developed. Even the massive use of chemical fertilisers, modern farm implements and irrigation machinery did not increase output by more than 100 per cent between the end of the nineteenth century and the 1960s, and the area under cultivation grew by no more than twenty per cent, the cropped area by some fifty per cent. Only the (second) Aswan Dam brought a further breakthrough.[210]

Unfortunately, it proves difficult if not impossible to establish precise figures for the volume of total annual output of individual crops for the time before the 1870s. None of the figures haphazardly reported for the first third of the nineeteenth century deserves much

---

[206] O'Brien (1968) 184. His calculation that under these circumstances, agricultural production in the 1870s would have amounted to 206 per cent of the volume in 1821 is of course incorrect, based as it is on seriously deficient figures for 1821 (see below, p. 229). The actual rates for 1821 remain unknown but the difference between 1821 and the 1870s must have been considerably smaller than he assumes.

[207] See Schamp (1968) 10, on the expansion of the cropped area, especially with the Delta barrage of 1884 and the first Aswan dam of 1902.

[208] Owen (1969) 252–3.

[209] Owen (1969) 253–4.

[210] O'Brien (1968) 184–5.

Table 3.9 Agricultural production in Egypt according to contemporary statistics (in 1,000 ardebs)[211]

Year	Wheat	Millet and maize	Barley	Beans	Rice
1821	1,156	912	576	1,176	141
1830–5	1,186	995	676	778	117
1872–8	3,780	6,113	1,277	2,520	127
converted into millions of litres					
1821	229	181	114	233	28
1830–5	235	197	134	154	23
1872–8	748	1,210	253	499	25

credence, notwithstanding the sometimes bewildering display of faith in these data in contemporary scholarship (Table 3.9).

These early statistics report a total cereal crop of 524 million litres in 1821, 566 million in the early 1830s, and 2,736 million in the mid-1870s. (If the ardeb was still less than 198 litres in the early nineteenth century, which cannot be ruled out, the early totals would be lower still.) However, 524 million litres of cereals cannot sustain more than 1.75 million people at 300 litres per year and person.[212] If the population was of the order of five million, even with some input from legumes and under the untenable assumption of zero exports, less than one-half of the population could have been fed. At that time, 600,000 to 700,000 ardebs, or 119 to 139 million litres, were said to be exported. This would not leave food for more than 1.5 million people. This figure is incompatible even with the census figure of 1821 of 2.5 million people that is itself invalidated by considerable underreporting (see above, section 4.1). The inevitable conclusion is that the figures for output suffer from the same deficiencies as the population counts, only more so. As a consequence, modern accounts that take these figures at face value to determine the rate of growth during the nineteenth century are so flawed as to be worthless.[213] In Table 3.10, I summarise what can be said about levels of

[211] From O'Brien (1968) 179 tab. 5.

[212] On grain intake levels, see below, section 5.6.

[213] This applies in particular to the elaborate indices of agricultural development from 1821 to the 1960s constructed by O'Brien (1968), esp. 179 tab. 6, 180 tab. 7, 185 tab. 9, 188 tab. 10. His reconstruction has been accepted at face value by Tignor (1984) 15. Richards (1982) 38 is also taken in by the 1821 data. The ear-

output from the 1840s to the 1880s. According to this breakdown, total output rose from 13,034,000 ardebs in 1844 to 14,038,000 in the 1870s, or by not more than 7.7 per cent. However, the total for 1844 is also given as 12,243,652 ardebs, implying an increase by 14.7 per cent. This discrepancy aside, we have to bear in mind that the figures for 1844 seem to indicate optimum output (following high flood levels) rather than that year's actual output.[214] This impression is also borne out by the model presented below (section 5.6).

Exports totalled 811,018 ardebs in 1844, averaged 1,065,117 in 1870/74 and 1,468,492 in 1875/79.[216] Thus, between 11,432,634 and 12,222,982 ardebs may have been available for local consump-

Table 3.10 Volume and indices of production of six staple crops in Egypt (in 1,000 feddans)[215]

Year	Wheat	Millett/ maize	Barley	Beans	Lentils	Rice
1844	2,534	4,495	3,109	2,243	163	490
1872–8	3,780	6,113	1,277	2,520	221	127
1886–7	4,393		1,504	1,852		
1844	100	100	100	100	100	100
1872–8	149	136	41	112	136	26
1886–7	173		48	83		

lier discussion by Rivlin (1961) is even more uncritical: not only does she accept the reported figures of output for 1821 and the 1830s, but she also criticises the 1844 count—the first plausible data—as inflated (158). She is even prepared to accept the figure for 1830 (a year of harvest failure) of 1,352,141 ardebs as Egypt's actual total output in that year. Of these cereals, according to a contemporary breakdown, 654,280 were sold in Cairo, 219,756 ardebs went to Alexandria, 112,505 to four other major cities, 296,952 to the armed forces, and 64,148 to the court and households of the ruling elite (159). These figures are roughly in keeping with the annual requirements of these recipients. However, if we were to believe this amount to be the total, *none* of this food would have been available for consumption by the peasants, or some 90 per cent or so of the population. Even the frugal *fallahin* would have found it difficult to go without any food whatsoever for an entire year. We must conclude that this count only records the cereals the government could lay its hand on to ensure the sustenance of its dependents and the major urban settlements.

[214] Rivlin (1961) 258 n. c, 261 tab. 15; O'Brien (1968) 173. The harvests of 1843 and 1844 were considered satisfactory, enabling generous exports: Rivlin (1961) 156.

[215] From Rivlin (1961) 261 tab. 15 (1844); O'Brien (1968) 179 tab. 5 (1872–8); Owen (1969) 251 tab. 47. The data for 1886–7 are estimates.

[216] Owen (1969) 127.

tion in 1844 (though probably less than either figure), and between 12,569,508 and 12,972,883 in the 1870s. Rich harvests would boost exports: in 1849/50 and 1852, 1,293,968 ardebs left the country every year, possibly excluding barley and maize. Egypt exported some two million ardebs per year in 1855 and in 1861/62.[217] In the same period, the population rose from perhaps 5.25 million to 7.25 million, or by thirty-five to forty per cent.[218]

There is no indication that the increase in exports was made possible by taking from the peasants who lived close to subsistence level to begin with.[219] We have to conclude that because of the previous disruption brought about by epidemics and other factors, the agricultural potential of Egypt in the 1840s, if properly exploited by sufficient manpower, exceeded the actual demand for food by a sizeable margin. It was only because of this that both the population and exports could grow at higher rates than the surface of arable land and the volume of agricultural output from the 1840s to the 1870s. Beyond that point, rising yields could still sustain the population but proved insufficient to keep exports from dropping, as we will see in the next section. Eventually, the population overran the country's potential and Egypt became dependent on imports.

5.5. *Exports of foodstuffs*

5.5.1. *Roman Egypt*

Throughout the Roman period, Egypt was a major exporter of grain. For our purposes, it is important to assess the gross volume of ancient exports compared to modern trade flows. Ancient texts offer but two figures of uncertain reliability: according to a fourth-century source, under Augustus Egypt annually sent twenty million *modii* (172 million litres) of grain to the city of Rome; and in the sixth century, Justinian put the total tax grain due from Egypt at eight million units, apparently artabas (310 million litres).[220] The former figure cannot bear much weight, amounting as it does to about two-thirds of the likely total annual rate of grain consumption in the capital.[221]

---

217 Owen (1969) 127 tab. 17.

218 Based on the mean in Tab. 3.4.

219 O'Brien (1968) 181–2.

220 *Epitome de Caesaribus* 1.6 (twenty million *modii*); Justinian, *Edict* 13.6 (eight million [artabas]).

221 As estimated by Garnsey (1983) 118, (1988) 231.

Even if Africa's contribution gradually became more important over the years, it would have provided a fair share of Rome's grain even under Augustus, as did Sicily and Sardinia.[222] Moreover, Rome must largely have relied on non-Egyptian sources of grain prior to 30 BCE, a situation that would be hard to reconcile with this high figure. On the other hand, the amount of imports may well have exceeded the amount of grain that was actually consumed, yet probably not by such a wide margin. We cannot avoid the conclusion that the fourth-century figure is exaggerated. Rathbone assumes that during the Principate, ten million *modii* may have been sent from Egypt to Rome (see below). Thus, Egypt would have provided roughly one-third of Rome's actual needs. This assumption tallies with a passage in Josephus according to which North African grain fed Rome for eight months and Egyptian imports for the remaining four. This split seems dubious, not least because it precludes imports from any other parts of the empire, and also conventional (with a possible parallel in Herodotus), but even so it need not be wide of the mark, if only by coincidence.[223]

The Justinianic figure is usually accepted as plausible,[224] even though it is worth bearing in mind that strictly speaking it represents nothing more than what Justinian publicily thought the revenue should be.[225] However, Rathbone has argued that this figure seems too high when applied to the early empire: if ten million *modii* (2.2 million artabas) went to Rome, more than three-quarters of the available Egyptian grain remained to be allocated. He speculates that six million *modii* may have gone to other cities and four million may have been distributed in Egypt. Subtracting one million for wastage, this still leaves a surplus of fifteen million *modii*, or one-third of the tax.[226] This surplus would have been even larger if we were to accept Duncan-Jones' recent recalculation of the annual amount of tax grain in Egypt during the Principate: reckoning with higher average tax revenue per aroura than is usually assumed, he arrives at a total

[222] Africa's share may have doubled from the Republic to the early empire, perhaps from five to ten million to ten to twenty million *modii*: cf. similarly Garnsey (1983) 120 and 201 n. 8. On Sicily, see Garnsey (1988) 231–2.

[223] Rathbone (1989) 172.

[224] Discussion in Durliat (1990) 257–60.

[225] A point made by Bagnall (1985) 305 n. 47.

[226] Rathbone (1989) 173. Note that Rathbone (1990) 108, with reference to his 1989 paper, erroneously speaks of exports of fifteen million artabas rather than *modii*.

levy of 17.5 million artabas per year, or more than twice the sixth-century figure. The unallocated surplus would grow accordingly. However, this revised figure appears to be too high.[227] Rathbone argues that a theoretical surplus of ten to fifteen million *modii* may not actually have been collected in grain but extracted in other forms of revenue, mostly in cash. Hopkins comes to a slightly different conclusion in arguing that some of the tax grain would have been sold in Egypt and thus converted into cash by the government (instead of by the tax-payer).[228] Both interpretations are mutually compatible and consistent with the high level of urbanisation in Roman Egypt that may well have been sustained in part by access to tax grain that did not leave the country.

What we are interested in here is of course how much grain actually did leave Egypt. With respect to exports to the city of Rome, we may establish a range between a minimum of ten million *modii*, or one-third of the grain required, and 20 million *modii*, the figure given by the *Epitome* which might just conceivably represent the total amount of Egyptian grain sent to Rome, part of which may have been left to rot.[229] I am inclined to suspect that the truth lies somewhere in between these two extremes: shipments to Rome may have considerably exceeded actual demand but hardly by as much as 100 per cent.

As for grain shipments to other cities, primarily on the littoral of the eastern Mediterranean, we are reduced to mere guesswork. Rathbone has argued that in the Hellenistic period, Egyptian grain exports in the eastern Mediterranean were on the whole surplus to basic requirements. That the reorientation of Egyptian surplus grain to

---

[227] He reckons with an average revenue of 2.23 artabas per aroura times 7,838,815 arouras (90 per cent the arable land estimated by Barois): Duncan-Jones (1994) 52–3. The tax is usually put at about 1.2 artabas/aroura: see, e.g., Bagnall (1985) 304 (with discussion); Rathbone (1989) 172; Durliat (1990) 258–9. I doubt that a global average can be calculated with sufficient precision. In any case, the Barois estimate is way too high (see above, section 5.2). If we reckon with 16,000 km^2 of arable in Roman Egypt, we get 5.78 million arouras and thus, at 2.23 artabas/aroura, a total of 12.9 million artabas, still more than one-and-a-half times the Justinianic figure. At 20,000 km^2, the tax revenues would amount to 16.1 million artabas. Hopkins (1995/96) 71 n. 56 doubts Duncan-Jones' estimate.

[228] Hopkins (1995/96) 56.

[229] The authorities would be keen to stockpile surplus: see *Historia Augusta, Life of Septimius Severus* 23, and cf. Garnsey (1983) 118; (1988) 232: 'The emperors made a virtue of necessity: far from setting a ceiling on grain imports, they brought in as much as they could'. See also Garnsey (1998) 236, who reckons with some spoilage of grain stored in Rome.

Rome did not cause severe disruption in the East supports this thesis.[230] Thus, we have no reason to assume that in the Roman period, large parts of the eastern provinces were dependent on massive Egyptian grain imports either. With respect to the sixth century, Durliat thinks that only a small fraction of the eight million artabas claimed by Justinian would go to provincial recipients.[231] As I mentioned above, Rathbone speculatively sets aside six million *modii* for such exports, enough to feed 200,000 people at 30 *modii* per year. A letter sent by an unknown second-century emperor to the citizens of Ephesus reminds them that 'first the imperial city should have a bounteous supply of wheat procured and assembled for its market, and then the other cities may also receive provisions in plenty'.[232] This suggests that there were a number of regular recipients of grain outside Rome,[233] whose numbers probably swelled in times of local or regional food crises caused by climatic fluctuations. Likely orders of magnitude of local demand are indicated by the allocation of 600,000 *modii* of (Sicilian) grain to the Rhodians in 169 BCE and the procuring of 60,000 *modii* by a grain commissioner of Tralles under Hadrian. During a drought in 24 BCE, Herod the Great used his friendship with the prefect C. Petronius to buy grain from Egypt.[234] Rare allusions in the Talmudic texts also refer to Egyptian grain imports to Palestine.[235]

The mean annual total of Egyptian grain exports to consumers outside Rome is impossible to establish with any certainty. In a schematic model, Hopkins reckons that ten per cent of minimum urban demand outside the mega-cities Rome, Alexandria, Antioch and Carthage was met by medium-range transport, i.e., fifteen million *modii* for ten per cent of five million non-metropolitan city-dwellers.[236] If one-half of this demand arose in the eastern Mediterranean, 7.5 million *modii* would have been needed there in an average year. On the reasonable assumption that most of these imports were supplied by Egypt, Rathbone's guess of six million *modii* seems quite plausible.

---

230 Rathbone (1983) 51–3. He maintains that exports of durum wheat replaced less popular cereals outside Egypt.

231 Durliat (1990) 259.

232 Wörrle (1971); cf. Pleket (1994) 120.

233 Thus also Garnsey (1988) 257.

234 For these three cases, see Garnsey (1988) 255–7.

235 Safrai (1994) 111.

236 Hopkins (1983) 93 tab. 2 (who gives 110,000 tonnes).

All I can do is to propose a range between a hypothetical minimum and a hypothetical maximum of Egyptian grain exports. The minimum may be put at ten million *modii* for Rome and five million for others, a total of 3.33 million artabas (129 million litres). The maximum may be thought to be twenty million for Rome and ten million for others, or 6.67 million artabas (258 million litres). We will see that relative to total output (see below, section 5.6), the discrepancy between these two figures is of little concern, and I find it hard to believe that the actual mean total could have been significantly below or above these limits.[237]

5.5.2. *Modern Egypt*

Egypt was considered the granary of the Ottoman empire, sending food to Istanbul, the Holy Places of Arabia, Rumelia, Anatolia and Syria.[238] Yet for all we can tell, the volume of grain exports under the Mamluks was modest compared both to the Roman period and the nineteenth century. On the eve of the French invasion, Egypt annually sent 40,000 to 50,000 ardebs of wheat (7.4 to 9.2 million litres at 184 litres per ardeb) to the Holy Cities in the Arabian peninsula, and 30,000 ardebs of rice to Syria.[239] Total grain exports could be put at 100,000 ardebs (18.4 million litres) a year.[240]

Before the onset of large-scale cotton production, Egypt increased its grain exports as a means of earning foreign currency. In 1822, it was estimated that from 1816, Egypt had exported 600–700,000 ardebs of grain per year.[241] In this respect, modern Egypt became increasingly more similar to Roman Egypt. The actual volume of exports in any given year depended above all on the quality of the previous year's inundation. While bumper harvests left huge surpluses for storage and sale, bad floods could curb exports or in rare cases even necessitate some imports to fend off starvation. Thus, bad floods in 1824 and 1825 led to a temporary prohibition of the export of foodstuffs and to imports of wheat. Emergency imports are also

[237] It is true that my maximum falls short of Justinian's eight million artabas. However, this amount—which was asked for but not documented—need not actually have been raised every year, and, more importantly, not all of it may have left the country (see above). At any rate, 100 million litres more or less would not significantly affect the models in section 5.6.

[238] Richards (1982) 6–7.

[239] Owen (1969) 15.

[240] Marsot (1984) 149.

[241] Marsot (1984) 149.

attested for 1837 and 1838.[242] As we have seen, the situation generally improved from the 1840s. However, even at the peak of the export boom Egypt was not immune to sudden reverses: in 1864, Ismail was forced to prohibit the export of wheat and flour and to suspend duties on imports of these goods. In this and the following year, Egypt temporarily turned into a net importer of grain, albeit on a small scale.[243] It is only reasonable to assume that in the Roman Egypt, every now and then the country would undergo similar crises, although we are almost entirely ignorant of these events and responses to food shortage.[244]

In Table 3.11, I chart the expansion of exports in basic foodstuffs that peaked in the late 1850s and early 1860s.[245] For comparative purposes, the totals are also expressed in ancient artabas (1 artaba = 38.745 litres).

Table 3.11 Exports of foodstuffs from Egypt (in ardebs)[246]

Year	Wheat	Beans	Barley	Maize	Total	artabas
1816	134,000	230,000	10,000	60,000	507,000	2,570,000
1829	150,000	160,000	80,000	30,000	480,000	2,440,000
1843	446,598	397,945	16,988	2,920	894,110	4,540,000
1844	287,502	430,489	57,051	–	811,018	4,120,000
1849/52	906,744	387,224	–	–	1,293,968	6,570,000
1855	1,674,852	445,246	–	–	2,120,098	10,770,000
1861–2	1,116,306	598,981	235,376	85,563	2,036,226	10,340,000
1866–9	579,403	513,409	75,566	65,983	1,234,361	6,270,000
1870–4	440,911	554,411	15,030	54,765	1,065,117	5,410,000
1875–9	–	688,731	732,652	47,109	1,468,492	7,460,000

[242] Rivlin (1961) 151, 154–5.

[243] Owen (1969) 102.

[244] In 99 CE Trajan ordered that grain be sent from Rome to Egypt to alleviate a food crisis (Plinius, *Panegyricus* 30–2); Garnsey (1988) 252 stresses that this is the only example of a relief operation of this kind. It is, however, merely the only *attested* example; we might speculate that serious crises triggered a range of responses from partial remission of taxes to the return of some tax grain to the country. In general, Egypt's lack of sovereignty and the precedence of Roman interests over local welfare would have put the country into a considerably less favourable position than it found itself in during much of the nineteenth century.

[245] The quality of the 1816 harvest is unknown; 1829 was an abundant harvest, while 1843 and 1844 were satisfactory years.

[246] From Rivlin (1961) 157 and Owen (1969) 127. The ardeb is put at 198 litres; ancient artabas are rounded off to 10,000s.

Figures 3.5–7 illustrate the decline of exports and the rise of imports in the late nineteenth and early twentieth centuries.[247] With this development, modern Egypt no longer resembled Roman Egypt. The moment when net exports began to drop beneath what the ancient rate was likely to have been (see above, section 5.5.1), its population must have exceeded the maximum figure that is conceivable for antiquity (see below, section 5.6). By the 1910s, the expansion of cerealiculture had run out of steam, if only for the time being. Egypt became a net importer of cereals around the year 1900,[248] when the population reached ten million. In the early 1900s, Egypt imported wheat and maize flour from USA and Australia but the country was still 'largely' able to feed itself.[249]

5.6. *Carrying capacity and population size: models for ancient and modern Egypt*

Given the dearth of reliable evidence, there are only two opportunities to construct quantitative models for a time when the demographic profile and the subsistence agriculture of modern Egypt were still reasonably similar to the Roman period, namely, for 1844 and the 1870s. First, I present calculations for nineteenth-century Egypt as it was. In a second step, with the necessary modifications, these data are applied to Roman Egypt. This exercise will suggest a range of possible scenarios for Roman Egypt which, if nothing else, will help define the margins of the plausible.

Some uncertainty is introduced into these reconstructions by the necessity, for computational purposes, to treat total output (of all basic food crops) as though it referred to wheat. However, we may derive some comfort from the fact that the evidence from 1870s Egypt suggests a close fit between total output and wheat equivalent (see below). Moreover, a substantial part of the cultivated area in Roman Egypt would have been devoted to the production of leguminous crops in addition to grain. Beans, which were so important in the early modern era, may have played a comparable role in antiquity.[250] There is also some evidence of bean exports from Egypt to Italy,[251] which might make us wonder whether the reported figures

[247] Source: Owen (1969) 308 tab. 58.
[248] Owen (1969) 309.
[249] Tignor (1984) 25, 27.
[250] Cf. Theophrastus, *Historia Plantarum* 11.3, on Egyptian beans.
[251] Garnsey (1998) 242.

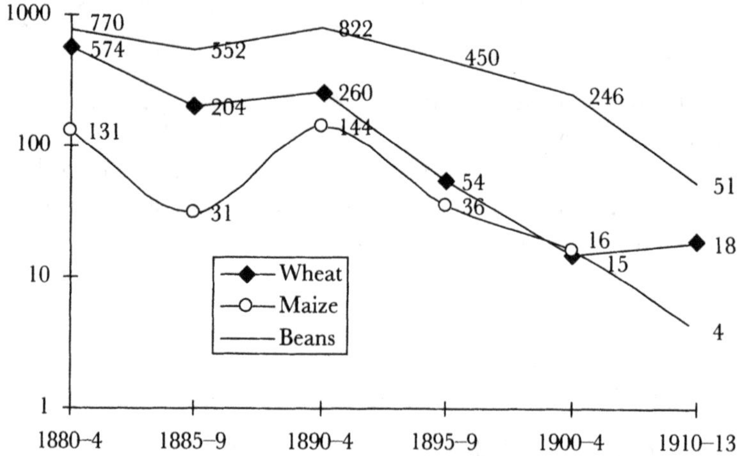

Figure 3.5 Value of Egyptian exports of wheat, maize and beans (in 1,000 Egyptian pounds; logarithmic scale)

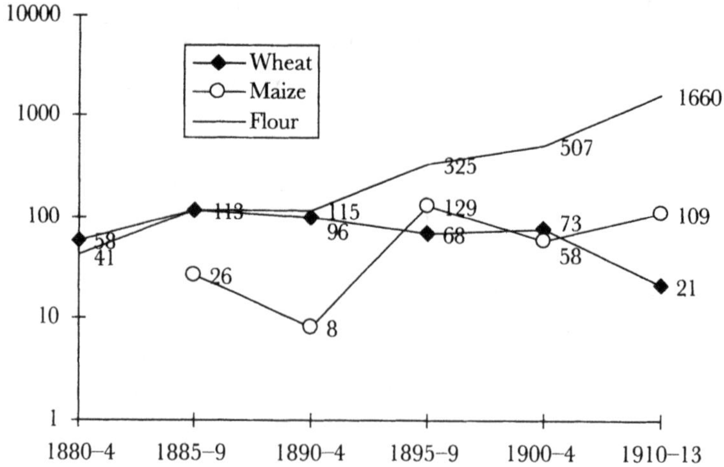

Figure 3.6 Value of Egyptian imports of wheat, maize and beans (in 1,000 Egyptian pounds; logarithmic scale)

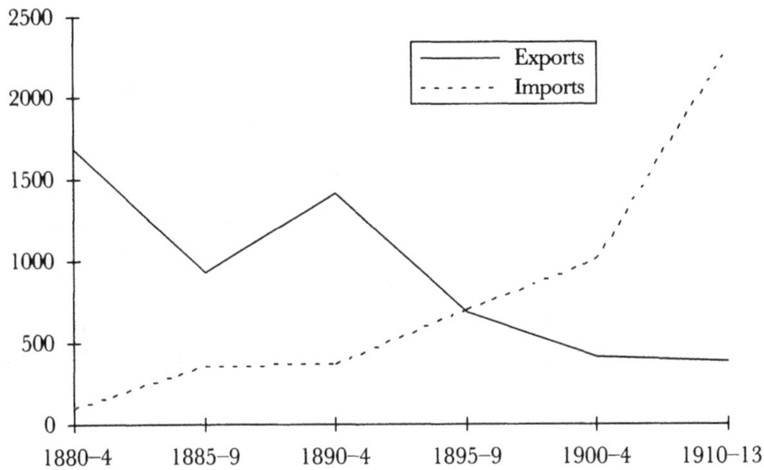

Figure 3.7 Value of Egyptian trade in cereals and flour (in 1,000 Egyptian pounds)

for wheat shipments to Rome actually exclusively pertained to grain or perhaps included a share of other crops as well.

According to the survey of 1844, Egypt produced, under optimum conditions, 12.25 to thirteen million ardebs of foodstuffs.[252] If ten per cent were set aside for seed and with annual exports of 0.8 to 0.9 million ardebs, between 10.125 and 10.9 million ardebs were available for local consumption, or 2.005 to 2.158 billion litres at 198 litres/ardeb. This was enough to feed 6.45 to 7.2 million people at 300 to 310 litres a year. If the population was about 5.25 million, between one-fifth and one-quarter of the available produce would have been disposable surplus, without, however, being exported.[253] This supports the assumption that the 1844 count does not reflect an average harvest. As a *mean* rate, it is more readily compatible with the situation around 1860 or so.

As we have seen, the situation in the middle of the nineteenth century was in crucial respects not greatly different from antiquity. Moreover, in 1844, 7.5 per cent of the total area under cultivation

[252] The difference between these two figures reflects the different reported totals; see above, section 5.4.

[253] It should be noted, however, that some of the surplus was stored for future export, such as the two million ardebs of grain reputedly kept in government warehouses in 1840: Rivlin (1961) 155.

was given over to cotton and rice. Assuming that part of this area was available for basin cultivation in the Roman period, the area of arable might have been slightly larger then. If we retain, for the sake of argument, the lower figure for 1844 Egypt of 12.25 million ardebs as a possible mean for Roman Egypt (taking into account the absence of cotton and rice but reckoning with lower yields per feddan), up to 16,100 km^2 (or 5.827 million arouras) may have been cultivated in antiquity,[254] and we arrive at the following results: 12.25 million ardebs equal 2.426 billion litres; subtracting ten per cent for seed and 130 to 260 million litres for export (see above, section 5.5.1), the people of Roman Egypt could have disposed of 1.923 to 2.053 billion litres of foodstuffs, enough to feed 6.2 to 6.85 million people at 300 to 310 litres a year.

The value of this calculation is dubious, mainly because we do not know how inflated the 1844 figures are. We must however remember that in any case, in 1844 the population was still in a state of depression owing to the severe demographic checks of the previous decade and that the carrying capacity of the land, given sufficient labour input, would therefore necessarily have been higher than the actual output of that year would suggest (if it were known). In other words, the situation ten, fifteen or even twenty years later, when the 1844 production figures would have more closely matched the actual size of the population of Egypt, may well have resembled that of Roman Egypt at the peak of its demographic development. At the very least, a figure of over five million is entirely compatible with this estimate, and a figure of over six million seems possible.

The more daring might want to go a step further. If we turn to Egypt in the mid-1870s, probably the last point in time when a comparison with ancient Egypt may still make sense, we find that at that time, the country produced some fourteen million ardebs, or 2.72 billion litres, of foodstuffs. Subtracting ten per cent for seed, we are left with 2.495 billion litres, 0.25 billion (1.267 million ardebs) of which were, on average, exported every year. The remaining 2.245 billion litres would have fed a population of 7.375 million people,[255] at a rate of 304 litres per person and year. As it happens, this calculation tends to corroborate both my population estimate for the 1870s and the reported figures of total output.

---

[254] 3,569,479 feddans arable plus 268,621 feddans under cotton and rice in 1844 = 3,838,100 feddans.

[255] The mean of my scenarios I and II above, Tab. 3.4.

304 litres of wheat equivalent correspond closely to the 8 artabas (310 litres) or so of wheat that may be taken to represent the annual dietary requirements of the average inhabitant of ancient Egypt.[256] This amount equals about 240 kg of wheat, roughly the minimum annual intake for hot regions.[257] 310 litres of wheat provide consumers with 2,090 calories a day; 304 litres yield 2,050 calories. This compares well with data from developing countries around 1960, such as 2,030 calories per day and person in Pakistan and 2,050 in India. Estimated daily rates could be as low as 1,875 calories (Haiti); Egypt, at that time, had improved to 2,340 calories, but was more developed than it had been in the nineteenth century.[258] In the nineteenth century, chronic malnourishment was far from unusual among Egyptian peasants and the poor;[259] conditions were hardly better in antiquity.[260]

By the mid-1870s, about one-sixth of the cultivated land had been taken over by cotton. If we raise actual output by twenty per cent to account for a hypothetical scenario in which all available land had been devoted to the production of foodstuffs, total possible output rises to 3.326 billion litres. Subtracting seed and (ancient) exports, 2.733 to 2.863 billion litres could have supported 8.8 to 9.55 million people at 300 to 310 litres a head. This gives us what one might call a 'theoretical absolute maximum' for Roman Egypt. Of course, not all the land available for cultivation in the 1870s need have been available in antiquity, especially in the northern Delta. Moreover, farmers operated a system of crop rotation that permitted them to grow cereals and cotton in alternating years. In this, cereal production would also benefit from irrigation, and produce higher yields than from inundation alone. Thus, perennial irrigation in the Delta probably gave a boost to cereal cultivation on a scale unknown to the Roman period.[261] As a result, total output in Roman times must

[256] See most recently van Minnen (1997) 21, with discussion. Rathbone (1990) 108 and 139 n. 18 reckons with an average annual intake of 8.3 artabas (322 litres), a daily requirement of 2,200 calories, possibly somewhat too much in the light of the comparative evidence cited below. Cf. also Crawford (1979) 144.

[257] Clark and Haswell (1970) 83.

[258] Clark and Haswell (1970) 81–2 tab. 15. Around 1930, the traditional ration for a widow yielded 2,672 to 2,848 calories a day in unprocessed cereals; after processing, the actual intake would have been lower: Jagailloux (1986) 265. For further comparative material from modern Egypt, cf. van Minnen (1997) 21 nn. 79–80.

[259] Cf. Jagailloux (1986) 266. For a general appraisal of chronic malnourishment in western Europe in the eighteenth and nineteenth centuries, cf. Fogel forthcoming.

[260] See Garnsey (1999) ch. 3–4.

[261] However, Kees (1955) 37 n. 5 notes that even in 1937, the maximum yield of

have fallen short of the 'theoretical absolute maximum' derived from the 1870s data.

In an attempt to correct for the likely discrepancy between ancient and modern landuse, we might adopt the actual output of foodstuffs in the mid-1870s as the maximum for the Roman period. In this scenario, 2.235 to 2.365 billion litres would have been available after subtracting seed and exports, providing sustenance for 7.2 to 7.9 million people. This result is about one million higher than the range established on the basis of the 1844 data, therein reflecting the intervening expansion of modern Egyptian agriculture.

Whether, in terms of the production of foodstuffs, Roman Egypt was more similar to Egypt in the 1840s, 1850s, 1860s or 1870s is hard to decide. Our ignorance of the conditions in antiquity is highlighted by the fact that on the basis of comparative evidence, we cannot tell whether the theoretical maximum was closer to seven than to nine million people. Margins of uncertainty like these are characteristic of estimates of maximum population size based on carrying capacity.

6. *From modern to ancient Egypt*

In what respects was ancient agriculture different from nineteenth-century farming? Did early modern land reclamation and perennial irrigation really make a significant difference? Basin irrigation had not changed from the Roman period.[262] Mechanical water-lifting devices were already known in the Roman period.[263] The most basic instrument, the *shaduf*, a counterweighted pole with a bucket suspended from the light end, had by then long been familiar. More sophisticated devices such as water-screws (Archimedian screws), compartmented wheels, bucket chains and pot garlands were also in

wheat on 'old' basin land was up to sixty per cent higher than average Egyptian yields. Thus, the overall benefits accruing from perennial irrigation should not be overrated.

[262] For a brief recent survey, see Bonneau (1989). Bonneau (1993) 119–234 discusses the administration of water management in Graeco-Roman Egypt; see 201–8 on basin irrigation. On the different types of irrigation in modern Egypt, see above, section 5.1.

[263] Oleson (1984) is the most comprehensive study to date; see 126–71 for an overview of the papyrological evidence. See also Bonneau (1993) 93–115.

use.[264] Even *saqiya*-driven water-lifting devices were known, often driven by animals.[265] Vineyards, orchards and vegetable gardens required perennial irrigation.[266]

Of course, the fact that such devices were in use tells us little about how common they were. Their efficiency would vary: papyrological sources suggest for individual irrigation devices an irrigated area from one-half of an aroura to twelve arouras.[267] The employment of human as opposed to animal labour made a great difference: in the late nineteenth century, according to one observer, a *saqiya* driven by a pair of oxen could irrigate two to two-and-a-half hectares, while one operated by two men working in spells only supplied half an hectare.[268] Barois estimated that in the late 1880s, 28,000 *saqiya* gear devices were in use in Lower Egypt.[269] The corresponding number for the Roman period is unknown, but it seems likely that in the absence of the profitable business of cotton cultivation (the main driving force behind these irrigation works), it would have been significantly smaller.[270] Moreover, by 1873, some 500 steam-pumps were in use in Egypt.[271]

The scope of agricultural development in the northern Delta and the Fayum is also of some importance. It seems that the relative share of the Delta in the population rose from the Ptolemaic period onward. The colonisation of the northernmost Delta and part of the littoral began under the Saites and the Ptolemies. Growth continued under the Romans and beyond but was finally checked and partly reversed in the early Middle Ages through the subsidence of the northernmost Delta by a rising sea level and autocompaction.[272] We may therefore assume that *some* (but how much?) of nineteenth-century

[264] For evidence and discussion, see Oleson (1984) 291–301, esp. 300 (water-screw), 325–50, esp. 349 (compartmented wheel), 350–70, esp. 369 (bucket chain and pot garland).

[265] Oleson (1984) 370–85, esp. 385. The *saqiya* gear is a drive system to be attached to compartmented wheels or bucket chains; it was expensive because of the personnel, livestock and parts required.

[266] Rowlandson (1996) 19.

[267] Oleson (1984) 368.

[268] Oleson (1984) 369.

[269] Barois (1889) 76–8.

[270] Bagnall (1993) 17 notes that in the Roman period, 'true canal irrigation' was limited to the Fayum.

[271] Owen (1981b) 534.

[272] See Butzer (1976) 95–6 on the development of the Delta.

land reclamation, which focused on the often saline, heavy clay soils of the northern Delta, merely recovered ground that had been lost since the Roman period.[273]

The situation in the Fayum is perhaps even more intriguing. The Ptolemies expanded cultivation to about 1,300 km^2 and the region clearly thrived in the early Roman period.[274] There is little doubt that in the eighteenth century, the Fayum had but a shadow of its former prosperity,[275] and even as late as in 1971, a study of the Hellenistic Fayum could refer to 'an extensive irrigation system in land now sanded over' and more generally evoke 'the circle of villages, abandoned to the desert, which surrounds the present area of cultivation'.[276] Because of the Fayum's dependence on irrigation, yields varied more than in the Nile valley; thus, while some land in the Fayum must have been the most productive in the Roman empire, other parts were never particularly profitable.[277]

In the Roman period, flood levels seem to have been high, and, as a result, farming was capable of sustaining a larger population than under less favourable ecological circumstances.[278] Evidence of three-year rotation systems with two years of cereals, and of multiple cropping, cited above, leaves no doubt that in some areas at least, ancient Egyptian agriculture was not inferior to nineteenth-century farming. However, it will never be possible to convert these qualitative impressions into a quantitative assessment which alone could narrow down our estimates of carrying capacity and population size. At most, they do not give us any strong reason to assume that total output in antiquity would necessarily have fallen short of

---

[273] Cf. Bagnall (1993) 19: 'Only the northernmost part of the Delta was uninhabitable. It is difficult to be sure how much of the Delta's total area was usable for agriculture, but in late antiquity it may have amounted to twice the arable land of the upper valley.'

[274] Butzer (1976) 93, who reckons with a population maximum in excess of 300,000. On agricultural innovation in the Fayum, see most recently Thompson (1999).

[275] Cf. the travel account by Pococke (1743) 55–67.

[276] Crawford (1971) 109. Kom Talit in the southwestern Fayum is a good example: excavations have revealed many wells and cisterns and a series of water supply and drainage channels dating from the Greco-Roman period in an area which was recently described as a 'lunar landscape' and is only now being cleared for farming: Kirby and Rathbone (1996).

[277] Bagnall (1985) 297, 306.

[278] Roman period: Said (1993) 152–55. The level of the Nile floods has been subject to long-term variation, studied by Popper (1951) and Said (1993) 127–69. Inundations levels were generally rather low from 700 to 1050 or so, with very low minima between 680 and 880: Popper (1951) 182 graph 5; cf. Said (1993) 162.

the rates attained around the middle of the nineteenth century.

This impression receives support from the demographic evidence, which tells against overly pessimistic appraisals of ancient population size. There is no doubt that the figures reported for much of the nineteenth century, and also some of the corrections advocated in modern scholarship, are too low. Even at a time of severe depression, the population of Egypt never dropped far below five million. Furthermore, given the extraordinary combination of plague, cholera, smallpox and physical dislocation that had checked population growth for a long time but markedly peaked in the 1830s, population figures during the first half of the nineteenth century, such as they can be determined, are *not* representative of the country under conditions of prolonged peace, good governance and a less severe epidemiologic regime. Other demographic parameters of ancient and early modern Egypt can be shown to be quite similar. Thus, we may conclude that *ceteris paribus*, the population of Roman Egypt could very well have been larger than it was at any point during the first half of the nineteenth century.

In this chapter, I have tried to show that it would be a mistake for modern observers to assume, on *a priori* grounds, that the earlier or smaller modern figures of population size are, the more likely they are to reflect conditions in the Roman period. There is also no reason to assume that prior to the last quarter of the nineteenth century or so, the rise of cotton production for export, the spread of perennial irrigation and economic growth in monetary terms had already changed the system of food production in a way that rendered it structurally different from ancient farming. Prior to the last quarter of the nineteenth century, neither the methods of farming, nor the food crops planted, nor the trade flows, nor, by implication, the total volume of output had been transformed sufficiently to set it firmly apart from what may have been achieved in the most prosperous periods of antiquity.

If there is one thing we can be sure of it is that we would be ill-advised to settle for a single figure for the population of Roman Egypt. The ancient numbers are clearly of little value: they are unlikely both to be right—implying as they do 170 per cent growth within 120 years[279]—and given their dubious origin, neither of them

[279] An emendation of Diodorus' figure from three to seven million would remove this problem, sensibly implying annual population growth of slightly over 0.1 per

inspires great confidence. Moreover, the modern evidence issues a stern warning to those who insist on clinging to isolated figures in ancient literature simply because such bits are all we have got: as I have tried to show in the previous sections, official census figures, not to mention quantitative assessments by supposedly well-informed individuals, for much of the nineteenth century regularly and often massively distort reality. These sources proffer conspicuously unrealistic values for population size and agricultural production. The burden of proof rests firmly on the shoulders of anyone who wishes to maintain that ancient numbers, arrived at under unknown circumstances and transmitted in a much more haphazard fashion than any of these modern data, are intrinsically more likely to be accurate than evidence from the early nineteenth century. If those modern counts which are seriously defective could not be tested against more reliable data from the following decades, it would be impossible to prove them wrong. No comparable means of testing ancient figures are available even to the most learned student of Roman Egypt.

Recent scholarship has been dominated by deliberately low estimates of the size of the population of Roman Egypt. In the commendable wish to eschew facile aggrandisement of the object under investigation and with a healthy scepticism towards Josephus' figure, the pendulum may, however, have swung too far in the opposite direction. Rathbone argues for a maximum of five million, whereas Bagnall and Frier settle for a range from four to five million, using 4.5 million for computational purposes.[280] Both studies contain the odd reference to modern data, but neither gives full weight to the implications raised by the demographic and agricultural evidence from the nineteenth century that I have discussed here.[281] Based on this discussion, a deliberately wide range from five to seven million seems a more adequate estimate. There is no reason to assume that

cent, but the very fact that a plausible result can only be obtained by tampering with the sources should in itself be sufficient to discourage us from approaching the question of population size through ancient texts.

[280] Rathbone (1990) 108; Bagnall and Frier (1994) 56, 103. Cf. Bagnall (1993) 175 n. 152, who considers seven million excessive. A preference for five million can be traced back to Beloch (1886) 258.

[281] This, however, is not true of the most recent discussion by van Minnen (1997) 8–62, esp. 34–43, which still awaits publication. After carefully considering the implications of the nineteenth-century evidence, he arrives at a maximum of 7.5 million for the Roman period, if only as 'a convenient model' (40). Lo Cascio (1999) also makes some use of comparative evidence.

the population of Roman Egypt at its apex was smaller than during or immediately after the crisis period from the 1780s to the 1830s. Taking account of a prolonged period of peace, absence of major epidemics and war, and undisrupted governance, the output in basic foodstuffs and the exploitation of marginal land in Roman Egypt need not have fallen short of the levels attested for the third quarter of the nineteenth century.[282] Indeed, it is at least conceivable that under conditions of high fertility, population pressure may have been mounting during the early Roman empire.[283] The strikingly high level of urbanisation in Roman Egypt could well be taken to corroborate this impression.

At the same time, the size of the ancient population is likely to have remained well below the theoretical absolute maximum, which, however, cannot be defined with precision. If pressed for a single figure for the actual population peak in Roman Egypt, six million may be as good a guess as any, if only for computational purposes. In terms of population density and agricultural output, Roman Egypt may well have resembled the country in the 1850s when the plague had already left for good, smallpox had begun to abate and peace and orderly governance had begun to sink in. At that time, the populations of Cairo and Alexandria combined very roughly equalled that of Roman Alexandria, but in the rest of the country, urbanisation had not even come close to ancient levels. With a total population size of six million, between 750,000 and 1,250,000 inhabitants of fifty-odd district capitals,[284] and 500,000 residents in Alexandria, the rate of urbanisation would have been around twenty-five per cent, which is still very considerable but not as forbiddingly high as the rate of thirty-five to forty per cent implied by the estimates of

---

[282] Compare Bowman (1995) 311 (close to seven million?). Issawi (1981) 377, 379 reckons with six to seven million people in Roman Egypt. Cf. also Carrié (1997) 139.

[283] See Frier (1999, 2000, 2001), partly based on Egyptian evidence, on the possibility of overpopulation in the Roman empire. This issue deserves more attention in the future, especially in the light of the abiding infatuation of many ancient historians with the supposed 'depopulation' of the Roman empire: see Scheidel (2001) 36–46, 64–70.

[284] The *metropoleis* of Roman Egypt will be discussed in the forthcoming Leiden doctoral thesis of L. E. Tacoma. His attempt to infer the size of the population of Upper Egypt from the ratio of the number of inhabitants of several nome capitals to the size of these cities' territories yields results that are broadly consistent with the notion of an aggregate urban population of around one million outside Alexandria. This theme will be fully developed in the first chapter of his work. I am grateful to L. E. Tacoma for his permission to refer to his findings in advance of publication.

Rathbone or Bagnall and Frier.[285] Excluding Alexandria, the rate of urbanisation drops to under twenty per cent.

Much hinges on the overall impact of land reclamation in the Delta and the expansion of perennial irrigation, and thus on the question of whether in the years after the death of Muhammad Ali, under the reign of his successors Abbas (1848–54) and Sait (1854–63), Lower Egypt had already become more developed than it had ever been in antiquity. If the answer to this question is affirmative, then we must bid farewell to Josephus' eight or rather nine million even as a merely theoretical option.[286] But even if this question were to remain unsettled, as it probably will, a total of up to nine million is in any case uncomfortably close to what I have found to be plausible absolute theoretical maxima and in excess of less extreme but still fairly optimistic estimates. Josephus' figure must be viewed above all in the specific context of his fictitious speech, which is prone to exaggeration for the purpose of persuading an agitated crowd in what this historian portrays as a matter of life and death for the Jewish people. The audience of King Agrippa, though initially impressed, ultimately remained unconvinced by his representations, and I propose that we follow their example.

7. *Epilogue*

As I have tried to show, agricultural productivity put fairly inelastic constraints on ancient Egyptian population growth. At the same time, and in much the same way as in the early nineteenth century, disease rather than economic performance may well have been the single most crucial determinant of *actual* population size, as opposed to its theoretical ceiling. While we cannot be sure whether by the mid-

[285] The exceptionally high rate of urbanisation advocated, *nolens volens*, by Rathbone and Bagnall and Frier *a priori* casts doubt on low population estimates. See Bowman (1995) 311 (who also considers *c.* twenty-five per cent 'more plausible'); van Minnen (1997) 40–1, esp. 41 n. 168, cf. 47–51; Lo Cascio (1999); cf. also Hopkins (1995/96) 64–5 n. 4.

[286] Josephus Flavius, *Bellum Judaicum* 2.385 claims to have derived his figure of 7.5 million Egyptians outside Alexandria from poll tax data. If that were true, we would need to add not only the population of Alexandria (500,000?) but also adjust the reported tally for the underregistration of male taxpayers as reflected in the village census returns and tax lists (see above, Chapter 2, pp. 156–60). Under those circumstances, a grand total of nine million would be the lowest reasonable estimate.

second century CE, population growth in Roman Egypt had begun to push against ecological limits, rendering its inhabitants vulnerable to Malthusian positive checks, there are strong indications that sudden exogenous changes in the disease environment disrupted any demographic-economic equilibrium that may by then have developed. Taken together, the apparent severity of the 'Antonine plague' of the 160s CE, the doubling of commodity prices between the 160s and the 190s CE, shifts from arable cultivation to arboriculture, and an increase in real wages coupled with a decline of real land rents and land prices after the 160s CE suggest that due to the pandemic, Roman Egypt experienced a demographic contraction that had still not been fully overcome an entire century after the first outbreak and/or was prolonged by subsequent epidemic events, above all in the 250s and 260s CE.[287] As a result, for at least part of the Roman period, actual Egyptian population size must have fallen short of its sustainable maximum by a considerable margin.

This observation underscores once more the pivotal role of mortality, and hence disease, in demographic development. On the basis of more recent comparative evidence, mortality has been identified as the most important exogenous determinant of demographic growth, which is itself inextricably intertwined with pre-industrial economic development in general.[288] In this book, I have arged that even under conditions of very high mortality overall, such as in Egypt from antiquity to the early twentieth century, patterns of infectious disease and therefore mortality can be expected to vary and did indeed vary significantly over time and space within a single region that has

[287] On the severity of the epidemic, see above, p. 162; for the epidemics of the mid-third century, see Zinsser (1935) 138–41. The 'structural doubling of prices'—as a sudden jump rather than a gradual increase—has been documented by Rathbone (1997), who relates it to 'unprecedented economic dislocation (. . .) caused by the Antonine plague' (215). Comparative evidence for the short-term repercussions of the 'Black Death' in fourteenth-century Europe supports this interpretation (e.g., Herlihy (1997) 46–7). For the contraction of arable land together with an expansion in wine and fruit cultivation in a village in the Fayum between 159 and 216 CE, see Sharp (1999). Again, similar developments are attested for late medival Europe (e.g., Gottfried (1983) 135–45). The development of real wages (in this case, the ratio of nominal daily and monthly wages to nominal grain, wine and oil prices) and of land rents and values from the second to the third centuries CE can tentatively be reconstructed from the data in Drexhage (1991) and Rathbone (1991, 1997), although the paucity and unbalanced geographical and chronological distribution of the evidence injects a fair amount of uncertainty into any such attempt: for a provisional model, see Scheidel (forthcoming b), responding to Bagnall (2000).

[288] Lee (1986).

traditionally best been known for its seemingly high degree of ecological uniformity and relatively slow pace of developmental change over several millennia. The fortunes of Egypt fluctuated accordingly.

What is true of Egypt is also likely to be true of other parts of the ancient Mediterranean world. Thus, in his study of malaria, Sallares has been able to relate changes in the character and prevalence of a single seasonal infectious disease to local and chronological variation in the social and economic development of central Italy.[289] Comparable studies of the dissemination and impact of other leading causes of morbidity and mortality are needed to further our understanding of the interaction between the invisible world of microorganisms and the so much more familiar world of human actors. Investigation of the physical reality of disease, instead of its cultural representation, is the only promising way forward.[290] The growing arsenal of biotechnology and the comparativist application of epidemiologic models will be of critical importance in compensating for the shortcomings of the textual sources. As I already observed at the end of an earlier book on ancient demography, the process of putting ancient history in a biological and thus truly interdisciplinary perspective has barely begun.[291]

[289] Sallares (forthcoming).

[290] The work of the late M. D. Grmek, especially Grmek (1989), highlights the potential of informed retrospective diagnosis. For criticism of this approach, see, e.g., Leven (1998). Hope and Marshall, eds. (2000) is a good example of the culturalist approach to the study of ancient mortality.

[291] Scheidel (1996a) 165.

APPENDIX ONE

MONTHS OF DEATH IN EPITAPHS FROM ANCIENT AND MEDIEVAL EGYPT AND NUBIA

1. *Upper Egypt and Nubia*

1.1. *Greek inscriptions*

Thoth: Lefebvre (1907) nos. 86, 102, 126, 133, 140, 292, 296, 322, 442, 612 (= *SB* V 8732); *SB* I 1600, III 6179.

Phaophi: Lefebvre (1907) nos. 96, 119, 123, 144, 220, 244, 256, 260–1, 290, 382 (= *SB* V 8718), 787; *SB* I 732, 3916, III 6186, 6197, 6235, VIII 10067/711.

Hathyr: Lefebvre (1907) nos. 129, 146, 184, 198, 238, 263, 287, 304, 415, 421, 480, 504, 506, 535, 573, 625 (= *SB* V 8721), 634 (= *SB* V 8726), 792, 805; *SB* I 90 = 1020, 1012 (= Bernand [1988] no. 43), 1442, 3912, III 6227, VI 9318 (I), VIII 10055/679, 10056/685.

Choiak: Lefebvre (1907) nos. 70, 94, 117, 242, 252, 271, 284, 300, 303, 319, 330, 346, 396, 398, 453, 478, 567, 622 (= *SB* 8736), 642, 648 (= *SB* V 8733), 650, 652 (= *SB* V 8737), 664–5; *SB* I 3908, 3949 (= *I.Fay.* I 43), III 6035 = V 8765, 6201, 6230, 6830, IV 7428, V 8241, 8758 = 8948, VIII 10056/684, 10059.

Tybi: Lefebvre (1907) nos. 80, 121, 125, 211, 239, 246, 259, 282, 294, 298, 308, 311, 345, 391, 410, 454, 457, 462, 467, 476, 482, 507, 564, 620, 623, 804; *SB* I 89 (= Bernand [1988] no. 106), 1561–2, 3911, 3913, 5758, V 8239, 8369, VIII 10022, 10055/680, XIV 12147.

Mecheir: Lefebvre (1907) nos. 97, 100, 103–04, 169, 248, 323–4, 349, 407, 437, 444, 495, 510, 578, 619, 795; *SB* I 118 (= Bernand [1988] no. 136), 724, 1197, 3907, 5467, V 8237–8.

Phamenoth: Lefebvre (1907) nos. 88, 101, 134, 150, 171, 173, 205, 265, 307, 309, 312, 332, 340, 445, 450, 459, 481, 511, 516, 525, 566, 575–7, 626, 629, 653, 659–60, 663, 666 (= *SB* I 5716), 668; *SB* I 4013 (= *I.Fay.* I 51), III 6190, 6192, V 7564, 7883, 8370, VIII 10047(g), 10058, X 10515, 10705.

Pharmouthi: Lefebvre (1907) nos. 76, 81, 85, 95, 107, 112, 151, 174, 176, 187, 195, 202, 217, 249, 253, 257, 297, 326, 336, 406, 426, 485, 489, 494, 503, 514, 517, 540, 582, 635–6, 649, 786; *SB* I 726 (= *I.Fay.* I 36), 1564, 3914, 5100, III 6133, 6188–9, 6198, VIII 10047(c–d), X 10517.

Pachon: Lefebvre (1907) nos. 135, 155, 177, 185, 190, 196, 208, 232, 258, 270, 275, 280, 316, 422, 466, 512, 520, 524, 541, 558, 581, 607 (= *SB* V 8730), 609, 621 (= *SB* V 8719); *SB* I 106 (= Bernand [1988] no. 124), 3915, III 6187, 6191, IV 7305, 7432, V 8316, VIII 10047(b, e), X 10516.

Pauni: Lefebvre (1907) nos. 77, 111, 137, 183, 194, 206, 215, 255, 273, 279, 289, 293, 301, 314–5, 402, 404, 432, 496, 624, 627, 655–6, 661–2; *SB* III 6193–4, 6199, 6229, V 8367; *SEG* XXXVIII 1689.

Epeiph: Lefebvre (1907) nos. 105, 136, 147, 251, 267, 276, 328, 381, 385, 427, 456, 491, 502, 549, 579, 606 (= *SB* 8729), 645 (= *SB* I 5826); *SB* I 121, 727 (= *I.Fay.* I 41), 3909, III 6200, 7190, V 8366, VIII 10055/681; *I.Fay.* III 198, 216.

Mesore: Lefebvre (1907) nos. 142, 170, 207, 213, 218, 266, 321, 335, 413, 479, 528, 568; *SB* I 107 (= Bernand [1988] no. 125), 1565, 5020, V 8763, 8937, VIII 10059, 10067/710; *I.Fay.* I 59.

Added days: Lefebvre (1907) nos. 240, 443; *SB* I 729, V 8368.

1.2. *Coptic inscriptions*

Thoth: *KSB* I 468, 483–4, 500, 503, 526–7, 538, 549, 570–1, 576, 581, 606, 609, 611, 685, 695, 705, 714, 722, 735, 764; Crum and Bell (1922) no. 31; Monneret de Villard (1933) nos. 16, 33, 42, 79, 81, 100, 105, 132, 145, 154, 189, 199; Kubinska (1974) nos. 7, 13.

Phaophi: *KSB* I 464, 468, 490, 512, 558, 629, 703, 737, 749, 776; Crum and Bell (1922) no. 46; Monneret de Villard (1933) nos. 5, 30, 66, 102, 111, 136, 182, 219; Bachatly (1965) no. 139.

Hathyr: *KSB* I 443, 460, 519, 524, 532, 542, 544, 547, 569, 573, 599, 614, 618, 717, 468, 736; Crum (1902) nos. 8442, 8571, 8652; Monneret de Villard (1933) nos. 2, 8, 14, 70, 95, 99, 116–17; Kubinska (1974) no. 8.

Choiak: *KSB* I 439, 452, 468, 470, 480–1, 504, 516, 550, 563, 578, 605, 620, 654, 696, 708, 718, 721, 741, 744, 757, 792, 794; Crum (1902) nos. 8459, 8462, 8499, 8505, 8578; Crum and Bell (1922) no. 42; Monneret de Villard (1933) nos. 32, 47, 50, 52, 62, 90, 104, 119–20, 122, 166, 169; Kubinska (1974) pp. 54–9 (not numbered).

Tybi: *KSB* I 458, 473, 475, 479–80, 520, 556, 568, 582, 590, 627, 750, 765, 768, 790; Crum (1902) nos. 8396, 8448; Monneret de Villard (1933) nos. 21, 24, 27, 31, 34, 53, 65, 96, 133, 148, 160, 171, 190, 195, 198; Bachatly (1965) no. 11; Kubinska (1974) nos. 4, 11.

Mecheir: *KSB* I 468, 471, 499, 513, 517, 525, 537, 551, 554, 557, 579–80, 587, 592, 610, 613, 631, 694, 697, 739, 743, 748; Crum (1902) nos. 8432, 8584; Crum and Bell (1922) no. 37; Monneret de Villard (1933) nos. 51, 82, 92, 108, 113, 118, 123, 126, 135, 138–9, 143, 147, 170; Bachatly (1965) no. 28.

Phamenoth: *KSB* I 427, 468, 476, 486–7, 505, 514–5, 528, 539, 559–60, 588, 600, 603, 612, 686, 734, 740, 745, 759, 766–7, 781; Crum and Bell (1922) nos. 35, 44 (?); Monneret de Villard (1933) nos. 9, 17, 80, 97, 101, 128–9, 150, 176, 202, 205.

Pharmouthi: *KSB* I 462, 468, 477, 506, 529, 535, 546, 552, 589, 596, 602, 610, 622, 677–8, 680, 683–4, 691, 696, 743, 747, 770, 773, 780, 782, 793; Crum (1902) nos. 8441, 8464, 8626–7, 8698; Crum and Bell (1922) nos. 29, 30, 38, 43, 44 (?), 63; Monneret de Villard (1933) nos. 10, 12, 28–9, 36, 63, 89, 93–4, 110, 121, 124, 131, 134, 155, 167, 196, 201, 207, 210, 218; Bachatly (1965) no. 43; Kubinska (1974) nos. 10, 12.

Pachon: *KSB* I 429, 455, 465, 472, 507, 522, 530, 564, 585, 601, 604, 617, 690, 746, 774, 791; Crum (1902) nos. 8325, 8607, 8632; Crum and Bell (1922) nos. 61, 64; Monneret de Villard (1933) nos. 3, 4, 6, 13, 15, 25, 45, 49, 61, 68, 72, 75, 78, 107, 125, 130, 142, 146, 152, 163, 185, 192, 212, 222; Kubinska (1974) pp. 54–9 (not numbered).

Pauni: *KSB* I 436, 463, 467–8, 478, 501, 545, 553, 555, 567, 572, 577, 597, 607, 682, 689, 760, 762, 771; Crum (1902) nos. 8423, 8481, 8490, 8510; Monneret de Villard (1933) nos. 1, 7, 20, 23, 38, 55–7, 60, 67, 69, 73, 84–6, 88, 91, 112, 140, 153, 156, 158–9, 172–3, 175, 177, 179–81, 183, 186, 188, 197, 203, 214, 221; Kubinska (1974) nos. 3, 9.

Epeiph: *KSB* I 426, 428, 469, 510–11, 518, 531, 533, 536, 584, 591, 614, 616, 687, 707, 719, 769, 772; Crum (1902) no. 8418; Monneret de Villard (1933) nos. 11, 16, 19, 26, 39–40, 46, 58, 64, 74, 77, 83, 98, 106, 109, 114, 127, 157, 168, 184, 187, 193, 215–16; Kubinska (1974) no. 6 and pp. 54–9 (not numbered).

Mesore: *KSB* I 434, 488, 502, 523, 534, 541, 548, 561, 575, 594, 608, 624, 637, 641, 695, 738, 761, 783, 793; Crum (1902) no. 8553; Monneret de Villard (1933) nos. 35, 37, 41, 43–4, 48, 54, 59, 71, 87, 103, 141, 151, 161–2, 200, 206, 220; Bachatly (1965) nos. 55, 82; Kubinska (1974) no. 5 and pp. 54–9 (not numbered).

1.3. *Mummy labels*

Thoth: *SB* I 3851 (4th), *SB* I 3462 (6th), *CEML* 131 (7th), *CEML* 169 (8th), *SB* V 7731 (8th), *CEML* 439 (12th), *CEML* 624 (22nd), *CEML* 193, 197 (24th), *CEML* 108 (27th).

Phaophi: *CEML* 955 (4th), *CEML* 1208 (20th), *CEML* 183 (24th), *SB* I 3876 (25th), *CEML* 210 (26th), *CEML* 209 (30th), *CEML* 697 (no day).

Hathyr: *CEML* 105 (5th), *CEML* 803 (15th), *SB* I 790 (25th), *CEML* 191 (28th).

Choiak: *SB* I 1203, 5487 (4th), *SB* X 10382 (8th), Wilfong (1995) no. 25 (11th), *SB* VI 9240 (12th), *CEML* 994 (21st), *SB* I 5538 (26th), *SB* I 2632 (no day).

Tybi: *SB* I 5699 (1st), *SB* VI 9240 = XIV 12104 (12th), *CEML* 1203 (18th), *SB* I 5482 (20th), *SB* I 784 (24th).

Mecheir: *SB* I 5467 (1st), *CEML* 329 (3rd), *CEML* 505 (10th), *SB* I 1197 (11th), *CEML* 173, 1029 (14th), *CEML* 196 (15th), *CEML* 230 (18th), *CEML* 345 (27th), *SB* III 7115 (29th), *SB* I 5772 (no day).

Phamenoth: *CEML* 1058 (4th), *SB* I 5060 (4th), *CEML* 1154 (5th), *CEML* 172 (14th), *CEML* 916 (26th).

Pharmouthi: *SB* X 10390 (2nd), *CEML* 164 (3rd), Wilfong (1995) no. 1 (8th), *CEML* 449 (9th), *SB* I 5387, 5394 = 5445, 5397 (21st), *SB* III 7124 (23rd), *CEML* 563 (24th), *CEML* 797 (25th), *CEML* 295 (29th), *SB* III 7043 (29th).

Pachon: Wilfong (1995) no. 21 (3rd), *SB* III 6007 (8th), *CEML* 184, 796 (11th), *CEML* 1039 (12th), *SB* I 5372 (12th), *CEML* 419 (20th), *CEML* 851 (22nd), *SB* I 3884 (22nd), *CEML* 139 (24th), *CEML* 1069 (26th), *CEML* 1135 (28th), *CEML* 188, 418 (no day), *SB* XIV 11990 (no day).

Pauni: *CEML* 280 (14th), *SB* III 7079 (16th), *CEML* 620 (24th), *SB* I 5623, III 7066 (25th), *SB* III 7101 (26th), *CEML* 159–60 (27th), *CEML* 143 (28th), *SB* I 3843 (28th), Walker and Bierbrier (1997) no. 241 (28th), *CEML* 288 (29th), *CEML* 470 (30th), *CEML* 117 (no day), *SB* I 4236, 5470, VI 9602/10 (no day).

Epeiph: *CEML* 147 (1st), *SB* I 3522 (8th), *CEML* 678, 693 (12th), *CEML* 664, 692 (15th), *CEML* 971 (21st), *SB* I 1194 (22nd), *CEML* 854 (23rd), *CEML* 149 (30th), *CEML* 70, 373 (no day), *SB* I 3553, 5425 (no day).

Mesore: *CEML* 213 (3rd), *SB* I 1198 (3rd), *CEML* 844, 1021 (4th), *CEML* 1188 (6th), *SB* X 10477 (6th), *CEML* 246 (9th), *SB* I 1196 (9th), *CEML* 168, 1006 (10th), *CEML* 145 (11th), *CEML* 251 (13th), *SB* I 1173, 1201, III 7058 (15th), *SB* I 802, 1202 (17th), *SB* I 1195 (25th), *CEML* 487, 688, 809 (no day), *SB* I 4185, 4238 (no day).

Added days: *SB* I 3931 (4th)

2. *Lower Egypt (Greek inscriptions)*

Thoth: Lefebvre (1907) nos. 11, 14, 50; *SB* I 11, 1415, III 6166, 6985, 7254, VIII 9996/861, 10162/533; *SFK* 35, 131; Hooper (1961) nos. 50, 118; Wagner (1996) no. 29.

Phaophi: Lefebvre (1907) nos. 3, 23–4; *SB* I 720, IV 7314, 7471, V 8099, 8101, 8792, VIII 9996/871, 10162/514. 519. 522–3; *SEG* XLII 1586, 1589, 1595; *SFK* 61, 115, 118, 126, 141; Hooper (1961) nos. 14, 46, 58, 89; El-Nassery and Wagner (1978) nos. 2, 31; Wagner (1994a) no. 23; Wagner (1996) no. 1.

Hathyr: Lefebvre (1907) nos. 6, 12, 58, 65; *SB* I 313, 695, III 6160–1, 6652, IV 7292, V 8102, VIII 9673(c), 9996/873. 875, 10162/527–8. 577–8.

589. 597. 601; *SEG* XL 1582, XLI 1664, XLII 1531; *SFK* 18, 92; Hooper (1961) nos. 21, 57, 70, 72, 78, 98, 124; Wagner (1972) no. 5; El-Nassery and Wagner (1978) nos. 30, 34, 43; Wagner (1996) nos. 46, 56, 103.

Choiak: Lefebvre (1907) nos. 13, 32; *SB* I 612, 703, 717, 5034, III 6167, 6170, 6250, 6255, 6646, 7255, V 7801, VIII 10162/515. 524. 534. 547; *SFK* 35, 37, 94; Hooper (1961) nos. 36, 62, 79, 88, 92; El-Nassery and Wagner (1978) nos. 3, 5, 53; Wagner (1996) nos. 19, 25, 69.

Tybi: Lefebvre (1907) nos. 4, 8, 16, 39, 68; *SB* I 619, 698, 704, 721, III 6162, 6165, IV 7295, VIII 9673(b), 9996/862, 10162/512. 520. 529. 536. 549. 560–1. 573; *SFK* 116–17; Hooper (1961) nos. 32, 38, 43, 66, 113–14, 188; El-Nassery and Wagner (1978) nos. 15, 32; Wagner (1994a) nos. 26, 33; Wagner (1996) no. 9.

Mecheir: Lefebvre (1907) nos. 1, 29, 62, 63 (= *SB* V 8720); *SB* I 707, 1163, 1641, 5013, 5025, 5035, 5056, III 6163, 6647, VIII 9996/863, 10162/513. 521. 525. 543. 562, 10698; *SFK* 140; Hooper (1961) nos. 107, 129, 139, 156; El-Nassery and Wagner (1978) nos. 1, 39, 41; Wagner (1996) nos. 12, 16, 21, 102.

Phamenoth: Lefebvre (1907) nos. 48 (= *SB* I 1540), 65, 66 (= *SB* I 2040); *SB* I 9, 337 = 389, 2646, 3944, III 6232, VIII 10162/530. 539. 552; *SEG* XXXVIII 1851, XLII 1600; *SFK* 2, 60, 67; Hooper (1961) nos. 47, 175, 189; Wagner (1996) no. 73.

Pharmouthi: Lefebvre (1907) nos. 2, 22; *SB* I 351, 1642, III 6233, IV 7296, 7311, VIII 9673(a), 10162/540. 559. 593; *SEG* XL 1585; *SFK* 33, 58, 91, 119; Hooper (1961) nos. 63, 108, 187; Wagner (1996) no. 64.

Pachon: Lefebvre (1907) no. 10; *SB* I 337 = 389, 2126, 5026, 5047, III 6234, 6249, 6656, VIII 9996/866, 10162/518. 537; *SFK* 127; Hooper (1961) nos. 10, 33; Wagner (1994a) no. 35.

Pauni: Lefebvre (1907) nos. 5, 59 (= *SB* IV 7372); *SB* I 409, 2028, 2131, 5019, III 6168, 6649, 6651, 7255, IV 7291, V 7781, 8960, VIII 10162/516. 531. 542. 544. 570. 599. 627; *SFK* 5; Hooper (1961) nos. 13, 30, 34, 82, 101, 159; Wagner (1972) nos. 9–10; El-Nassery and Wagner (1978) nos. 6, 56; Wagner (1996) nos. 3, 34, 87, 89.

Epeiph: Lefebvre (1907) nos. 7, 56; *SB* I 609, 692, 696–7, III 6164, 6657, 7255, V 8125, VIII 10045, 10162/545–6. 550. 628; Hooper (1961) nos. 55, 112, 120, 178; El-Nassery and Wagner (1978) no. 8; Wagner (1994a) nos. 6, 22; Wagner (1996) no. 91.

Mesore: Lefebvre (1907) no. 9; *SB* III 6169, 6987, IV 7294, V 7837, 8103, VIII 10162/517. 538. 551; *SFK* 149; Hooper (1961) nos. 44, 59; El-Nassery and Wagner (1978) no. 7; Wagner (1996) no. 100, 101.

Jewish epitaphs have been republished by Horbury and Noy (1992).

APPENDIX TWO

PERSONS WITH EXACT AGES IN THE CENSUS RETURNS

	Females			Males			Uncertain sex			All		
Age	Vill	Met	All	Vill	Met	All	Vill	Met	All	Vill	Met	All
0	3	1	4	1	4	5	2	–	2	6	5	11
1	5	2	7	8	10	18	–	–	–	13	12	25
2	3	2	5	5	3	8	–	–	–	8	5	13
3	8	3	11	5	6	11	1	–	1	14	9	23
4	9	–	9	6	5	11	–	1	1	15	6	21
5	3	4	7	4	6	10	–	2	2	7	12	19
6	3	3	6	5	6	11	–	–	–	8	9	17
7	–	2	2	1	3	4	–	1	1	1	6	7
8	10	6	16	3	7	10	–	–	–	13	13	26
9	2	2	4	3	8	11	–	–	–	5	10	15
10	6	3	9	3	4	7	–	1	1	9	8	17
11	1	1	2	–	4	4	–	–	–	1	5	6
12	7	1	8	–	2	2	–	–	–	7	3	10
13	6	4	10	–	2	2	1	–	1	7	6	13
14	4	5	9	4	5	9	–	–	–	8	10	18
15	4	4	8	1	3	4	–	–	–	6	6	12
16	8	1	9	3	4	7	–	–	–	12	4	16
17	1	6	7	3	6	9	–	–	–	4	12	16
18	6	2	8	2	5	7	–	–	–	8	7	15
19	3	1	4	4	5	9	–	2	2	7	8	15
20	8	8	16	5	6	11	1	1	2	14	15	29
21	4	2	6	4	7	11	–	–	–	8	9	17
22	1	4	5	3	1	4	–	–	–	4	5	9
23	–	5	5	1	1	2	–	–	–	1	6	7
24	2	2	4	–	4	4	–	1	1	2	7	9
25	6	3	9	1	1	2	–	–	–	7	4	11
26	1	5	6	4	3	7	–	–	–	5	8	13
27	1	1	2	2	1	3	–	–	–	3	2	5
28	–	4	4	2	3	5	–	–	–	2	7	9
29	7	5	12	5	4	9	2	1	3	14	10	24

Table *(cont.)*

	Females			Males			Uncertain sex			All		
Age	Vill	Met	All	Vill	Met	All	Vill	Met	All	Vill	Met	All
30	6	2	8	6	3	9	–	–	–	12	5	17
31	3	1	4	1	4	5	–	–	–	4	5	9
32	5	1	6	3	5	8	–	–	–	8	6	14
33	3	3	6	5	5	10	–	–	–	8	8	16
34	2	1	3	2	2	4	1	2	3	5	5	10
35	7	4	11	5	–	5	–	–	–	12	4	16
36	3	3	6	3	3	6	1	–	1	7	6	13
37	–	–	–	1	1	2	–	–	–	1	1	2
38	7	2	9	1	1	2	–	–	–	8	3	11
39	5	1	6	–	1	1	–	–	–	5	2	7
40	4	2	6	4	3	7	–	–	–	8	5	13
41	–	1	1	1	1	2	–	–	–	1	2	3
42	2	2	4	2	–	2	–	–	–	4	2	6
43	1	2	3	2	2	4	–	–	–	3	4	7
44	2	2	4	4	1	5	–	–	–	6	3	9
45	3	–	3	4	2	6	–	–	–	7	2	9
46	–	–	–	1	2	3	–	–	–	1	2	3
47	2	1	3	4	2	6	–	–	–	6	3	9
48	4	–	4	5	5	10	–	–	–	9	5	14
49	2	2	4	1	1	2	–	–	–	3	3	6
50	2	1	3	4	3	7	–	–	–	6	4	10
51	1	1	2	–	2	2	–	–	–	1	3	4
52	1	1	2	2	–	2				3	1	4
53	2	1	3	–	–	–	–	–	–	2	1	3
54	7	1	8	1	2	3	–	–	–	8	3	11
55	2	1	3	2	–	2	–	–	–	4	1	5
56	1	–	1	3	1	4	–	–	–	4	1	5
57	1	2	3	3	2	5	–	–	–	4	4	8
58	–	–	–	1	–	1	–	–	–	1	–	1
59	1	–	1	2	–	2	–	–	–	3	–	3
60	6	2	8	1	–	1	–	–	–	7	2	9
61	–	–	–	2	2	4	–	–	–	2	2	4
62	–	–	–	–	1	1	–	1	1	–	2	2
63	–	–	–	–	1	1	–	–	–		1	1
64	–	1	1	–	–	–	–	–	–	–	1	1
65	1	1	2	2	–	2	–	–	–	3	1	4
66	–	–	–	2	1	3	–	–	–	2	1	3
67	–	–	–	–	–	–	–	–	–	–	–	–

Table *(cont.)*

Age	Females Vill	Met	All	Males Vill	Met	All	Uncertain sex Vill	Met	All	All Vill	Met	All
68	1	–	1	–	1	1	–	1	1	1	2	3
69	1	–	1	1	–	1	–	–	–	2	–	2
70	3	1	4	3	1	4	–	–	–	6	2	8
71	–	–	–	1	–	1	–	–	–	1	–	1
72	1	1	2	1	1	2	–	–	–	2	2	4
73	–	–	–	1	–	1	–	–	–	1	–	1
74	1	–	1	–	1	1	–	–	–	1	1	2
75	1	–	1	1	–	1	–	–	–	2	–	2
76	–	–	–	1	–	1	–	–	–	1	–	1
77	–	–	–	–	–	–	–	–	–	–	–	–
78	–	1	1	–	–	–	–	1	1	–	2	2
79	–	–	–	–	–	–	–	–	–	–	–	–
80	–	–	–	–	1	1	–	–	–	–	1	1
	216	135	351	179	193	372	9	15	24	403	344	747

Source: This tabulation is based on Bagnall and Frier (1994) 334–6, table A (710 data, corrected according to Bagnall, Frier and Rutherford (1997) 113), with thirty-seven additional data from the addendum to the catalogue of census returns in Bagnall and Frier (1994) 309–12; Nelson (1995) 131–2; Sijpesteijn (1995); Duttenhöfer (1997); *P.Prag.* II 127.

BIBLIOGRAPHY

Abd el-Hafeez abd el-Al, Grenier, J.-C. and Wagner, G. (1985) *Stèles funéraires de Kom Abu Bellou.* Paris

Abd el-Halim Nur el-Din and Pestman, P. W. (1978) 'Demotic mummy labels containing permission for burial', in Boswinkel and Pestman, eds. (1978): 171–89

Abdel-Wahab, M. F. (1982) *Schistosomiasis in Egypt.* Boca Raton

Ablin, R. J., Gonder, M. J. and Immerman, R. S. (1985) 'AIDS: a disease of ancient Egypt?', *New York State Journal of Medicine* 85, 5: 200–01

Adamson, P. B. (1976) 'Schistosomiasis in antiquity', *Medical History* 20: 176–88

—— (1982) 'Human diseases and deaths in the ancient Near East', *Die Welt des Orients* 13: 5–14

—— (1988) 'Dracontiasis in antiquity', *Medical History* 32: 204–09

Alleaume, G. (1999) 'An industrial revolution in agriculture? Some observations on the evolution of rural Egypt in the nineteenth century', in Bowman and Rogan, eds. (1999): 331–45

Allen, P. (1979) 'The "Justinianic" plague', *Byzantion* 49: 5–20

Alpin, P. (1980) *La médecine des Egyptiens par Prosper Alpin 1581–1584.* Paris

Alston, R. (2001) 'Urban population in late Roman Egypt and the end of the ancient world', in Scheidel, ed. (2001): 161–204

Alter, G. and Carmichael, A. (1996) 'Studying causes of death in the past: problems and models', *Historical Methods* 29: 44–8

——, eds. (1997) *Classification of causes of death*, special issue of *Continuity and Change* 12, 2

Andorlini Marcone, I. (1993) 'L'apporto dei papiri alla conoscenza della scienza medica antica', in *Aufstieg und Niedergang der Römischen Welt* II.37.1: 458–562

Andreau, J., Briant, P. and Descat, R., eds. (1997) *Économie antique: prix et formations des prix dans les économies antiques.* Saint-Bertrand-de-Comminges

Antes, J. (1801) *Observations on the manners and customs of the Egyptians, the overflowing of the Nile, with remarks on the plague, and other subjects.* Dublin

Anti-Malarial Commission (1919) *Preliminary report of the Anti-Malarial Commission*, ed. Egyptian Government. Cairo

Anti-Malaria Commission (1928) *Report No. 1 of the Anti-Malaria Commission for the period from 1919 to March 1925*, ed. Anti-Malaria Commission. Cairo

—— (1933) *Report No. 8 of the Anti-Malaria Commission for the fiscal year 1931–32*, ed. Anti-Malaria Commission. Cairo

Anti-malarial work (1939) *Report No. 13 on the anti-malarial work in Egypt, 1936*, ed. Egyptian Government. Cairo

Appleby, A. B. (1980) 'The disappearance of plague: a continuing problem', *Economic History Review* 33: 161–73

Area handbook (1970) *Area handbook for the United Arab Republic (Egypt).* Washington DC

Arlacchi, P. (1983) *Mafia, peasants and great estates: society in traditional Calabria.* Cambridge

Armitage, P. L. (1994) 'Unwelcome companions: ancient rats reviewed', *Antiquity* 68: 231–40

Arnold, D. (1989) 'Cholera mortality in British India, 1817–1947', in Dyson, ed. (1989): 261–84

Atiya, A. S., ed. (1991) *The Coptic encyclopedia, vols. 1–8.* New York

Aykroyd, R. G., Lucy, D., Pollard, A. M. and Roberts, C. A. (1999) 'Nasty, brutish, but not necessarily short: a reconstruction of the statistical methods used to calculate age at death from adult human skeletal and dental age indicators', *American Antiquity* 64: 55–70

Bachatly, C. (1965) *Le monastère de Phoebammon dans la Thébaide, II: graffiti, inscriptions et ostraca.* Cairo

Baer, G. (1969) 'The beginnings of urbanization', in id., *Studies in the social history of modern Egypt.* Chicago and London: 133–48

—— (1982) 'Continuity and change in Egyptian rural society, 1805–1882', in *L'Egypte au XIXe siècle.* Paris: 231–46

Bagnall, R. S. (1985) 'Agricultural productivity in later Roman Egypt', *Transactions of the American Philological Association* 115: 289–308

—— (1993) *Egypt in late antiquity.* Princeton

—— (1997a) 'Missing females in Roman Egypt', *Scripta Classica Israelica* 16: 121–38

—— (1997b) 'The Fayum and its people', in Walker and Bierbrier (1997): 17–20

—— (1997c) Review of Scheidel (1996a), *Bryn Mawr Classical Review* 8: 871–8

—— (2000) '*P.Oxy* 4527 and the Antonine plague in Egypt: death or flight?', *Journal of Roman Archaeology* 13: 288–92

—— and Frier, B. W. (1994) *The demography of Roman Egypt.* Cambridge

——, Frier, B. W. and Rutherford, I. C. (1997) *The census register P.Oxy 984: the reverse of Pindar's Paeans.* Brussels

Bairoch, P. (1989) 'Urbanization and the economy in preindustrial societies: the findings of two decades of research', *Journal of European Economic History* 18: 239–90

Baker, B. J. and Armelagos, G. J. (1988) 'The origin and antiquity of syphilis: paleopathological diagnosis and interpretation', *Current Anthropology* 29: 703–37

——, Kealhofer, L. K. and Richards, J. E. (1989) 'Death and disease in ancient Egypt: the Northern Cemetery at Abydos', *American Journal of Physical Anthropology* 78: 187

Balfour, M. (1936) 'Some features of malaria in Greece and experience with its control', *Rivista di Malariologia* 15: 114–31

Ball, J. (1939) *Contributions to the geography of Egypt.* Cairo

Barber, M. A. and Rice, J. B. (1937) 'A survey of malaria in Egypt', *American Journal of Tropical Medicine* 17: 413–36

Barbès (1800) 'Notes sur les maladies qui ont régné en frimaire an 7, recueillies dans l'hôpital militaire du vieux Kaire', *La décade égyptienne: Journal littéraire et d'économie politique* 2: 201–8

Barclay, G. W., Coale, A. J., Stoto, M. A. and Trussell, T. J. (1976) 'A reassessment of the demography of traditional rural China', *Population Index* 42: 606–35

Barois, J. (1889) *Irrigation in Egypt.* Washington DC

Barrett-Lennard, R. J. S. (1987) 'Request for prayer for healing', in G. H. R. Horsley, ed., *New documents illustrating early Christianity,* 4: 245–50

Barsoum, S. (1938) *Le paludisme en Egypte.* Lyon

Beloch, J. (1886) *Die Bevölkerung der griechisch-römischen Welt.* Leipzig

Beloch, K. J. (1937) *Bevölkerungsgeschichte Italiens, I.* Berlin

Benedictow, O. J. (1987) 'Morbidity in historical plague epidemics', *Population Studies* 41: 401–31

—— (1993) *Plague in the late medieval Nordic countries.* 2nd ed. Oslo

Benenson, A. S. (1976) 'Smallpox', in A. S. Evans, ed., *Viral infections of humans: epidemiology and control.* London: 429–55

Bernand, E. (1975) *Recueil des inscriptions grecques du Fayoum, I.* Leiden

—— (1981) *Recueil des inscriptions grecques du Fayoum, III.* Paris

—— (1988) *Inscriptions grecques et latines d'Akôris.* Paris

Bertier, J. (1990) 'Enfants malades et maladies des enfants dans le Corpus hippocratique', in P. Potter *et al.*, eds. (1990) *La maladie et les maladies dans la Collection hippocratique.* Québec: 209–20

—— (1996) 'La médicine des enfants à l'époque impériale', in *Aufstieg und Niedergang der römischen Welt* II.37.3: 2147–227

Béthemont, J. (1987) 'L'irrigation en Egypte: éléments pour une controverse', in *L'homme et l'eau* (1987): 95–101

Betz, H. D. (1992) *The Greek magical papyri in translation including the demotic spells.* 2nd ed. Chicago and London

Bideau, A., Desjardins, B. and Pérez Brignoli, eds. (1997) *Infant and child mortality in the past.* Oxford

Bingen, J. (1987) 'La série *Kappa* des stèles de Térenouthis', in C. Saerens, R. de Smet and H. Melaerts, eds., *Studia varia Bruxellensia ad orbem Graeco-Latinum pertinentia.* Leuven: 3–14

—— (1996) 'Une nouvelle stèle de la "série Kappa" de Térénouthis', *Chronique d'Egypte* 71: 331–4

Biraben, J.-N. (1975) *Les hommes et la peste en France et dans les pays européens et méditerranées, I: la peste dans l'histoire.* Paris and La Haye

—— (1988) 'L'hygiène, la maladie, la mort', in *Histoire de la population francaise 1—des origines à la Renaissance.* Paris: 421–62

—— (1989) 'La peste du VIe siècle dans l'empire byzantin', in *Hommes et richesses dans l'Empire byzantin, I: IVe–VIIe siècle.* Paris: 121–5

—— and Le Goff, J. (1969) 'La peste dans le Haut Moyen Age', *Annales: Economie, Sociétés, Civilisations* 24: 1484–510

Bocquet-Appel, J.-P. and Masset, C. (1982) 'Farewell to paleodemography', *Journal of Human Evolution* 11: 321–33

—— (1996) 'Paleodemography: expectancy and false hopes', *American Journal of Physical Anthropology* 99: 571–83

Boddington, A. (1987) 'From bones to population: the problem of numbers', in A. Boddington, A. N. Garland and R. C. Janaway, eds., *Death, decay and reconstruction: approaches to archaeology and forensic science.* Manchester: 180–97

Bolognesi, D. (1980) 'Demografia ed economia del Ravennate nel Settecento', in *La popolazione italiana nel settecento.* Bologna: 263–83

Bonneau, D. (1982) 'Le *drymos*, marais du Fayoum, d'après la documentation papyrologique', in *L'égyptologie en 1979: axes prioritaires de recherches, I.* Paris: 181–90

—— (1989) 'L'Egypte dans l'histoire de l'irrigation antique (de l'époque hellénistique à l'époque arabe)', in Criscuolo and Geraci, eds. (1989): 301–13

—— (1993) *La régime administratif de l'eau du Nil dans l'Egypte grecque, romaine et byzantine.* Leiden, New York and Cologne

Borza, E. N. (1979) 'Some observations on malaria and the ecology of central Macedonia in antiquity', *American Journal of Ancient History* 4: 102–24

Boswinkel, E. and Pestman, P. W., eds. (1978) *Textes grecs, démotiques et bilingues (P.L. Bat. 19).* Leiden

Bowman, A. K. (1990) *Egypt after the Pharaohs: 332 BC–AD 642, from Alexander to the Arab conquest.* Oxford

—— (1995) Review of Bagnall and Frier (1994), *Journal of Roman Studies* 85: 310–11

—— and Rogan, E., eds. (1999) *Agriculture in Egypt: from Pharaonic to modern times.* Oxford

Boyaval, B. (1975) 'Remarques à propos des indications d'âges des etiquettes de momies', *Zeitschrift für Papyrologie und Epigraphik* 18: 49–74

—— (1976a) *Corpus des etiquettes des momies.* Lille

—— (1976b) 'Remarques sur les indications d'âges de l'épigraphie funéraire d'Egypte', *Zeitschrift für Papyrologie und Epigraphik* 21: 217–43

—— (1980) 'La mortalité saisonnière dans l'Egypte gréco-romaine', in J. Vercoutter, ed., *Institut francais d'archéologie orientale du Caire: Livre du centenaire 1880–1980*, Cairo: 281–6

—— (1981) 'La date sur les etiquettes de momies', *Bulletin of the American Society of Papyrologists* 18, 3–4: 101–18

—— (1988) 'Datation du décès dans l'épigraphie funéraire de l'Egypte gréco-romaine', *Kentron* 4, 3: 65–70

—— (1991) 'L'apport des étiquettes de momies grecques à l'histoire', *Kentron* 7, 4: 103–24

—— (1992) 'L'âge au décès dans l'Egypte chrétienne', *Kentron* 8, 4: 177–80

Brahin, J. L. and Fleming, S. J. (1982) 'Children's health problems: some guidelines for their occurrence in ancient Egypt', *MASCA Journal* 2, 3: 75–81

Bratton, T. L. (1981) 'The identity of the plague of Justinian', *Transactions and Studies of the College of Physicians of Philadelphia*, ser. 5, 3: 113–24, 174–80

Braunert, H. (1964) *Die Binnenwanderung: Studien zur Sozialgeschichte Ägyptens in der Ptolemäer- und Kaiserzeit.* Bonn

Breitwieser, R. (1995) 'Virunum und die "Antoninische Pest"', *Grazer Beiträge* 21: 149–56

Brewer, D. J. (1991) 'Temperatures in predynastic Egypt inferred from the remains of the Nile perch', *World Archaeology* 22: 288–303

Brown, N. (1995) *The impact of climate change: some indications from history, AD 250–1250.* Oxford

Bruant (1800) 'Observations sur les maladies, et en particulier la dysenterie, qui ont regné en fructidor an 6, dans l'armée d'Orient', *La décade egyptienne: Journal littéraire et d'économie politique* 2: 51–62

Brulé, P. (1990) 'Enquête démographique sur la famille grecque antique: étude de listes de politographie d'Asie mineure d'époque hellénistique (Milet et Ilion)', *Revue des études anciennes* 92: 233–58

—— (1992) 'Infanticide et abandon d'enfants: pratiques grecques et comparaisons anthropologiques', *Dialogues d'histoire ancienne* 18: 53–90

Brunsch, W. (1991) 'Bemerkungen zu koptischen und griechischen Inschriften aus Kairo', *Orientalia* 60: 92–108

—— (1992) 'Verzeichnis der 1982 aufgenommenen koptischen und griechischen Inschriften aus dem Koptischen Museum in Alt-Kairo', *Archiv für Papyrusforschung* 38: 47–60

—— (1993) 'Koptische und griechische Inschriften in Kairo', *Aegyptus* 73: 127–96

Brunt, P. A. (1971) *Italian manpower 225 BC–AD 14.* Oxford (repr. 1987)

Brunton, D. (1992) 'Smallpox inoculation and demographic trends in eighteenth-century Scotland', *Medical History* 36: 403–29

Buikstra, J. E., Baker, B. J. and Cook, D. C. (1993) 'What diseases plagued ancient Egyptians? A century of controversy considered', in Davies and Walker, eds. (1993): 24–53

—— and Konigsberg, L. W. (1985) 'Paleodemography: critiques and controversies', *American Anthropologist* 97: 316–33

Burke, P. F., Jr. (1996) 'Malaria in the Greco-Roman world: a historical and epidemiological study', in *Aufstieg und Niedergang der Römischen Welt* II.37.3: 2252–81

Burns, J. R. and Denness, B. (1985) 'Climate and social dynamics: the Tripolitanian example', in D. J. Buck and D. J. Mattingly, eds., *Town and country in Roman Tripolitania: papers in honour of Olwen Hackett.* Oxford: 201–25

Butzer, K. W. (1976) *Early hydraulic civilization in Egypt: a study in cultural ecology.* Chicago and London

[Campbell, J.] (1739) *The travels and adventures of Edward Brown.* London

Capasso, L. (1985) *L'origine delle malattie.* Chieti

Carrié, J.-M. (1997) 'L'arithmétique de l'économie agraire: prix de la terre, rente foncière et prix des céréales dans l'Egypte romano-byzantine', in Andreau, Briant and Descat, eds. (1997): 121–46

Casanova, G. (1984) 'Epidemie e fame nella documentazione greco d'Egitto', *Aegyptus* 64: 163–201

—— (1985) 'Le epigrafi di Terenouthis e la peste', *Yale Classical Studies* 28: 145–54

Casarico, L. (1985) *Il controllo della popolazione nell'Egitto romano, 1: le denunce di morte.* Azzate

Casini, M. (1990/91) 'La valle del Nilo e il Sahara: la rappresentazione, l'ambiente, i rapporti reciproci', *Origini* 15: 321–36

Chambers, R., Longhurst, R. and Pacey, A., eds. (1981), *Seasonal dimensions to rural poverty.* London

Chenival, F. de (1972) *Les associations religieuses en Egypte d'après les documents démotiques*. Cairo

Clark, A. W. (1989) 'Mortality, fertility, and the status of women in India, 1881–1931', in Dyson, ed. (1989): 119–49

Clark, C. and Haswell, M. (1970) *The economics of subsistence agriculture*. 4th ed. London and Basingstoke

Clauss, M. (1973) 'Probleme der Lebensalterstatistik aufgrund römischer Grabinschriften', *Chiron* 3: 395–417

Cleland, W. (1936) *The population problem in Egypt: a study of population trends and conditions in modern Egypt*. Lancaster PA

Clot-Bey, A.-B. (1840) *Aperçu général sur l'Egypte*. 2 vols. Paris

Clutton-Brock, T. H. (1991) *The evolution of parental care*. Princeton

Coale, A. J. and Demeny, P. (1983) *Regional model life tables and stable populations*. 2nd ed. New York and London

Cockburn, A. (1981) 'Ancient parasites on the West Bank of the Nile', *The Lancet* no. 8252, October 24: 938

Cohen, J. E. (1995) *How many people can the earth support?* New York and London

Collari, S. (1932) 'Rapporti tra malaria e tuberculosi dal punto di vista epidemiologico, clinico e biologico', *Rivista di Malariologia* 11: 308–35

Congourdeau, M.-H. (1993) 'La société byzantine face aux grandes pandémies', in E. Patlagean, ed., *Maladie et société à Byzance*. Spoleto: 21–41

Conrad, L. (1981) 'The plague in the early medieval Near East'. Ph.D. thesis Princeton

—— (1982) '*Ta'un* and *waba'*: conceptions of plague and pestilence in early Islam', *Journal of the Economic and Social History of the Orient* 25: 268–307

—— (1994) 'Epidemic disease in central Syria in the late sixth century: some new insights from the verse of Hassan ibn Thabit', *Byzantine and Modern Greek Studies* 18: 12–58

Contis, G. and David, A. R. (1996) 'The epidemiology of bilharzia in ancient Egypt: 5000 years of schistosomiasis', *Parasitology Today* 12: 253–5

Conway, D. and Hulme, M. (1993) 'Recent fluctuations in precipitation and runoff over the Nile sub-basins and their impact on main Nile discharge', *Climatic Change* 25: 127–51

Cook, G. C. (1996) 'The Asiatic cholera: an historical determinant of human genomic and social structure', in B. S. Drasar and B. D. Forrest, eds., *Cholera and the ecology of* Vibrio cholerae. London: 18–53

Cooper, D. B. (1965) *Epidemic disease in Mexico City 1761–1813: an administrative, social, and medical study*. Austin

Corsini, C. (n.d.) 'Problemi di utilizzazione dei dati desunti dai registri di sepolture e morti', in *Problemi di utilizzazione delle fonti di demografia storica, II*. Rome: 93–136

Corvisier, J.-N. (1994) 'Eau, paludisme et démographie en Grèce péninsulaire', in *L'eau, la santé et la maladie dans le monde grec*. Paris: 297–319

—— and Suder, W. (1996) *Polyanthropia—oliganthropia: bibliographie de la démographie du monde grec*. Wroclaw

Craig, J. I. (1908) 'Mortality in Cairo and relative humidity', *Cairo Scientific Journal* 2: 101–4

—— (1912) 'Meteorological factors of mortality in Cairo and Alexandria', *Cairo Scientific Journal* 6: 246–50

Crawford, D. J. (1971) *Kerkeosiris: an Egyptian village in the Ptolemaic period*. Cambridge

—— (1979) 'Food: tradition and change in Hellenistic Egypt', *World Archaeology* 11: 136–46

Crecelius, D. (1981) 'Archival sources for demographic studies of the Middle East', in Udovitch, ed. (1981): 349–74

Cribiore, R. (1997) 'A stele from Terenouthis', *Bulletin of the American Society of Papyrologists* 34: 5–10

Criscuolo, L. and Geraci, G., eds. (1989) *Egitto e storia antica dall'ellenismo all'età araba: bilancio di un confronto.* Bologna

Crum, W.-E. (1902) *Catalogue général des antiquités égyptiennes du Musée du Caire, nos. 8001–8741: Coptic monuments.* Cairo

—— and Bell, H. I. (1922) *Wadi Sarga: Coptic and Greek texts.* Copenhagen

Cuno, K. M. (1992) *The Pasha's peasants: land, society, and economy in Lower Egypt, 1740–1858.* Cambridge

Curschmann, H. (1902) *Typhoid fever and typhus fever*, ed. W. Osler. Philadelphia and London.

Curtin, P. D. (1989) *Death by migration: Europe's encounter with the tropical world in the nineteenth century.* Cambridge

Cuvigny, H. (1992) 'La mort et la maladie', in *Mons Claudianus: ostraca graeca et latina, I (O.Claud. 1 à 190).* Cairo: 75–109

—— (1997) 'La mort et la maladie (191–223)', in *Mons Claudianus: ostraca graeca et latina, II: O.Claud. 191 à 416.* Cairo: 19–41

Davies, W. V. and Walker, R., eds. (1993) *Biological anthropology and the study of ancient Egypt.* London

Davoli, P. (1998) *L'archeologia urbana nel Fayyum di età ellenistica e romana.* n.p.

De Chamberet, R. (1909) *Enquête sur la condition du fellah égyptien au triple point de vue de la vie agricole, de l'éducation de l'hygiène et de l'assistance publique.* Dijon

Deelder, A. M., Miller, R. L., de Jonge, N. and Krijger, F. W. (1990) 'Detection of schistosome antigen in mummies', *The Lancet* 335: 724–5

Delia, D. (1988) 'The population of Roman Alexandria', *Transactions of the American Philological Association* 118: 275–92

Del Panta, L. (1989) *Malaria e regime demografico: la maremma grossetana nell'ottocento pre-unitario.* Messina

Desgenettes, R. (1800) 'Tables nécrologiques du Kaire, l'an 7, recueillies d'après les rapports des commandants de sections, adressés au général commandante de cette place', *La décade égyptienne: Journal littéraire et d'économie politique* 2: 287–97

—— (1812) 'Tables nécrologiques du Kaire, pendant les années VII, VIII et IX', in *Description de l'Egypte: état moderne, vol. 2.* Paris: 311–20

De Vries, J. (1984) *European urbanization 1500–1800.* London

DeWolfe Miller, F., Hussein, M., Mancy, K. H. and Hilbert, M. S. (1978) *Schistosomiasis in rural Egypt: a report of U.S.-Egyptian River-Nile and Lake Nasser-Research Project.* Athens GA

Dikaios (1862) 'Des maladies prédominantes dans la colonie grecque d'Alexandrie', *Mémoires ou travaux originaux présentés et lus à l'Institut Egyptien* 1: 499–503 (French summary)

Dobson, M. J. (1997) *Contours of death and disease in early modern England.* Cambridge

Dols, M. W. (1974) 'Plague in early Islamic history', *Journal of the American Oriental Society* 94: 371–83

—— (1977) *The Black Death in the Middle East.* Princeton

—— (1979) 'The second plague pandemic and its recurrence in the Middle East: 1347–1894', *Journal of the Economic and Social History of the Orient* 22: 162–89

—— (1981) 'The general mortality of the Black Death in the Mamluk empire', in Udovitch, ed. (1981): 397–428

Dong, L., Xi, M. and Thann, F. (1996) *Les maux épidémiques dans l'empire chinois.* Paris

Dreizehnter, A. (1978) *Die rhetorische Zahl: Quellenkritische Untersuchungen anhand der Zahlen 70 und 700.* Munich

Drexhage, H.-J. (1991) *Preise, Mieten/Pachten, Kosten und Löhne im römischen Ägypten bis zum Regierungsantritt Diokletians: Vorarbeiten zu einer Wirtschaftsgeschichte des römischen Ägypten I.* St. Katharinen

—— (1994) 'Einige Bemerkungen zum Mumientransport und den Bestattungskosten im römischen Ägypten', *Laverna* 5: 167–75

Duncan-Jones, R. P. (1979) 'Age-rounding in Greco-Roman Egypt', *Zeitschrift für Papyrologie und Epigraphik* 33: 169–77

—— (1982) *The economy of the Roman empire: quantitative studies.* 2nd ed. Cambridge

—— (1990) *Structure and scale in the Roman economy.* Cambridge

—— (1994) *Money and government in the Roman empire.* Cambridge

—— (1996) 'The impact of the Antonine plague', *Journal of Roman Archaeology* 9: 108–36

—— (1997) 'Numerical distortion in Roman writers', in Andreau, Briant and Descat, eds. (1997): 147–59

Durliat, J. (1989) 'La peste du VIe siècle: pour un nouvel examen des sources byzantines', in *Hommes et richesses dans l'Empire byzantin, I: IVe–VIIe siècle.* Paris: 107–19

—— (1990) *De la ville antique à la ville byzantine: le problème des subsistances.* Paris

Duttenhöfer, R. (1997) 'Five census returns in the Beinecke Library', *Bulletin of the American Society of Papyrologists* 34: 53–78

Dyson, T., ed. (1989) *India's historical demography: studies in famine, disease and society.* London

Dzierzykray-Rogalski, T. (1980) 'Paleopathology of the Ptolemaic inhabitants of Dakleh Oasis (Egypt)', *Journal of Human Evolution* 9: 71–4

Ebbell, B. (1946) 'La variole dans l'Ancien Testament et dans le papyrus Ebers', *Nordiskt medicinskt arkiv* 39: 1–58

—— (1967) *Beiträge zur ältesten Geschichte einiger Infektionskrankheiten.* Oslo

Eid, A. (1907) *La fortune immobilière de l'Egypte et sa dette hypothécaire.* Paris

El Baz, A. and Orabey, N. (1975) 'Causes of death in Egypt 1963–1969', *Population Researches and Studies* 10: 7–20

El-Nassery, S. A. A. and Wagner, G. (1978) 'Nouvelles stèles de Kom Abu Bellou', *Bulletin de l'Institut Francais d'Archéologie Orientale* 78: 231–58

El-Sawy, A., Bouzek, J. and Vidman, L. (1980) 'New stelae from the Terenouthis cemetery in Egypt', *Archiv Orientální* 48: 330–55

Ennabli, L., ed. (1975) *Les inscriptions funéraires chrétiennes de la basilique dite de Sainte-Monique à Carthage.* Paris

—— (1982) *Les inscriptions funéraires chrétiennes de Carthage II: la basilique de Mcidfa.* Rome

—— (1991) *Les inscriptions funéraires chrétiennes de Carthage III. Carthage intra et extra muros.* Rome

Erichsen, W. (1956) *Eine neue demotische Erzählung.* Wiesbaden

Ery, K. K. (1969) 'Investigations on the demographic source value of tombstones originating from the Roman period', *Alba Regia* 10: 51–67

Estimation (1982) *The estimation of recent trends in fertility and mortality in Egypt.* Washington DC

Etienne, R. (1973) 'La conscience médicale antique et la vie des enfants', *Annales de Démographie Historique 1973*: 15–61

Evans, J. A. S. (1991) 'The Faiyum and the Lake of Moeris', *Ancient History Bulletin* 5: 66–74

Fahmy, K. (1997) *All the Pasha's men: Mehmed Ali, his army and the making of modern Egypt.* Cambridge

Farris, W. W. (1985) *Population, disease, and land in early Japan, 645–900.* Cambridge MA and London

Fauve-Chamoux, A. (1994) 'Female surplus and pre-industrial work: the French urban experience', in A. Fauve-Chamoux and S. Sogner, eds., *Socio-economic perspectives of sex-ratios in historical perspective, 1500–1900. Proceedings Eleventh International Economic History Congress, Milan, September 1994, B5.* Milan: 31–50

Fehling, D. (1990) *Herodotus and his "sources": citation, invention, and narrative art.* Leeds

Fenner, F., Henderson, D. A., Arita, I., Jezek, Z. and Ladnyi, I. D. (1988) *Smallpox and its eradication.* Geneva

Ferrari, G. and Livi Bacci, M. (1985) 'Sulle relazione tra temperatura e mortalità nell'Italia Unita, 1861–1914', in *La popolazione italiana nell'ottocento: continuità e mutamenti.* Bologna: 273–98

Finlay, R. (1981) *Population and metropolis: the demography of London 1580–1650.* Cambridge
Flinn, M. W. (1979) 'Plague in Europe and the Mediterranean countries', *Journal of European Economic History* 8: 131–48
Fogel, R. W. (forthcoming) *The escape from hunger and early death.* Cambridge
Frank, L. (1820) *De peste, dysenteria et ophthalmia aegyptica.* Vienna
Frank, T. (1924) 'Roman census statistics from 225 to 28 BC', *Classical Philology* 19: 329–41
Frier, B. W. (1982) 'Roman life expectancy: Ulpian's evidence', *Harvard Studies in Classical Philology* 86: 213–51
—— (1983) 'Roman life expectancy: the Pannonian evidence', *Phoenix* 37: 328–44
—— (1994) 'Natural fertility and family limitation in Roman marriage', *Classical Philology* 90: 318–33
—— (1997) 'Demographic analysis', in Bagnall, Frier and Rutherford (1997): 89–113
—— (1999) 'Roman demography', in D. S. Potter and D. J. Mattingly, eds., *Life, death, and entertainment in the Roman empire.* Ann Arbor: 85–109
—— (2000) 'Demography', in *The Cambridge Ancient History*, 2nd ed., vol. 11. Cambridge: 787–816
—— (2001) 'More is worse: some observations on the population of the Roman empire', in Scheidel, ed. (2001): 139–59
Gage, T. B. (1988) 'Mathematical hazard models of mortality: an alternative to model life tables', *American Journal of Physical Anthropology* 76: 429–41
Garbrecht, G., ed. (1986) *Staat und landwirtschaftliche Bewässerungssysteme Ägyptens in vorrömischer Zeit.* Braunschweig
—— and Jaritz, H. (1990) 'Forschungsvorhaben Ga 183/28-1. Untersuchungen antiker Anlagen zur Wasserspeicherung im Fayum, Ägypten', *Mitteilungen Leichtweiss-Institut für Wasserbau der Technischen Universität Braunschweig* 107: 1–216
Garnsey, P. (1983) 'Grain for Rome', in P. Garnsey, K. Hopkins and C. R. Whittaker, eds., *Trade in the ancient economy.* Cambridge: 118–30
—— (1988) *Famine and food supply in the Graeco-Roman world: responses to risk and crisis.* Cambridge
—— (1998) *Cities, peasants and food in classical antiquity: essays in social and economic history* (ed. W. Scheidel). Cambridge
—— (1999) *Food and society in classical antiquity.* Cambridge
—— and Whittaker, C. R., eds. (1983) *Trade and famine in classical antiquity.* Cambridge
Giglioli, G. (1972) 'Changes in the pattern of mortality following the eradication of hyperendemic malaria from a highly susceptible community', *Bulletin of the World Health Organisation* 46: 181–202
Gilles, H. M. and Warrell, D. A. (1993) *Bruce-Chwatt's essential malariology.* 3rd ed. London
Gilliam, J. F. (1961/86) 'The plague under Marcus Aurelius', in *Roman army papers.* Amsterdam: 227–53
Ginter, B. and Kozlowski, J. K. (1986) 'Kulturelle und paläoklimatische Sequenz in der Fayum-Depression—eine zusammenfassende Darstellung der Forschungsarbeiten in den Jahren 1979–1981', *Mitteilungen des Deutschen Archäologischen Instituts Abteilung Kairo* 42: 9–23
Golden, M. (2000) 'A decade of demography: recent trends in the study of Greek and Roman populations', in P. Flensted-Jensen, T. H. Nielsen and L. Rubinstein, eds., *Polis and politics: studies in ancient Greek history presented to Mogens Herman Hansen on his sixtieth birthday, August 20, 2000.* Copenhagen: 23–40
Goldman, N. (1980) 'Far Eastern patterns of mortality', *Population Studies* 34: 5–19
Gottfried, R. S. (1983) *The Black Death: natural and human disaster in medieval Europe.* New York and London
Gragnolati, M., Elo, I. T. and Goldman, N. (1999) 'New insights into the Far Eastern pattern of mortality', *Population Studies* 53: 81–95

Greene, D. L., van Gerven, D. P. and Armelagos, G. J. (1985) 'Life and death in ancient populations: bones of contention in paleodemography', *Human Evolution* 1: 193–207

Greenhill, W. A., transl. (1848) *A treatise on the small-pox and measles by Abú Becr Mohammed Ibn Zacaríyá Ar-Rázi (commonly called Rhazes)*. London

Grégoire, M. (1862) 'Du khamsin et de ses effets; du blé retrait', *Mémoires ou travaux originaux présentés et lus à l'Institut Egyptien* 1: 369–400

Griffith, F. L. (1900) *Stories of the High Priests of Memphis: the Sethon of Herodotus and the demotic tale of Khamuas*. Oxford

—— (1909) *Catalogue of the demotic papyri in the John Rylands Library Manchester, III, 1*. Manchester and London

Grmek, M. D. (1989) *Diseases in the ancient Greek world*. Baltimore and London

Groves, A. N. (1832) *Journal of a residence at Bagdad, during the years 1830 and 1831*. London

Guillaumont, A. (1991) 'Monasticism, Egyptian', in Atiya, ed. (1991), vol. 5: 1661–4

Günther, W. (1988) 'Milesische Bürgerrechts- und Proxenieverleihungen der hellenistischen Zeit', *Chiron* 18: 383–419

Habachi, L. (1947) 'A statue of Osiris made for Ankhefenamun, prophet of the house of Amun in Khapu and his daughter', *Annales du Service des Antiquités de l'Egypte* 47: 261–82

Hansen, M. H. (1985) *Demography and democracy: the number of Athenian citizens in the fourth century BC*. Herning

—— (1988) *Three studies in Athenian demography*. Copenhagen

—— (1994) 'The number of Athenian citizens *secundum* Sekunda', *Echos du Monde Classique/Classical Views* 38: 299–310

Harer, W. B. (1993) 'Health in Pharaonic Egypt', in Davies and Walker, eds. (1993): 19–23

Hartmann, F. (1923) *L'agriculture dans l'ancienne Egypte*. Paris

Hasitzka, M. R. M. (1993) *Koptisches Sammelbuch I*. Vienna

Hassan, F. A. (1981a) *Demographic archaeology*. New York

—— (1981b) 'Historical Nile floods and their implications for climatic change', *Science* 212: 1142–5

—— (1986a) 'Desert environment and origins of agriculture in Egypt', *Norwegian Archaeological Review* 19: 63–76

—— (1986b) 'Holocene lakes and prehistoric settlements of the western Faiyum, Egypt', *Journal of Archaeological Science* 13: 483–501

—— (1988) 'The Predynastic of Egypt', *Journal of World Prehistory* 2: 135–85

Hatcher, J. (1986) 'Mortality in the fifteenth century: some new evidence', *Economic History Review* 39: 19–38

Hawwass, Z. A. (1979) 'Preliminary report on the excavations at Kôm Abou Bellou', *Studien zur altägyptischen Kultur* 7: 75–87

Hellmann, G. (1916) 'Über die ägyptischen Witterungsangaben im Kalender von Claudius Ptolemaeus', *Sitzungsberichte der Königlich Preussischen Akademie der Wissenschaften 1916*: 332–41

Henige, D. (1998) *Numbers from nowhere: the American Indian contact population debate*. Norman

Herlihy, D. (1997) *The Black Death and the transformation of the West*. Cambridge MA and London

—— and Klapisch-Zuber, C. (1978) *Les Toscans et leurs familles: un étude du catasto florentin de 1427*. Paris

—— and —— (1985) *Tuscans and their families: a study of the Florentine catasto of 1427*. New Haven and London

Hewison, R. N. (1989) *The Fayoum: a practical guide*. 2nd ed. Cairo

Higgins, A. R. and Floyd, T. M. (1955) 'Studies in shigellosis', *American Journal of Tropical Medicine and Hygiene*, 58: 166–8

Hillson, S. W. (1980) 'Chronic anaemias in the Nile valley', *MASCA Journal mummification supplement*. Philadelphia: 172–4
Hinard, F. ed. (1987) *La mort, les morts et l'au-delà dans le monde romain: actes du colloque de Caen, 20–22 novembre 1985*. Caen
Hinnebusch, B. J. (1997) 'Bubonic plague: a molecular genetic case history of the emergence of an infectious disease', *Journal of Molecular Medicine* 75: 645–52
Hirsch, A. (1881–6) *Handbuch der historisch-geographischen Pathologie*. 3 vols. 2nd ed. Stuttgart
Hodkinson, S. (1989) 'Inheritance, marriage and demography: perspectives upon the success and decline of Sparta', in A. Powell, ed., *Classical Sparta: techniques behind her success*. London: 79–121
Hooper, F. A. (1961) *Funerary stelae from Kom Abou Billou*. Ann Arbor
Hope, V. M. and Marshall, E., eds. (2000) *Death and disease in the ancient city*. London and New York
Hopkins, D. R. (1983) *Princes and peasants: smallpox in history*. Chicago and London
Hopkins, K. (1966) 'On the probable age structure of the Roman population', *Population Studies* 20: 245–64
—— (1978) *Conquerors and slaves: sociological studies in Roman history 1*. Cambridge
—— (1980) 'Brother-sister marriage in Roman Egypt', *Comparative Studies in Society and History* 22: 303–54
—— (1983) 'Models, ships and staples', in Garnsey and Whittaker, eds. (1983): 84–109
—— (1987) 'Graveyards for historians', in Hinard, ed. (1987): 113–26
—— (1995/96) 'Rome, taxes, rents and trade', *Kodai* 6/7: 41–75
Hoppa, R. and Saunders, S. (1998) 'The MAD legacy: how meaningful is mean age-at-death in skeletal samples', *Human Evolution* 13: 1–14
Horbury, W. and Noy, D. (1992) *Jewish inscriptions of Graeco-Roman Egypt*. Cambridge
Hornick, R. B. (1982) 'Typhoid fever', in A. S. Evans and H. A. Feldman, eds., *Bacterial infections of humans: epidemiology and control*. New York and London: 659–76
Howell, N. (1976) 'Toward a uniformitarian theory of human paleodemography', in R. H. Ward and K. M. Weiss, eds., *The demographic evolution of human populations*. London, New York and Los Angeles: 25–40
—— (1986) 'Demographic anthropology', *Annual Review of Anthropology* 15: 219–46
Huckstep, R. L. (1962) *Typhoid fever and other salmonella infections*. Edinburgh and London
Hummel, C. (1999) *Das Kind und seine Krankheiten in der griechischen Medizin: Von Aretaios bis Johannes Aktuarios (1. bis 14. Jahrhundert)*. Frankfurt a. M.
Imhof, A. E. (1990) *Lebenserwartungen in Deutschland vom 17. bis 19. Jahrhundert*. Weinheim
Infectious diseases handbook (1922) *Infectious diseases handbook*. Cairo
Issar, A. S. and Yakir, D. (1997) 'The Roman period's colder climate', *Biblical Archaeologist* 60: 101–06
Issawi, C. (1981) 'The area and the population of the Arab empire: an essay in speculation', in Udovitch, ed. (1981): 375–96
Jackes, M. (1992) 'Paleodemography: problems and techniques', in: Saunders and Katzenberg, eds. (1992): 189–224
Jackson, R. (1988) *Doctors and diseases in the Roman empire*. London
Jagailloux, S. (1986) *La médicalisation de l'Egypte au XIXe siècle (1798–1918)*. Paris
—— (1996) *La médecine traditionelle égyptienne du XIXème siècle à nos jours*. Paris
James, S. P. (1920) *Malaria at home and abroad*. London
Jarcho, S. (1987) 'A history of semitertian fever', *Bulletin of the History of Medicine* 61: 411–30
Johansson, S. R. (1994a) 'Food for thought: rhetoric and reality in modern mortality history', *Historical Methods* 27: 101–25
—— (1994b) Review of O. J. Benedictow, *The medieval demographic system of the Nordic countries* (Oslo 1993), *Population Studies* 48: 527–34
—— and Horowitz, S. (1986) 'Estimating mortality in skeletal populations: influence

of the growth rate on the interpretation of levels and trends during the transition to agriculture', *American Journal of Physical Anthropology* 71: 233–50

John, A. M. (1988) *The plantation slaves of Trinidad, 1783–1816: a mathematical and demographic enquiry*. Cambridge

Jongman, W. (1990) 'Het romeins imperialisme en de verstedelijking van Italie', *Leidschrift* 7, 1: 43–58

Kamel, I. (1987) *Catalogue général des antiquités du Musée Copte, nos. 1–253: Coptic funerary stelae*. Cairo

Kane, P. (1989) 'Famine in China 1959–61: demographic and social implications', in L. Ruzicka, G. Wunsch and P. Kane, eds., *Differential mortality: methodological issues and biosocial factors*. Oxford: 231–53

Keeley, L. H. (1996) *War before civilization*. New York and Oxford

Kees, H. (1955) *Das alte Ägypten: eine kleine Landeskunde*. Berlin

Khattab, A. (1982) *Das Ägyptenbild in den deutschsprachigen Reisebeschreibungen der Zeit von 1285–1500*. Frankfurt a. M. and Bern

Kirby, C. and Rathbone, D. (1996) 'Kom Talit: the rise and fall of a Greek town in the Faiyum', *Egyptian Archaeology* 8: 29–31

Kirkpatrick, T. W. (1925) *The mosquitoes of Egypt*. Cairo

Kolta, K. S. (1984) 'Neue Erkenntnisse zur Medizin der Kopten', *Sudhoffs Archiv* 68: 157–72

Konen, H. (1999) 'Reis im Imperium Romanum: Bemerkungen zu seinem Anbau und seiner Stellung als Bedarfs- und Handelsartikel in der Römischen Kaiserzeit', *Münstersche Beiträge zur Antiken Handelsgeschichte* 18: 23–47

Konigsberg, L. W. and Frankenberg, S. R. (1992) 'Estimation of age structure in anthropological demography', *American Journal of Physical Anthropology* 89: 235–56

—— (1994) 'Paleodemography: "not quite dead"', *Evolutionary Anthropology* 3: 92–105

Krause, M. (1991) 'Inscriptions', in Atiya, ed. (1991), vol. 4: 1293–6

Kubinska, J. (1974) *Faras IV: Inscriptions grecques chrétiennes*. Warsaw

Kuhnke, L. (1971) 'Resistance and response to modernization: preventive medicine and social control in Egypt, 1825–1850'. Ph.D. thesis University of Chicago

—— (1990) *Lives at risk: public health in nineteenth-century Egypt*. Berkeley, Los Angeles and Oxford

Kunitz, S. J. (1983) 'Speculations on the European mortality decline', *Economic History Review* 36: 349–64

Lamb, H. H. (1977) *Climate: present, past and future, 2: climate history and the future*. London and New York

—— (1995) *Climate, history and the modern world*. 2nd ed. London and New York

Lancaster, H. O. (1990) *Expectations of life: a study in the demography, statistics, and history of world mortality*. New York

Landers, J. (1993) *Death and the metropolis: studies in the demographic history of London 1670–1830*. Cambridge

—— and Mouzas, A. (1988) 'Burial seasonality and causes of death in London 1670–1819', *Population Studies* 42: 59–83

Lanphear, K. M. (1989) 'Testing the value of skeletal samples in demographic research: a comparison with vital registration samples', *International Journal of Anthropology* 4: 185–93

Laronde, A. (1989) 'La vie agricole en Libye jusqu'à l'arrivée des Arabes', *Libyan Studies* 20: 127–34

Larsen, C. S. (1997) *Bioarchaeology: interpreting behaviour from the human skeleton*. Cambridge

Learmonth, A. (1988) *Disease ecology: an introduction*. Oxford and New York

Leca, A.-P. (1971) *La médicine égyptienne au temps des Pharaons*. Paris

Ledermann, S. (1969) *Nouvelles tables-types de mortalité*. Paris

Lee, J. Z. and Campbell, C. D. (1997) *Fate and fortune in rural China: social organization and population behavior in Liaoning 1774–1873*. Cambridge

——, Wang, F., and Campbell, B. (1994) 'Infant and child mortality among the Qing nobility: implications for two types of positive check', *Population Studies* 48: 395–411

Lee, R. (1986) 'Population homeostasis and English demographic history', in R. I. Rotberg and T. K. Rabb, eds., *Population and economy: population and history from the traditional to the modern world.* Cambridge: 74–100

Lefebvre, G. (1907) *Recueil des inscriptions grecques chrétiennes d'Egypte.* Cairo

Leven, K.-H. (1998) 'Krankheiten – historische Deutung versus retrospektive Diagnose', in N. Paul and T. Schlich, eds., *Medizingeschichte: Probleme und Perspektiven.* Frankfurt a. M.: 153–85

Lewis, N. (1994) 'Olyra = triticum', *Chronique d'Egypte* 69: 138–9

L'homme et l'eau (1987) *L'homme et l'eau en Méditerranée et au Proche Orient, IV: l'eau dans l'agriculture.* Lyon

Lippi, D. and Lippi, G. (1985) 'L'ematuria parassitaria nell'antico Egitto: interpretazione alla luce degli ultimi studi', *Minerva Medica* 76: 587–9

Littman, R. J. and Littman, M. L. (1973) 'Galen and the Antonine plague', *American Journal of Philology* 94: 243–53

Livi-Bacci, M. (1991) *Population and nutrition: an essay on European demographic history.* Cambridge

Lloyd, A. B. (1976) *Herodotus book II: commentary 1–98.* Leiden

Lo Cascio, E. (1994a) 'La dinamica della popolazione in Italia da Augusto al III secolo', in *L'Italie d'Auguste à Dioclétien.* Rome: 91–125

—— (1994b) 'The size of the Roman population: Beloch and the meaning of the Republican census figures', *Journal of Roman Studies* 84: 23–40

—— (1999) 'La popolazione dell'Egitto romano', in M. Bellancourt-Valdher and J.-N. Corvisier, eds., *La démographie historique antique.* Arras: 153–69

—— (2000) 'The population of Roman Italy in town and country', in J. Bintliff and K. Sbonias, eds., *Reconstructing past population trends in Mediterranean Europe (3000 BC–AD 1800).* Oxford: 161–71

—— (2001) 'Recruitment and the size of the Roman population from the third to the first century BCE', in Scheidel, ed. (2001): 111–37

MacDonald, G. (1957) *The epidemiology and control of malaria.* Oxford

Macke, A. and Macke-Ribet, C. (1993) 'Paléopathologie osseuse de la population égyptienne d'époque romaine provenant de la Vallée des Reines', in *Sesto congresso internazionale di Egittologia: Atti, II.* Turin: 299–306

Maddicott, J. R. (1997) 'Plague in seventh-century England', *Past and Present* 156: 7–54

Maharatna, A. (1996) *The demography of famines: an Indian historical perspective.* Delhi

Manchester, K. (1986) 'Tuberculosis and leprosy in antiquity: an interpretation', *MASCA Journal* 4: 22–30

Manniche, L. (1989) *An ancient Egyptian herbal.* London

Marasco, G. (1998) 'Cléopatre et les sciences de son temps', in G. Argoud and J.-Y. Guillaumin, eds., *Sciences exactes et sciences appliquées à Alexandrie,* St Etienne: 39–53

Marcus, A. (1989) *The Middle East on the eve of modernity: Aleppo in the eighteenth century.* New York

Marganne, M.-H. (1991) 'L'Égypte médicale de Pline l'Ancien', *Mémoires Centre Jean Palerne* 10: 155–71

Marganne-Mélard, M.-H. (1996) 'La médicine dans l'Egypte romaine: les services et les méthodes', in *Aufstieg und Niedergang der römischen Welt* II.37.3: 2709–40

Mari Bhat, P. N. (1989) 'Mortality and fertility in India, 1881–1961: a reassessment', in Dyson, ed. (1989): 73–118

Marsot, A. L. Al-S. (1984) *Egypt in the reign of Muhammad Ali.* Cambridge

Mata, L., Kromal, R. A. and Villegas, H. (1980) 'Diarrheal diseases: a leading world health problem', in Ö. Ouchterlony and J. Holmgren, eds., *Cholera and related diarrheas.* Basle: 1–14

Maury, P. (1987) 'Irrigation et agriculture en Egypte à la fin du XVIIIe siècle', in *L'homme et l'eau* (1987): 77–93

Mays, S., Taylor, G. M., Legge, A. J., Young, D. B. and Turner-Walker, G. (2001) 'Paleopathological and biomolecular study of tuberculosis in a medieval skeletal collection from England', *American Journal of Physical Anthropology* 114: 298–311

McCarthy, J. A. (1976) 'Nineteenth-century Egyptian population', *Middle Eastern Studies* 12, 3: 1–39

McCormick, M. (1998) 'Bateaux de vie, bateaux de mort: maladie, commerce, transports annonaires et le passage économique du Bas-Empire au Moyen Âge', in *Morfologie sociali e culturali in Europa fra tarda antichità e alto medioevo*. Spoleto: 35–118

McNeill, W. S. (1977) *Plagues and peoples*. Oxford

Mercer, A. J. (1985) 'Smallpox and epidemiological-demographic change in Europe: the role of vaccination'; *Population Studies* 39: 287–307

—— (1990) *Disease, mortality and population in transition: epidemiological-demographic change in England since the eighteenth century as part of a global phenomenon*. Leicester, London and New York

Miller, R. L., Armelagos, G. J., Ikram, S., de Jonge, N., Krijger, F. W. and Deelder, A. M. (1992) 'Palaeoepidemiology of Schistosoma infection in mummies', *British Medical Journal* 304: 555–6

——, Ikram, S., Armelagos, G. J., Walker, R., Harer, W. B., Shiff, C. J., Baggett, D., Carrigan, M. and Maret, S. M. (1994) 'Diagnosis of Plasmodium falciparum infections in mummies using the rapid manual *Para*Sight™-F test', *Transactions of the Royal Society of Tropical Medicine and Hygiene* 88: 31–2

——, de Jonge, N., Krijger, F. W. and Deelder, A. M. (1993) 'Predynastic schistosomiasis', in Davies and Walker, eds. (1993): 54–60

Milner, G. R., Humpf, D. A. and Harpending, H. C. (1989) 'Pattern matching of age-at-death distributions in paleodemographic analysis', *American Journal of Physical Anthropology* 80: 49–58

Mittler, D. M. and van Gerven, D. P. (1994) 'Developmental, diachronic, and demographic analysis of cribra orbitalia in the medieval Christian populations of Kulubnarti', *American Journal of Physical Anthropology* 93: 287–97

Mollaret, H. H. (1989) 'Le cas de la peste', *Annales de Démographie Historique 1989*: 101–10

Möller, G. (1913) *Demotische Texte aus den Königlichen Museen zu Berlin, Erster Band: Mumienschilder*. Leipzig

Monneret de Villard, U. (1933) *Le iscrizioni del cimitero di Sakinya (Nubia)*. Cairo

Montserrat, D. (1997) 'Death and funerals in the Roman Fayum', in M. L. Bierbrier, ed., *Portraits and masks: burial customs in Roman Egypt*. London: 33–44

Morley, N. (1996) *Metropolis and hinterland: the city of Rome and the Italian economy 200 BC-AD 200*. Cambridge

Morris, I. (1992) *Death-ritual and social structure in classical antiquity*. Cambridge

Morsy, T. A., el Kadery, A. A., Salama, M. M., Sabry, A. H., Kotb, M. M. and el Sharkawy, I. M. (1995), 'Studies in anopheline larvae in El Faiyum Governorate, Egypt', *Journal of the Egyptian Society of Parasitology* 25, 2: 329–53

Morsy, T. A., el Kadery, A. A., Salama, M. M., Sabry, A. H. and el Sharkawy, I. M. (1995) 'Studies on the bionomics and vector competence of adult anopheline mosquitoes in El Faiyum Governorate, Egypt', *Journal of the Egyptian Society of Parasitology* 25, 1: 213–44

Munier, H. (1930/31) 'Les stèles coptes du Monastère de Saint-Siméon à Assouan', *Aegyptus* 11: 257–300, 433–84

Muniruzzaman, A. N. M. (1966a) *Demographic survey in East Pakistan, 1961–62, part 2, chapter 1: basic demographic characteristics*. Dacca

—— (1966b) *Demographic survey in East Pakistan, 1961–62, part 3, chapters 1+2: field problems: the interview and the response*. Dacca

Murray, W. M. (1987) 'Do modern winds equal ancient winds?', *Mediterranean Historical Review* 2: 139–67

Muzzolini, A. (1985) 'Les climats au Sahara sur ses bordures, du Pleistocène final à l'aride actuel', *Empúries* 47: 8–27

Nelson, C. A. (1995) 'Four papyri from the Berlin collection', *Bulletin of the American Society of Papyrologists* 32: 123–32

Neugebauer, O. and Parker, R. A. (1960) *Egyptian astronomical texts, I: the early decans*. London

Neumann, J. (1991) 'Climate of the Black Sea region around 0 CE', *Climatic Change* 18: 453–65

—— and Parpola, S. (1987) 'Climatic change and the eleventh-century eclipse of Assyria and Babylonia', *Journal of Near Eastern Studies* 46: 161–82

Nicholson, S. E. (1981) 'The historical climatology of Africa', in Wigley, Ingram and Farmer, eds. (1981): 249–70

Nordberg, H. (1963) *Biometrical notes: the information on ancient Christian inscriptions from Rome concerning the duration of life and the dates of birth and death*. Helsinki

Norden, F. L. (1757) *Travels in Egypt and Nubia, I–II*. London

North, W. (1896) *Roman fever*. London

Nunn, J. F. (1996) *Ancient Egyptian medicine*. London

Nutton, V. (2000) 'Medical thoughts on urban pollution', in Hope and Marshall, eds. (2000): 65–73

O'Brien, P. (1968) 'The long-tern growth of agricultural production in Egypt: 1821–1962', in P. M. Holt, ed., *Political and social change in modern Egypt: historical studies from the Ottoman conquest to the United Arab Republic*. London: 162–95

Oleson, J. P. (1984) *Greek and Roman mechanical water-lifting devices: the history of a technology*. Toronto, Buffalo and London

Oliver, J. E. (1991) 'Al-Biruni's chronology: a source for historical climatology', *Climatic Change* 18: 437–52

Omran, A. R. (1971) 'The epidemiological transition: a theory of the epidemiology of population change', *Milbank Memorial Fund Quarterly* 49: 509–38

—— (1973a) 'The population of Egypt', in id., ed. (1973): 3–38

—— (1973b) 'The mortality profile', in id., ed. (1973): 39–72

——, ed. (1973) *Egypt: population problems and prospects*. Chapel Hill

Ortner, D. J. and Putschar, W. G. J. (1981) *Identification of pathological conditions in human skeletal remains*. Washington DC

Owen, E. R. J. (1969) *Cotton and the Egyptian economy 1820–1914*. Oxford

—— (1981a) *The Middle East in the world economy 1800–1914*. London and New York

—— (1981b) 'The development of agricultural production in nineteenth-century Egypt: capitalism of what type?', in Udovitch, ed. (1981): 521–46

Paine, R. R. (1989) 'Model life table fitting by maximum likelihood estimation: a procedure to reconstruct paleodemographic characteristics from skeletal age distributions', *American Journal of Physical Anthropology* 79: 51–61

—— and Harpending, H. C. (1998) 'Effect of sample bias on paleodemographic fertility estimates', *American Journal of Physical Anthropology* 105: 231–40

—— and Storey, G. R. (1997) 'Latin funerary inscriptions: (yet) another attempt at demographic analysis', in *Preatti, XI international congress of Greek and Latin epigraphy*. Rome: 847–54

Palanque, C. (1903) *Le Nil à l'époque pharaonique: son rôle et son culture en Egypte*. Paris

Pampana, E. (1963) *A textbook of malaria eradication*. Oxford

Panzac, D. (1978) 'Alexandrie: évolution d'une ville cosmopolite au XIXe siècle', *Annales Islamologiques* 14: 195–215

—— (1981) 'La population de l'empire ottoman et de ses marges du XV au XIXe siècle: bibliographie (1941–1980) et bilan provisoire', *Revue de l'Occident musulman et de la Mediterranée* 31: 119–37

—— (1982) 'Endémies, épidémies et population en Egypte au XIXe siècle', in *L'Egypte au XIXe siècle: Aix-en-Provence 4–7 juin 1979*. Paris: 83–100

—— (1985) *La peste dans l'empire ottoman 1700–1850*. Leuven

—— (1987) 'The population of Egypt in the nineteenth century', *Asian and African Studies* 21: 11–32

Parkin, T. G. (1992) *Demography and Roman society*. Baltimore and London

Parlasca, K. (1970) 'Zur Stellung der Terenuthis-Stelen—eine Gruppe römischer Grabreliefs aus Ägypten in Berlin', *Mitteilungen des Deutschen Archäologischen Instituts in Kairo* 26: 173–98

Patlagean, E. (1977) *Pauvreté économique et pauvreté sociale à Byzance: 4e–7e siècles*. Paris and La Haye

Perrenoud, A. (1979) *La population de Genève du seizième au début du dix-neuvième siècle: étude démographique, I: structures et mouvements*. Genève and Paris

Petraccone, C. (1974) *Napoli dal cinquecento all'ottocento: problemi di storia demografica e sociale*. Naples

Petrioli, L. (1982) *Nouvelles tables-types de mortalité: application et population stable*. Siena

Petropoulou, A. (1985) *Beiträge zur Wirtschafts- und Gesellschaftsgeschichte Kretas in hellenistischer Zeit*. Frankfurt a.M.

Pilet, C. and Alduc-Le Bagousse, A. (1987) 'Les vivants et les morts en Gaule romaine', in Hinard, ed. (1987): 13–31

Piontek, J. and Weber, A. (1990) 'Controversy on paleodemography', *International Journal of Anthropology* 5: 71–83

Pleket, H. W. (1994) 'The Roman state and the economy: the case of Ephesus', in J. Andreau, P. Briant and R. Descat, eds., *Economie antique: les échanges dans l'antiquité: le rôle de l'État*. St-Bertrand-de-Comminges: 115–26

Pococke, R. (1743) *A description of the East and some other countries, I: Observations on Egypt*. London

Podzorski, P. V. (1990) *Their bones shall not perish: an examination of predynastic human skeletal remains from Naga-ed-Dêr in Egypt*. New Malden

Pollitzer, R. (1954) *Plague*. Geneva

Pomeroy, S. B. (1983) 'Infanticide in Hellenistic Greece', in A. Cameron and A. Kuhrt, eds., *Images of women in antiquity*. London: 207–22

Popper, W. (1951) *The Cairo Nilometer: studies in Ibn Taghrî Birdî's Chronicles of Egypt, I*. Berkeley and Los Angeles

Preston, S. H., McDaniel, A. and Grushka, C. (1993) 'New model life tables for high-mortality populations', *Historical Methods* 26: 149–59

Prominska, E. (1972) *Investigations on the population of Muslim Alexandria: anthropological-demographic study*. Warsaw

Pruner, F. (1847) *Die Krankheiten des Orients vom Standpunkte der vergleichenden Nosologie*. Erlangen

Prusakov, D. B. (1997) '"Old dunes" in Middle Egypt', *Vestnik Drevnej Istorii* 221: 95–9

Puranen, B. (1991) 'Tuberculosis and the decline of mortality in Sweden', in R. Schofield, D. Reher and A. Bideau, eds., *The decline of mortality in Europe*. Oxford: 97–117

Quaegebeur, J. (1972) 'Contribution à la prosopographie des prêtres memphites à l'époque ptolémaique', *Ancient Society* 3: 77–109

—— (1978) 'Mummy labels: an introduction', in Boswinkel and Pestman, eds. (1978): 232–59

Quirke, S. (1988) 'Mummy labels', in S. D'Auria, P. Lavocara and C. H. Roehrig, *Mummies and magic: the funerary arts of ancient Egypt*. Boston: 229

Rabie, H. (1981) 'Some technical aspects of agriculture in medieval Egypt', in Udovitch, ed. (1981): 59–90

Raikes, R. L. and Palmieri, A. (1972) 'Environmental conditions in the Nile valley over the past 10,000 years', *Journal of Human Evolution* 1: 147–54

Rathbone, D. W. (1983) 'The grain trade and grain shortages in the Hellenistic East', in Garnsey and Whittaker, eds. (1983): 45–55

—— (1989) 'The ancient economy and Graeco-Roman Egypt', in Criscuolo and Geraci, eds. (1989): 159–76

—— (1990) 'Villages, land and population in Graeco-Roman Egypt', *Proceedings of the Cambridge Philological Society* 36: 103–42

—— (1991) *Economic rationalism and rural society in third-century AD Egypt: the Heroninos archive and the Appianus estate.* Cambridge

—— (1996) 'Towards a historical topography of the Fayum', in D. M. Bailey, ed., *Archaeological research in Roman Egypt.* Ann Arbor: 50–6

—— (1997) 'Prices and price formation in Roman Egypt', in Andreau, Briant and Descat, eds. (1997): 183–244

Raymond, A. (1972) 'Les grandes épidémies de peste au Caire aux XVIIe et XVIIIe siècles', *Bulletin d'études orientales* 25: 203–10

—— (1981) 'The economic crisis in Egypt in the eighteenth century', in Udovitch, ed. (1981): 687–707

Regöly-Mérei, G. (1966) 'Paläopathologische und epigraphische Angaben zur Frage der Pocken in Altägypten', *Sudhoffs Archiv* 50: 411–17

Rehm, A., ed. (1914) *Milet: Ergebnisse der Ausgrabungen und Untersuchungen seit dem Jahre 1899, I, 3: Das Delphinion von Milet. Die Inschriften.* Berlin

Renati (1800) 'Topographie physique et médicale du vieux Kaire', *La décade égyptienne: Journal littéraire et d'économie politique* 2: 180–90

Reymond, E. A. E. (1981) *From the records of a priestly family from Memphis, I.* Wiesbaden

Richards, A. (1982) *Egypt's agricultural development, 1800–1980: technical and social change.* Boulder

Riley, J. C. and Alter, G. (1989) 'The epidemiologic transition and morbidity', *Annales de Démographie Historique* 1989: 199–213

Risse, G. B. (1997) 'Cause of death as a historical problem', *Continuity and Change* 12 (= Alter and Carmichael, eds. [1997]): 175–88

Rivlin, H. A. B. (1961) *The agricultural policy of Muhammad 'Ali in Egypt.* Cambridge MA

Rogers, L. (1913) *Dysenteries: their differentiation and treatment.* London

Rose, J. C., Armelagos, G. J. and Perry, L. S. (1993) 'Dental anthropology of the Nile valley', in Davies and Walker, eds. (1993): 61–74

Röser, B. (1837) *Über einige Krankheiten des Orients.* Augsburg

Ross, R. (1903) *Report on malaria at Ismailia and Suez.* London and New York

Rossi, P. F., Bondioli, L., Geusa, G. and Macchiarelli, R. (n.d.) 'Osteodental biology of the people of *Portus Romae* (Necropolis of Isola Sacra, 2nd–3rd cent. AD), I: enamel microstructure and developmental defects of the primary dentition'. CD-ROM. Rome

Roth, E. A. (1992) 'Applications of demographic models to paleodemography', in Saunders and Katzenberg, eds. (1992): 175–88

Rowlandson, J. (1996) *Landowners and tenants in Roman Egypt: the social relations of agriculture in the Oxyrhynchite nome.* Oxford

Rubin, R. (1989) 'The debate over climatic changes in the Negev, fourth-seventh centuries CE', *Palestine Exploration Quarterly* 121: 71–8

Rubincam, C. (1991) 'Casualty figures in the battle descriptions of Thucydides', *Transactions of the American Philological Association* 121: 181–98

Russell, J. C. (1966) 'The population of medieval Egypt', *Journal of the American Research Center in Egypt* 5: 69–82

—— (1968) 'That earlier plague', *Demography* 5: 174–84

—— (1985) *The control of late ancient and medieval population.* Philadelphia

Safrai, Z. (1994) *The economy of Roman Palestine.* London and New York

Said, R. (1993) *The river Nile: geology, hydrology and utilization.* Oxford

Saito, O. (1997) 'Infant mortality in pre-transition Japan: levels and trends', in Bideau, Desjardins and Pérez Brignoli, eds. (1997): 135–53

Sakamoto-Momiyama, M. (1977) *Seasonality in human mortality: a medico-geographical study.* Tokyo

Sallares, R. (1991) *The ecology of the ancient Greek world*. London
—— (1995) 'The ecology of the ancient world: problems and approaches', *Vestnik Drevnei Istorii* 3: 80–103 (in Russian)
—— (forthcoming) *Malaria and Rome: a history of malaria in central Italy in antiquity*. Oxford
—— and Gomzi, S. (forthcoming) 'Biomolecular archaeology of malaria', *Ancient Biomolecules*
Saller, R. P. (1994) *Patriarchy, property and death in the Roman family*. Cambridge
—— (forthcoming) 'Framing the debate over growth in the ancient economy', in J. Manning and I. Morris, eds., *The ancient economy: evidence and models*. Stanford
Salem, T., Soliman, S. and el Sayed, S. (1973) 'Seasonal Variation of Deaths in A.R.E. (1961–1970)', *Population Researches and Studies* 6: 34–48
Salmon, P. (1974) *Population et dépopulation dans l'empire romain*. Brussels
—— (1992) 'La contamination des eaux et son impact sur la démographie du monde greco-romain', in G. Argoud *et al.*, eds., *L'eau et les hommes en Méditerranée et en Mer Noire dans l'antiquité de l'époque mycénienne au règne de Justinien*. Athens: 541–55
Sandford-Smith, J. (1997) *Eye diseases in hot climates*. 3rd ed. Oxford
Sandison, A. T. (1972) 'Evidence of infective disease', *Journal of Human Evolution* 1: 213–24
—— (1980) 'Diseases in ancient Egypt', in A. Cockburn and E. Cockburn, eds., *Mummies, disease, and ancient cultures*. Cambridge: 29–44
Sandwith, F. M. (1905) *The medical diseases of Egypt*. London
Saunders, S. R., Herring, D. A. and Boyce, G. (1995) 'Can skeletal samples accurately represent the living populations they come from? The St. Thomas' Cemetery Site, Belleville, Ontario', in A. L. Grauer, ed., *Bodies of evidence: reconstructing history through skeletal analysis*. New York: 69–89
—— and Hoppa, R. D. (1996) 'Growth deficit in survivors and non-survivors: biological mortality bias in subadult skeletal samples', *Yearbook of Physical Anthropology* 36: 127–51
—— and Katzenberg, M. A., eds. (1992) *The skeletal biology of past peoples: research methods*. New York
Savaresi, A. (1800a) 'Essai sur la topographie physique et médicale de Damiette', *La décade égyptienne: Journal littéraire et d'économie politique* 2: 85–90
—— (1800b) 'Observations sur les maladies qui ont regné à Damiette dans le premier semestre de l'an 7', *La décade égyptienne: Journal littéraire et d'économie politique* 2: 122–7
Saxena, P. C., Verma, R. K. and Sharma, A. K. (1986) 'Errors in age-reporting in India: a socio-cultural and psychological explanation', *Indian Journal of Social Work* 47: 127–35
Schamp, H. (1968) *Ägypten (Vereinigte Arabische Republik): das Land am Nil im wirtschaftlichen und sozialen Umbruch*. 2nd ed. Frankfurt
Scheidel, W. (1994) 'Libitina's bitter gains: seasonal mortality and endemic disease in the ancient city of Rome', *Ancient Society* 25: 151–75
—— (1995) 'Incest revisited: three notes on the demography of sibling marriage in Roman Egypt', *Bulletin of the American Society of Papyrologists* 32: 143–55
—— (1996a) *Measuring sex, age and death in the Roman empire: explorations in ancient demography*. Ann Arbor
—— (1996b) 'Brother-sister and parent-child marriage outside royal families in ancient Egypt and Iran: a challenge to the sociobiological view of incest avoidance?', *Ethology and Sociobiology* 17: 319–40
—— (1996c) 'Finances, figures and fiction', *Classical Quarterly* 46: 222–38
—— (1996d) 'What's in an age? A comparative view of bias in the census returns of Roman Egypt', *Bulletin of the American Society of Papyrologists* 33: 25–59
—— (1997a) 'Brother-sister marriage in Roman Egypt', *Journal of Biosocial Science* 29: 361–71

—— (1997b) 'Twins in Roman Egypt: postscript to *BASP* 33 (1996)', *Bulletin of the American Society of Papyrologists* 34: 35–7

—— (1998) 'The meaning of dates on mummy labels: seasonal mortality and mortuary practice in Roman Egypt', *Journal of Roman Archaeology* 11: 285–92

—— (1999a) 'Emperors, aristocrats and the Grim Reaper: towards a demographic profile of the Roman élite', *Classical Quarterly* 49: 254–81

—— (1999b) 'The death declarations of Roman Egypt: a re-appraisal', *Bulletin of the American Society of Papyrologists* 36: 53–70

—— (2001) 'Progress and problems in Roman demography', in Scheidel, ed. (2001): 1–81

—— (forthcoming a) 'Germs for Rome', in C. Edwards and G. Woolf, eds., *Rome the cosmopolis.* Cambridge

—— (forthcoming b) 'A model of demographic and economic change in Roman Egypt after the 'Antonine plague''

—— (forthcoming c) 'Demography', in I. Morris, R. Saller and W. Scheidel, eds., *The Cambridge economic history of the Greco-Roman world.* Cambridge

——, ed. (2001) *Debating Roman demography.* Leiden

Scheper-Hughes, N. (1992) *Death without weeping: the violence of everyday life in Brazil.* Berkeley, Los Angeles and London

Schlott, A. (1969) *Die Ausmasse Ägyptens nach altägyptischen Texten.* Tübingen

Schnebel, M. (1925) *Die Landwirtschaft im hellenistischen Ägypten.* Munich

Schnepp, M. B. (1861) 'Observations recueìlliés à Alexandrie d'Egypte, du Ier octobre 1858 au 30 septembre 1860', *Comptes rendus hebdomadaires des séances de l'Académie des Sciences* 52: 641–4

—— (1862a) 'Etudes sur les climat de l'Egypte', *Mémoires ou travaux originaux présentés et lus à l'Institut Egyptien* 1: 177–368

—— (1862b) 'Considérations sur le mouvement de la population en Egypte', *Mémoires ou travaux originaux présentés et lus à l'Institut Egyptien* 1: 525–600

Scobie, A. (1986) 'Slums, sanitation and mortality in the Roman world', *Klio* 68: 399–433

Scott, J. A. (1937) 'The incidence and distribution of human schistosomes in Egypt', *American Journal of Hygiene* 25: 566–614

Segal, M., Alpert, P., Stein, U., Mandel, M. and Mitchell, M. J. (1994) 'Some assessments of the potential 2 × CO_2 climatic effects on water balance components in the eastern Mediterranean', *Climatic Change* 27: 351–71

Sgarlata, M. (1991) *Ricerche di demografia storica: le iscrizioni tardo-imperiali di Siracusa.* Vatican City

Sharlin, A. (1978) 'Natural decrease in early modern cities: a reconsideration', *Past and Present* 79: 126–38

Sharp, M. (1999) 'The village of Theadelphia in the Fayyum: land and population in the second century', in Bowman and Rogan, eds. (1999): 159–92

Shaw, B. D. (1981) 'Climate, environment, and history: the case of Roman North Africa', in Wigley, Ingram and Farmer, eds. (1981): 379–403

—— (1991) 'The cultural meaning of death: age and gender in the Roman family', in D. I. Kertzer and R. P. Saller, eds., *The family in Italy from antiquity to the present.* New Haven and London: 66–90

—— (1996) 'Seasons of death: aspects of mortality in imperial Rome', *Journal of Roman Studies* 86: 100–38

—— (1997) 'Agrarian economy and the marriage cycle of Roman women', *Journal of Roman Archaeology* 10: 57–76

—— (2001) 'The seasonal birthing cycle of Roman women', in Scheidel, ed. (2001): 83–110

Shore, A. F. (1992) 'Human and divine mummification', in A. B. Lloyd, ed., *Studies in Pharaonic religion and society in honour of J. Gwyn Griffiths.* London: 226–35

—— and Smith, H. S. (1960) 'A demotic embalmers' agreement (Pap. dem. B.M. 10561)', *Acta Orientalia* 25: 277–94

Shousha, A. T. (1948) 'Species-eradication: the eradication of Anopheles gambiae from Upper Egypt 1942–1945', *Bulletin of the World Health Organization* 1: 309–52

Sideras, A. (1994) 'Rufus von Ephesos und sein Werk im Rahmen der antiken Medizin', in *Aufstieg und Niedergang der Römischen Welt* II.37.2: 1077–1253, 2036–62

Sijpesteijn, P. J. (1967) *The Wisconsin papyri I.* Leiden

—— (1995) 'Three papyri concerning census', *Zeitschrift für Papyrologie und Epigraphik* 107: 271–6

Siven, C.-H. (1991) 'On estimating mortalities from osteological age data', *International Journal of Anthropology* 6: 97–110

Slack, P. (1981) 'The disappearance of plague: an alternative view', *Economic History Review* 34: 469–76

—— (1985) *The impact of plague in Tudor and Stuart England.* Oxford

Smith, D. C. (1982) 'The rise and fall of typhomalarial fever: I. Origins. II. Decline and fall', *Journal of the History of Medicine and Allied Sciences* 37: 182–220, 287–321

Smith, M. (1987) *Catalogue of demotic papyri in the British Museum, III: the mortuary texts of Papyrus BM 10507.* London

Smith, R. M. (1991) 'Demographic development in rural England, 1300–48: a survey', in B. M. S. Campbell, ed., *Before the Black Death: studies in the 'crisis' of the early fourteenth century.* Manchester and New York: 25–78

Sonnini, C. S. (1799) *Travels in Upper and Lower Egypt, II.* London

Sperduti, A. (1995) 'I resti scheletrici umani della necropoli di età romano-imperiale di Isola Sacra (I–III sec. d. C.): analisi paleodemografica'. Tesi di dottorato di ricerca, Università di Roma 'La Sapienza'

—— and Manzi, G. (1990) 'Hyperostosis frontalis interna in a cranial sample from the Roman population of Portus (Isola Sacra necropolis, I–III century AD)', *Rivista di Antropologia* 68: 279–86

Spiegelberg, W. (1923) 'Die Beisetzung des Patriarchen Jakob (Gen. 50, 2ff.) im Lichte der ägyptischen Quellen', *Orientalistische Literaturzeitung* 26, 9: 421–4

Spurr, M. S. (1986) *Arable cultivation in Roman Italy* c. *200 BC*–c. *AD 100.* London

Strouhal, E. (1989) 'Palaeopathology of the Christian population at Sayala (Egyptian Nubia, 5th–11th cent. AD)', in L. Capasso, ed., *Advances in paleopathology.* Chieti: 191–6

Stuart-Macadam, P. (1985) 'Porotic hyperostosis: representative of a childhood condition', *American Journal of Physical Anthropology* 66: 391–8

—— (1992) 'Anaemia in past human populations', in P. Stuart-Macadam and S. Kent, eds., *Diet, demography, and disease: changing perspectives on anaemia.* New York: 151–70

Suder, W. (1988) *Census populi: bibliographie de la démographie de l'antiquité romaine.* Bonn

—— (1990) *A study of the age and sex structure of population in the western provinces of the Roman empire.* Wroclaw

Thieme, M. and Pestman, P. W. (1978a) 'Inscribed cloths from mummies', in Boswinkel and Pestman, eds. (1978): 131–3

—— (1978b) 'Inscribed mummy linen of the Roman period', in Boswinkel and Pestman, eds. (1978): 225–31

Thompson, D. (1999) 'New and old in the Ptolemaic Fayyum', in Bowman and Rogan, eds. (1999): 123–38

Thüry, G. E. (1977) 'Zur Infektkette der Pest in hellenistisch-römischer Zeit', in *75 Jahre Anthropologische Staatssammlung München 1902–1977.* Munich: 275–83

Tietze, A. (1975) *Mustafa 'Ali's description of Cairo of 1599: text, transliteration, translation, notes.* Vienna

Tignor, R. L. (1984) *State, private enterprise, and economic change in Egypt, 1918–1952.* Princeton

Till, W. C. (1951) *Die Arzneikunde der Kopten*. Berlin

Toledano, E. R. (1990) *State and society in mid-nineteenth century Egypt*. Cambridge

Traina, G. (1988) *Paludi e bonifiche del mondo antico*. Rome

Udovitch, A. L., ed. (1981) *The Islamic Middle East, 700–1900: studies in economic and social history*. Princeton

United Nations (1982) *Unabridged model life tables corresponding to the new United Nations model life tables for developing countries*. New York

Valaoras, V. G. (1972) *Population analysis of Egypt, 1935–1970 (with special reference to mortality)*. Cairo

Valassopoulo, A., Parodi, D. and Lévy, I. (1912) *La tuberculose en Egypte et l'oeuvre de la Ligue contre la tuberculose*. Alexandria

Valensi, L. (1969) 'Calamités démographiques en Tunisie et en Mediterranée orientale aux XVIIIe et XIXe siècles', *Annales: Economies, Sociétés, Civilisations* 24: 1540–61

van der Horst, P. W. (1991) *Ancient Jewish epitaphs: an introductory survey of a millennium of Jewish funerary epigraphy (300 BCE–700 CE)*. Kampen

van Minnen, P. (1997) *Roman Hermopolis: a study of the social and economic history of an Egyptian town in the first four centuries AD*. Leuven

Vercoutter, J. (1962) *Textes biographiques du Sérapéum de Memphis: contribution à l'étude des stèles votives du Sérapéum*. Paris

Vergote, J. (1959) *Josephe en Egypte: Gènese chap. 37–50 à la lumière des études égyptologiques récentes*. Louvain

Volney, M. C. (1788) *Travels through Syria and Egypt, in the years 1783, 1784, and 1785, I–II*. 2nd ed. London

Voyage (1971) *Voyage en Egypte de Jean Palerne Forésien 1581*. Paris

Voyages (1971) *Voyages en Egypte de Jean Coppin 1638–1639, 1643–1646*. Paris

Voyages (1973a) *Voyages en Egypte des années 1611 et 1612: George Sandys. William Lithgow*. Paris

Voyages (1973b) *Voyages en Egypte de Johann Wied 1606–1610*. Paris

Voyage (1977) *Voyage en Egypte du Père Antonius Gonzales 1665–1666*. Paris

Voyages (1981) *Voyages en Egypte pendant les années 1678–1701*. Paris

Wagner, G. (1972) 'Inscriptions grecques d'Egypte', *Bulletin de l'Institut Francais d'Archéologie Orientale* 72: 139–67

—— (1993) 'L'épigraphie du village dans l'Egypte grecque et romaine', in A. Calbi, A. Donati and G. Poma, eds., *L'epigrafia del villaggio*. Faenza: 101–16

—— (1994a) 'Les stèles funéraires de Kom Abu Bellou (BSAA 44, 1991, 169–200)', *Zeitschrift für Papyrologie und Epigraphik* 101: 113–9

—— (1994b) 'Une épigramme funéraire de Kom Abu Bellou: l'épitaphe métrique de Marcella, morte à 6 ans', *Zeitschrift für Papyrologie und Epigraphik* 103: 177–80

—— (1996) 'Nouvelles inscriptions funéraires grecques de Kom Abu Bellou', *Zeitschrift für Papyrologie und Epigraphik* 114: 115–40

Wagstaff, J. M. (1985) *The evolution of Middle Eastern landscapes: an outline to AD 1840*. London and Sydney

Walker, P. L., Johnson, J. R. and Lambert, P. M. (1988) 'Age and sex biases in the preservation of human skeletal remains', *American Journal of Physical Anthropology* 76: 183–8

Walker, R., Parsche, F., Bierbrier, M. and McKerrow, J. H. (1987) 'Tissue identification and histologic study of six lung specimens from Egyptian mummies', *American Journal of Physical Anthropology* 72: 43–8

Walker, S. and Bierbrier, M. (1997) *Ancient faces: mummy portraits from Roman Egypt*. London

Watkins, S. C. and Menken, J. (1985) 'Famines in historical perspective', *Population and Development Review* 11: 647–75

Watts, S. (1998) 'An ancient scourge: the end of dracunculiasis in Egypt', *Social Science and Medicine* 46: 811–19

Weiss, K. M. (1973) *Demographic models for anthropology*. Washington DC
Wendorf, F. and Schild, R. (1976) *Prehistory of the Nile valley*. New York, San Francisco and London
Whitby, M. (1995) 'Recruitment in Roman armies from Justinian to Heraclius (*ca*.565–615)', in A. Cameron, ed., *The Byzantine and early Islamic Near East, II: states, resources and armies*. Princeton: 61–124
White, K. M. (1999) 'Cardiovascular and tuberculosis mortality: the contrasting effects of changes in two causes of death', *Population and Development Review* 25: 289–302
Whitley, G. (1864) 'Sixth report of the Medical Officer of the Privy Council, as to the quantity of ague and other malarious diseases now prevailing in the principal marsh districts of England', *Reports and Commissioners (13), Public Health Records* 28: 430–54
Wietheger, C. (1992) *Das Jeremias-Kloster zu Saqqara unter besonderer Berücksichtigung der Inschriften*. Altenberge
Wigley, T. M. L., Ingram, M. J. and Farmer, G., eds. (1981) *Climate and history: studies in past climates and their impact on man*. Cambridge
——, Jones, P. D. and Kelly, P. M. (1980) 'Scenario for a warm, high-CO_2 world', *Nature* 283: 17–21
Wilcken, U. (1901) 'Heidnisches und Christliches aus Ägypten', *Archiv für Papyrusforschung* 1: 396–436
Wilcocks, C. (1962) *Aspects of medical investigations in Africa*. London and New York
Wilfong, T. G. (1995) 'Mummy labels from the Oriental Institute's excavations at Medinet Habu', *Bulletin of the American Society of Papyrologists* 32, 3–4: 157–81
Wilson, R. T. (1803) *History of the British expedition to Egypt*. 2nd ed. London
Winkler, E.-M. and Wilfing, H. (1991) *Tell El-Dab'a VI: anthropologische Untersuchungen an den Skelettresten der Kampagnen 1966–69, 1975–80, 1985*. Vienna
Winnicki, J. K. (1992) 'Demotische Stelen aus Terenuthis', in J. H. Johnson, ed., *Life in a multi-cultural society: Egypt from Cambyses to Constantine and beyond*. Chicago: 351–60
Winter, M. (1992) *Egyptian society under Ottoman rule 1517–1798*. London and New York
Woenig, F. (1886) *Die Pflanzen im alten Ägypten*. Leipzig
Woods, R. (1993) 'On the historical relationship between infant and adult mortality', *Population Studies* 47: 195–219
Woodward, S. (1996) 'Commoners' graves', *Archaeology* September/October 1996: 46
Worrell, W. H. (1935) 'Coptic magical and medical texts', *Orientalia* 4: 1–37, 184–94
Wörrle, M. (1971) 'Ägyptisches Getreide für Ephesos', *Chiron* 1: 325–40
Wrigley, E. A. (1978) 'A simple model of London's importance in changing English society and economy 1650–1750', in P. Abrams and E. A. Wrigley, ed., *Towns in societies: essays in economic history and historical sociology*. Cambridge: 215–43
——, Davies, R. S., Oeppen, J. E. and Schofield, R. S. (1997) *English population history from family reconstitution 1580–1837*. Cambridge
—— and Schofield, R. S. (1981) *The population history of England 1541–1871: a reconstruction*. London
Yates, D. N. and Strzepek, K. M. (1998) 'An assessment of integrated climate change impacts on the agricultural economy of Egypt', *Climatic Change* 38: 261–87
Yates, W. H. (1843) *The modern history and condition of Egypt, its climate, diseases, and capabilities, I–II*. London
Zagiell, I. T. (1863) *Des maladies des yeux régnantes en Afrique, en Egypte et en Nubie*. Paris
Zeki, A. (1898) 'Une description arabe du Fayoum au VIIe siècle de l'hégire', *Bulletin de la Société Khédivale de Géographie*, ser. 5, 1: 253–95
Zhao, Z. (1997) 'Long-term mortality patterns in Chinese history: evidence from a recorded clan population', *Population Studies* 51: 117–27
Zimmermann, M. R. (1979) 'Pulmonary and osseous tuberculosis in an Egyptian mummy', *Bulletin of the New York Academy of Medicine* 55: 604–8
Zinsser, H. (1935) *Rats, lice, and history*. London

INDEX

Abbas, 201, 248
Abydos, 59, 92
Africa, tropical, 53, 102, 128
Age distribution, *see* Life tables, Mortality
Age-rounding, 175
Agriculture, in hellenistic Egypt, 220, 225, in Roman Egypt, 223, 225, in medieval Egypt, 220, in nineteenth-century Egypt, 217–19, 221–31, of ancient compared to nineteenth-century Egypt, 242–4; *see also* Carrying capacity, Farming techniques, Food, Irrigation, Land, Yields
Agrippa II, 184, 248
Ahrun, 95
AIDS, 105
al-Biruni, 54
Aleppo, 190
Alexandria, Roman, 19–21, 25, 51, 54–5, 78–9, 95, 112, 142–3, 184, 234, 247, modern, 42–5, 64, 66–7, 73–4, 81–2, 92–3, 96, 105–09, 112, 188, 191, 194, 198, 202, 208, 247
Alpinus, Prosper, 59–61, 63, 78, 95, 98, 111
Al-Razi, 96
Ankylostomiasis, 103
Anopheles, see Mosquitoes
Antes, J., 64, 98
Antioch, 234
Antonine plague, 95–6, 127, 162–6, 171, 249
Arabia, 235
Aretaios, 66, 104
Aristotle, 56
Arsinoe (city), 84, 149, 156, 171, population of, 173
Arsinoite nome, *see* Fayum
Asia Minor, 200, 235
Asthma, 104
Aswan, 6–10, 57, 103, 228
Athens, XXIV, 95, 179, 181
Augustus, 182, 231–2
Australia, 237
Baer, G., 205–07
Bagnall, R. S., XXII–V, XXVII–III, 1, 118–20, 141–4, 151, 153, 156, 160, 162, 164, 166, 172–3, 176–8, 246, 248
Baghdad, 189
Bahr Yussuf, 77, 82–3
Bangladesh, 149
Barber, M. A., 81
Barley, 222, 224–6, 229–30, 236
Beans, 222, 224–6, 229–30, 236–7
Beijing, 133–5
Beloch, K. J., 182
Bilharzia, *see* Schistosomiasis
Birket Qarun, 4, 82–3, 85–6
Birth rate, 57, 165, 170, 197, 213–14; *see also* Fertility
Blindness, 104
Bonneau, D., 87
Boyaval, B., 3
Brother-sister marriage, XXV, 171

Cairo, 4, 41–45, 61, 66–7, 69, 72–4, 82, 92, 94–5, 98–9, 103–09, 112, 166, 187–91, 194, 198, 201–02, 208, 214, 247
Campbell, J., 95, 111
Canterbury, 98
Carrying capacity, 237–42
Carthage, 21–2, 234
Cemetery populations, 121–2, 135–41; *see also* Paleodemography, Skeletal evidence
Census, in Roman Republic and early empire, 182, in Roman Egypt, 118, 123, 183, in modern Egypt, 203–06
Census lists, from Ptolemaic Egypt, XXV
Census returns, from Roman Egypt, XXIV–V, XXVII–III, 1, 118, 123, 142–3, from metropoleis, 118, 143–56, from villages, 118, 143, 156–62, from Upper Egypt, 153–4, compared to tax lists, 158–61, and Antonine plague, 162–6, from Asia, 157

Chicago, 62–3
Children, in census returns, 119, 149–50, on epitaphs, 26–32, mortality of, 26–30, 41, 58, 94, 108–09, 196–7, vaccination of, 198–9; *see also* Infant mortality
China, XXIII, 114, 129–31, 133–5, 157
Cholera, 101, 194–5, 209, 213
Cities, *see* Metropoleis, Mortality, Population size, Urbanisation
Clark, A. W., 127
Clarysse, W., XXV
Climate, in Egypt, 54–7, 60
Clot Bey, A.-B., 64, 92, 194, 197–8
Coale, A. J., 123–6, 131, 140
Coale-Demeny models, 120, 123–6, 156, 175
Colchester, 188
Commemorative practices, 100, in Roman Egypt, 30–35, 111–12
Conscription, in modern Egypt, 199–201
Constipation, 65
Coppin, J., 61
Cotton, 218–19, 227, 240–1
Craig, J. I., 65
Cribra orbitalia, 104, 138–40
Crocodilopolis, *see* Arsinoe

Damietta, 64
Death declarations, from Roman Egypt, 3
Death rate, in nineteenth-century Egypt, 49, 195–6, 212–14; *see also* Mortality
Demeny, P., 123–6, 131, 140
Denderah, 77
Diaconus, Marcus, 60
Diarrhoea, 60, 62–6
Diet, *see* Nutrition
Diodorus Siculus, 184
Diphtheria, 104
Disease, 51–116, classification of, 105–09, and demography, XXII, 195–6, in pre-Roman Egypt, 59, 76, 92, 95, Roman Egypt, 77, 95–6, 99–100, 103–04, in early modern Egypt, 59–61, 64, 78, 94–5, 97–8, in nineteenth-century Egypt, 64, 66–9, 72–3, 78–9, 92–3, 98, 101–09, 186–99, in twentieth-century Egypt, 65, 69–70, 72, 80–2, 84–6, 89, 92, 102–03, 107–09, relative prevalence of, 105–09, seasonal incidence of, 60–1, 64–5, 67–9, 72–4, 78–81, 89, 96, 97–8, 110, change in Egypt, 114–15; *see also* Epidemics, and entries for particular diseases
Dobson, M., XXVI, 58
Dols, M. W., 187
Dracunculiasis (dracontiasis), 103
Drainage, 85, 87, 89
Duncan-Jones, R. P., 232
Durliat, J., 234
Dysentery, 53, 63–6, 106

Economic development, 183–4, 218–31, 236–9, 242–4, 249
Edfu, 220
Egypt, *passim*, pre-Roman, 59, 76, 83, 92, 95, 99, 220, Roman 3–35, 54–5, 77–9, 86–9, 92, 95, 99–100, 103–04, 118–20, 142–78, 183–6, 231–5, 246–9, medieval, 54–5, 84, 96–7, 100, 187, 220, early modern, 59–61, 63–4, 78, 94–5, 97–8, 104, 188–90, in the nineteenth century, 41–45, 48–9, 64, 66–7, 69, 72–4, 78–9, 92–3, 98, 101, 105–09, 190–215, 218–19, 221–31,235–6, 243, in the twentieth century, 39–41, 49, 65, 67, 69–70, 72, 80–2, 84–6, 92, 102–03, 107–09, 237, size of, 220; *see also* Fayum, Lower Egypt, Middle Egypt, Upper Egypt
Embalmment, in ancient Egypt, 13, 15; *see also* Mummies
England, early modern, 53, 98, 128, 179, 197, nineteenth-century, 69, 91
Ephesus, 234
Epidemics, 24, 61, 64, 67, 94–5, 97–101, 126–7, 162–6, 187–93, 207, 249; *see also* Antonine Plague
Epizootic, 199
Essex, 132–3
Europe, 124, northwestern, 36
Export, of food, from Egypt, 231–6, 240–1
Ezbet El Sham-ekh Masoud, 86

Famine, 126, 188
Farming techniques, 217–18, 222, 225, 228, 241–4
Fayum, 4, 70, 76, 82–3, 90, pre-Roman 83, 244, Roman, 16–19, 51, 77, 86–9, 175, 177, 244, medieval, 70, 84, 87, modern, 40–1, 70, 84–6, modern city of, 84–5

Females, in Egyptian census returns, 119–20, 147, 149–50, 160–2, 174–5, migration of, 166–7, in villages, 160–1, 174–5; *see also* Life expectancy, Mortality, Sex ratio
Fertility, 176, 213; *see also* Birth rate
Fleas, 99
Florence and Tuscany, 126
Food, *see* Agriculture, Barley, Beans, Export, Import, Maize, Millet, Nutrition, Rice, Sorghum, Wheat
Food poisoning, 62–3
Frank, L., 64
French forces in Egypt, 41, 60, 64, 72, 190
Frier, B. W., XXII–V, XXVII–III, 1, 118–22, 141–4, 151, 153, 156, 160, 162, 164, 166, 172–3, 176–8, 246, 248

Gastro-enteritis, 53, 105–06; *see also* Diarrhoea, Dysentery, Typhoid, Typhus
Geneva, 94, 196
Germany, 69
Gonzales, Father, 64, 78, 104
Grmek, M. D., XXII–V, 92, 104
Grosseto, 132, 156
Guinea-worm disease, *see* Dracunculiasis

Haiti, 241
Hatcher, J., 98
Hawara, 19, 82
Hepatitis, 72, 111
Herlihy, D., 126
Hermopolis Magna, 77, 149, 173
Herod, 234
Herodotus, 58–9, 76, 82–3, 232
Hippocratics, 60
Hirsch, A., 93
Hopkins, M. K., XXII, 120, 123, 176, 233–4
Households, in Roman Egypt, 147–9, in modern Egypt, 201–02
Hungary, 131
Hyksos, 59

Ibion Argaiou, 87
Ibrahim, 201
Import, of food, to Egypt, 235–7
India, 63, 101, 127, 129, 194, 241
Infant mortality, 30–2, 41, 45, 49, 58, 63, 89, 108, 133–4, 214, and relationship to adult mortality, 128–30
Infanticide, 150
Irrigation, in Egypt, 76, 81, 83, 89, 199–201, 217–19, 222, 241–4
Ismail, 219, 236
Ismail Bey, 189
Ismailia, 88
Istanbul, 235
Italy, Roman, XXIX, 37–8, 181–3, 250, in the nineteenth century, 45–6, 131, 183

Japan, 52, 130, 157
Jaundice, *see* Hepatitis
Jomard, 201–02
Josephus Flavius, 184, 232, 246, 248
Justinian, 231–2, 234

Karanis, 86
Kent, 58
Kerkeosiris, 88
Khamseen, 61, 90, 92, 98, 111
Klapisch-Zuber, C., 126
Kom Abu Bellou, *see* Terenouthis
Kom Talit, 88
Kulubnarti, 138–9

Land, cultivated, 220–4
Landers, J., 3, 58
Lane, E. W., 98, 194
Leontopolis, 19–20, 24, 35, 48, 90–1, 93, 97, 112
Leprosy, XXV, XXIX, 115, 178
Liaoning, *see* Manchuria
Libya, 99
Life expectancy, Roman, 121–3, 176–8, in Roman Egypt, XXVII, 120, 178, female, 120, 174–5, male, 120, in modern Egypt, 176, 214, in cemetery populations, 137–40, in China, 133–4, in Italy, 132; *see also* Life tables, Mortality
Life tables, anthropological, 137–8, historical, 124–5, model, 30, 120–42; *see also* Ulpianic life table
Livia, 88
Lo Cascio, E., XXIII
Lodgers, 146–7, 154, 171
London, early modern, 3, 53, 58, 94
Lower Egypt, 4, 19–25, 26–33, 39–40, 48–9, 54, 61, 72, 76, 78, 80, 90, 93, 97, 102–03, 112–13, 142, 178, 188, 190, 218–20, 225–8, 243, 248
Luxor, 76
Lykopolis, 153–4, 167–9

Maize, 226, 228, 236–7
Malaria, 75–6, in Egypt, 76–91, 115, in pre-Roman Egypt, 76, in Roman Egypt, 77, in early modern Egypt, 78–9, in twentieth-century Egypt, 80–2, in the Roman Fayum, 77, 88–9, 175, in the medieval Fayum, 84, in the modern Fayum, 84–6, in Roman Italy, XXV, XXIX, 250, in modern Italy, 132, in modern England, 132–3, seasonality of, 78, 80–2, 89, and other diseases, 71, 75
Males, in Egyptian census returns, 119–20, 148, 156–62, in tax lists, 158–61, migration of, 166–8; *see also* Life expectancy, Mortality, Sex ratio
Malnutrition, 34, 57, 104, 140; *see also* Famine, Nutrition
Manchuria, 134–6
Mareotis (Mariut), Lake, 79, 81
Mari Bhat, P. N., 129
Marseille, 189
Marshes, in Egypt, 76, 79, 87–8
McCarthy, J. A., 190, 193–5, 201–09
Measles, 102, 114
Medicine, ancient Egyptian, 65, 92, in modern Egypt, 198–9, 215
Mediterranean region, 116, mortality in 25, 36, 47–8, winds in, 56
Memphis, 6
Men, *see* Males
Metropoleis (nome capitals), census returns from, 118, 144–56, growth of, 169–71, sex ratio in, 167–9, size of, 247
Middle Egypt, 142–53, 155–68, 173, 177, 218–19
Migration, 126–8, to hellenistic Egypt, 80, 83, in Roman Egypt, 146–9, 151, 156, 160, 166–71
Miletus, 150
Millet, 225–6
Minya, 201
Moab, late Roman, 36–7
Models, *see* Life tables
Moeris, Lake, *see* Birket Qarun
Monasteries, Coptic, 6–10, 34–5, 93
Monks, *see* Monasteries
Mortality, age-specific, 25–35, 38, 41–6, 67–9, 91, 116–17, 125–6, 128–41, 165, causes of 3–4, 51, 66, 139–40, 156, 195, 197, change in, 53, crises, 10, 23–4, 126–7, 162, 187–96, 207, 249, sex-specific, 120, 134, 136, urban, 155–6, 172–4, 176, variation in, 179; *see also* Death rate, Epidemics, Infant mortality, Life Tables, Seasonal mortality
Mosquitoes, 75, in Egypt, 76–7, 80, 82, 86
Mouzas, A., 3
Muhammad Ali, 198–200, 203–05, 213, 218, 248
Mummies, 76, 91, 99, 104; *see also* Embalmment
Mummy labels, XXVII, 3, 10–16, 28, 30, 32, meaning of dates on, 12–15
Mustafa Ali, 59

Nabulsi, 84, 87
Napoleon, 166
Naples, 188
Nile, inundation of, 57, 76–7, 81, 217, 244
Nile Delta, 19–20, 48, 76, 81, 103, 112, 142, 177–8, 225–6, 243–4; *see also* Lower Egypt
Nordberg, H., 2
Normandy, 122
North Africa, Roman, 122–3, 232; *see also* Carthage
North Argin, 76
Norway, 91
Nubia, 4–10, 34, 76, 113, 138–40
Numbers, in ancient texts, 1, 181, 246
Nutrition, 225–7, 235–6, 239–42

Omran, A. R., 127
Oxyrhynchus, 77, 149, 173

Pagolo Morelli, G. di, 150
Pakistan, 241
Paleodemography, 121–2, 135–40
Palestine, 234, late Roman, 36–7, 47, 60, 117
Palladius, 78
Pannonia, 121–2
Panzac, D., 190, 193–4, 205–09, 213–14
Papyrus, cultivation of, 87
Paratyphoid, *see* Typhoid
Parkin, T. G., XXII, 121
Paulus of Aegina, 103
Penrith, 188
Perrenoud, A., 94, 114, 127, 196
Plague, bubonic, 97, in antiquity, 99–101, 115, 179, Justinianic, 10, 100, 115, in medieval Egypt, 97,

114–15, 187, in modern Egypt, 97–9, 115, 187–94, 209, 213, in medieval Italy, 126
Plasmodium falciparum, 75, 77–8, 81
Plasmodium malariae, 75, 77
Plasmodium vivax, 75, 77
Pococke, R., 61, 98
Poll tax, 151, 156–7, 203
Population, density, 53–4, 115, 178, growth, 154–5, 170–1, 195–7, 203–05, 207–13, 245, 248–9; *see also* Population size
Population pressure, 171, 249
Population size, in Roman Egypt, XXVIII, 170–1, 183–6, 239–42, 245–8, in cities of Roman Egypt, 173, 247, in modern Egypt, 201–15, 247, in Roman Italy, 182–3
Prices, 219, 249
Pruner, F., 43, 64
Ptolemais, 153–4, 167–9
Ptolemy, (I) 83, (II) 83, (V) 220
Ptolemy (Claudius Ptolemaeus), 54

Qing, 133–5

Rachitis, 104
Rathbone, D. W., 184, 232–4, 246, 248
Rats, 99–100
Ravenna, 71
Raymond, A., 189
Relapsing fever, 71–2, 111
Rhodes, 234
Rice, 81, 226, 229–30, 235, 240
Rice, J. B., 81, 86
Richards, A., 226
Roman citizens, number of, 181–3
Rome, ancient city of, 2, 37–8, 45–7, 113, 116–17, 179, 183, 231–5
Röser, B., 66
Ross, R., 87
Rufus of Ephesus, 99, 103

Sait, 248
Sakinya, 6–7, 9–10, 38
Sallares, R., XXV–VI, XXIX, 47, 178, 250
Saller, R. P., XXII
Sandwith, F. M., 66–7, 69, 72, 98, 102
Saqqara, 6–7, 9–10, 38
Sardinia, 232
Savaresi, A., 78
Scandinavia, 131
Scarlet fever, 53
Schistosomiasis, 102–03
Schnepp, M. B., 42, 49, 69, 73, 78, 92, 101, 105, 198
Schofield, R., XXIV
Scorpions, 104–05
Seasonal mortality, XXVII, 1–117 *passim*, in Roman Egypt, 3, 50–1, 113, 174, in Roman and early medieval Upper Egypt and Nubia, 5–10, in Roman Upper Egypt, 10–16, in the Roman Fayum, 16–19, in Roman Lower Egypt, 19–25, in modern Egypt, 39–45, 49–50, 73–4, 89–90, in Roman Palestine, 36–7, in ancient Rome, 2, 37–8, 45–7, 113, in Roman Italy, 37–8, 113, in modern Italy, 45–6, in Carthage, 21–2, in early modern London, 3, in Japan, 52, age-specific, 25–35, 38, and causes of death, 51, and climate, 36
Sex ratio, 149–50, 167–9
Shaw, B. D., XXII–III, 2–3, 37, 113
Sicily, 232
Skeletal evidence, for demography, 121–2, for disease, 138–40; *see also* Mummies
Slaves, 34, 146–7, 154, 183, freed, 146–7
Smallpox, 94, in ancient Egypt, 10, 95–6, 162, 165, 196, in modern Egypt, 94–5, 114, 196–9, 213, in early modern China, 133–4
Solitary persons, 147
Sonnini, C. S., 59, 64, 104
Sorghum, 225–6
Sparta, 181
Strabo, 78–9, 112
Streptococcal infection, 53
Sweden, 69
Syphilis, 104
Syria, 99, 104, 200, 235

Taxation, *see* Poll tax
Tax grain, from Roman Egypt, 231–4
Tax lists, from Roman Egypt, 158–61
Tebtunis, 77, 88
Tendernden, 58
Terenouthis, 3, 19–24, 26–9, 32–3, 35, 38, 48, 90–1, 93, 97, 112
Theadelphia, 88
Thebaid, 64, 194
Theophrastus, 56

Thompson, D., XXV
Tombstones, Greek, in Egypt and Nubia, XXVII, 5–10, 16–19, 26–35, Coptic, in Egypt and Nubia, XXVII, 3, 5–10, 34, in Rome, 2, ancient Christian, 2, 37, Roman, 1, 122–3, cost of, 34
Tralles, 234
Transition, epidemiologic, 114, 127
Tuberculosis, 91–3, 105, 111, 115, 128, 131, 134
Tunisia, 189
Tuscany, *see* Florence
Typhoid, 66–75, 101, 111
'Typhomalarial fever', 71
Typhus, 66–8, 112

Ulpianic life table, 121
Uniformitarianism, in demographic modelling, 125–6
United States of America, 237
Upper Egypt, 4–16, 28, 30–2, 34, 39–40, 47, 49, 57, 80, 82, 90, 92, 97–8, 113, 153–4, 167–9, 178, 190, 193, 218–20, 226
Urbanisation, of Roman Egypt, 115–16, 119, 143, 170, 183, 247–8, of Roman Italy, 182–3

Venice, 189
Villages, in Roman Egypt, 35, 146, in the Roman Fayum, 86–7, in modern Egypt, 193, census returns from, 118, 156–62, growth of, 169–71, population of, 174, sex ratio in, 167–9
Volney, M. C., 94, 98, 104

War, 126, 200
Weiss, K. M., 137–8
Western Oases (of Egypt), 49–50, 81, 90–1, 112
Wheat, 222, 224–6, 229–30, 235–7, 241
Wild, J., 104
Women, *see* Females
Woods, R., 128
Wrigley, E. A., XXIV

Yates, W. H., 61, 64
Yields, agricultural, 224–5, 228–31, 239–42

Zeki, Abu, 84

SUPPLEMENTS TO MNEMOSYNE

EDITED BY H. PINKSTER, H.S. VERSNEL,
D.M. SCHENKEVELD, P.H. SCHRIJVERS AND S.R. SLINGS

Recent volumes in the series

149. VINOGRADOV, J.G.& S.D. KRYŽICKIJ (eds.). *Olbia.* Eine altgriechische Stadt im Nordwestlichen Schwarzmeerraum. 1995. ISBN 90 04 09677 9
150. MAURER, K. *Interpolation in Thucydides.* 1995. ISBN 90 04 10300 7
151. HORSFALL, N. (ed.) *A Companion to the Study of Virgil.* 1995 ISBN 90 04 09559 4
152. KNIGHT, V.H. *The Renewal of Epic.* Responses to Homer in the *Argonautica* of Apollonius. 1995. ISBN 90 04 10386 4
153. LUSCHNIG, C.A.E. *The Gorgon's Severed Head.* Studies of *Alcestis*, *Electra*, and *Phoenissae.* 1995. ISBN 90 04 10382 1
154. NAVARRO ANTOLÍN, F. (ed.). *Lygdamus.* Corpus Tibullianum III. 1-6: Lygdami elegiarum liber. Translated by J.J. Zoltowski. 1996. ISBN 90 04 10210 8
155. MATTHEWS, V.J. *Antimachus of Colophon.* Text and Commentary. 1996. ISBN 90 04 10468 2
156. TREISTER, M.Y. *The Role of Metals in Ancient Greek History.* 1996. ISBN 90 04 10473 9
157. WORTHINGTON, I. (ed.). *Voice into Text.* Orality and Literacy in Ancient Greece. 1996. ISBN 90 04 10431 3
158. WIJSMAN, H.J.W. *Valerius Flaccus,* Argonautica, *Book V.* A Commentary. 1996. ISBN 90 04 10506 9
159. SCHMELING, G. (ed.). *The Novel in the Ancient World.* 1996. ISBN 90 04 09630 2
160. SICKING, C.M.J. & P. STORK. *Two Studies in the Semantics of the Verb in Classical Greek.* 1996. ISBN 90 04 10460 7
161. KOVACS, D. *Euripidea Altera.* 1996. ISBN 90 04 10624 3
162. GERA, D. *Warrior Women.* The Anonymous Tractatus *De Mulieribus.* 1997. ISBN 90 04 10665 0
163. MORRIS, I. & B. POWELL (eds.). *A New Companion to Homer.* 1997. ISBN 90 04 09989 1
164. ORLIN, E.M. *Temples, Religion and Politics in the Roman Republic.* 1997.ISBN 90 04 10708 8
165. ALBRECHT, M. VON. *A History of Roman Literature.* From Livius Andronicus to Boethius with Special Regard to Its Influence on World Literature. 2 Vols.Revised by G.Schmeling and by the Author. Vol. 1: Translated with the Assistance of F. and K. Newman, Vol. 2: Translated with the Assitance of R.R. Caston and F.R. Schwartz. 1997. ISBN 90 04 10709 6 (Vol. 1), ISBN 90 04 10711 8 (Vol. 2), ISBN 90 04 10712 6 (Set)
166. DIJK, J.G.M. VAN. Αἶνοι, Λόγοι, Μῦθοι. Fables in Archaic, Classical, and Hellenistic Greek Literature. With a Study of the Theory and Terminology of the Genre. 1997. ISBN 90 04 10747 9
167. MAEHLER, H. (Hrsg.). *Die Lieder des Bakchylides.* Zweiter Teil: Die Dithyramben und Fragmente. Text, Übersetzung und Kommentar. 1997. ISBN 90 04 10671 5
168. DILTS, M. & G.A. KENNEDY (eds.). *Two Greek Rhetorical Treatises from the Roman Empire.* Introduction, Text, and Translation of the Arts of Rhetoric Attributed to Anonymous Seguerianus and to Apsines of Gadara. 1997. ISBN 90 04 10728 2
169. GÜNTHER, H.-C. *Quaestiones Propertianae.* 1997. ISBN 90 04 10793 2
170. HEINZE, T. (Hrsg.). *P. Ovidius Naso. Der* XII. *Heroidenbrief: Medea an Jason.* Einleitung, Text und Kommentar. Mit einer Beilage: Die Fragmente der Tragödie *Medea.* 1997. ISBN 90 04 10800 9

171. BAKKER, E.J. (ed.). *Grammar as Interpretation.* Greek Literature in its Linguistic Contexts. 1997. ISBN 90 04 10730 4
172. GRAINGER, J.D. *A Seleukid Prosopography and Gazetteer.* 1997. ISBN 90 04 10799 1
173. GERBER, D.E. (ed.). *A Companion to the Greek Lyric Poets.* 1997. ISBN 90 04 09944 1
174. SANDY, G. *The Greek World of Apuleius.* Apuleius and the Second Sophistic. 1997. ISBN 90 04 10821 1
175. ROSSUM-STEENBEEK, M. VAN. *Greek Readers' Digests?* Studies on a Selection of Subliterary Papyri. 1998. ISBN 90 04 10953 6
176. McMAHON, J.M. *Paralysin Cave.* Impotence, Perception, and Text in the *Satyrica* of Petronius. 1998. ISBN 90 04 10825 4
177. ISAAC, B. *The Near East under Roman Rule.* Selected Papers. 1998. ISBN 90 04 10736 3
178. KEEN, A.G. *Dynastic Lycia.* A Political History of the Lycians and Their Relations with Foreign Powers, c. 545-362 B.C. 1998. ISBN 90 04 10956 0
179. GEORGIADOU, A. & D.H.J. LARMOUR. *Lucian's Science Fiction Novel* True Histories. Interpretation and Commentary. 1998. ISBN 90 04 10667 7
180. GÜNTHER, H.-C. *Ein neuer metrischer Traktat und das Studium der pindarischen Metrik in der Philologie der Paläologenzeit.* 1998. ISBN 90 04 11008 9
181. HUNT, T.J. *A Textual History of Cicero's* Academici Libri. 1998. ISBN 90 04 10970 6
182. HAMEL, D. *Athenian Generals.* Military Authority in the Classical Period. 1998. ISBN 90 04 10900 5
183. WHITBY, M. (ed.). *The Propaganda of Power.* The Role of Panegyric in Late Antiquity. 1998. ISBN 90 04 10571 9
184. SCHRIER, O.J. *The* Poetics *of Aristotle and the* Tractatus Coislinianus. A Bibliography from about 900 till 1996. 1998. ISBN 90 04 11132 8
185. SICKING, C.M.J. *Distant Companions.* Selected Papers. 1998. ISBN 90 04 11054 2
186. P.H. SCHRIJVERS. *Lucrèce et les Sciences de la Vie.* 1999. ISBN 90 04 10230 2
187. BILLERBECK M. (Hrsg.). *Seneca.* Hercules Furens. Einleitung, Text, Übersetzung und Kommentar. 1999. ISBN 90 04 11245 6
188. MACKAY, E.A. (ed.). *Signs of Orality.* The Oral Tradition and Its Influence in the Greek and Roman World. 1999. ISBN 90 04 11273 1
189. ALBRECHT, M. VON. *Roman Epic.* An Interpretative Introduction. 1999. ISBN 90 04 11292 8
190. Hout, M.P.J. van den. *A Commentary on the Letters of M. Cornelius Fronto.* 1999. ISBN 90 04 10957 9
191. Kraus, C. Shuttleworth (ed.). *The Limits of Historiography.* Genre and Narrative in Ancient Historical Texts. 1999. ISBN 90 04 10670 7
192. Lomas, K. & T. Cornell. *Cities and Urbanisation in Ancient Italy.* ISBN 90 04 10808 4 *In preparation*
193. Tsetskhladze, G.R. (ed). *History of Greek Colonisation and Settlement Overseas.* 2 vols. ISBN 90 04 09843 7 *In preparation*
194. Wood, S.E. *Imperial Women.* A Study in Public Images, 40 B.C. - A.D. 68. 1999. ISBN 90 04 11281 2
195. Ophuijsen, J.M. van & P. Stork. *Linguistics into Interpretation.* Speeches of War in Herodotus VII 5 & 8-18. 1999. ISBN 90 04 11455 6
196. Tsetskhladze, G.R. (ed.). *Ancient Greeks West and East.* 1999. ISBN 90 04 11190 5
197. Pfeijffer, I.L. *Three Aeginetan Odes of Pindar.* A Commentary on *Nemean* V, *Nemean* III, & *Pythian* VIII. 1999. ISBN 90 04 11381 9
198. Horsfall, N. *Virgil,* Aeneid 7. A Commentary. 2000. ISBN 90 04 10842 4
199. Irby-Massie, G.L. *Military Religion in Roman Britain.* 1999. ISBN 90 04 10848 3
200. Grainger, J.D. *The League of the Aitolians.* 1999. ISBN 90 04 10911 0
201. Adrados, F.R. *History of the Graeco-Roman Fable.* I: Introduction and from the Origins to the Hellenistic Age. Translated by L.A. Ray. Revised and Updated by the Author and Gert-Jan van Dijk. 1999. ISBN 90 04 11454 8
202. Grainger, J.D. *Aitolian Prosopographical Studies.* 2000. ISBN 90 04 11350 9
203. Solomon, J. *Ptolemy* Harmonics. Translation and Commentary. 2000. ISBN 90 04 115919

204. WIJSMAN, H.J.W. *Valerius Flaccus,* Argonautica, *Book VI.* A Commentary. 2000. ISBN 90 04 11718 0
205. Mader, G. *Josephus and the Politics of Historiography.* Apologetic and Impression Management in the *Bellum Judaicum.* 2000. ISBN 90 04 11446 7
206. Nauta, R.R. *Poetry for Patrons.* Literary Communication in the Age of Domitian. 2001. ISBN 90 04 10885 8
207. Adrados, F.R. *History of the Graeco-Roman Fable.* II: The Fable during the Roman Empire and in the Middle Ages. Translated by L.A. Ray. Revised and Updated by the Author and Gert-Jan van Dijk. 2000. ISBN 90 04 11583 8
208. James, A. & K. Lee. *A Commentary on Quintus of Smyrna,* Posthomerica V. 2000. ISBN 90 04 11594 3
209. Derderian, K. *Leaving Words to Remember.* Greek Mourning and the Advent of Literacy. 2001. ISBN 90 04 11750 4
210. Shorrock, R. *The Challenge of Epic.* Allusive Engagement in the *Dionysiaca* of Nonnus. 2001. ISBN 90 04 11795 4
211. Scheidel, W. (ed.). *Debating Roman Demography.* 2001. ISBN 90 04 11525 0
212. Keulen, A.J. *L. Annaeus Seneca* Troades. Introduction, Text and Commentary. 2001. ISBN 90 04 12004 1
213. Morton, J. *The Role of the Physical Environment in Ancient Greek Seafaring.* 2001. ISBN 90 04 11717 2
214. Graham, A.J. *Collected Papers on Greek Colonization.* 2001. ISBN 90 04 11634 6
215. Grossardt, P. *Die Erzählung von Meleagros.* Zur literarischen Entwicklung der kalydonischen Kultlegende 2001. ISBN 90 04 11952 3
216. Zafiropoulos, C.A. *Ethics in Aesop's Fables: The* Augustana *Collection.* 2001. ISBN 90 04 11867 5
217. Rengakos, A. & T.D. Papanghelis (eds.). *A Companion to Apollonius Rhodius.* 2001. ISBN 90 04 11752 0
218. Watson, J. *Speaking Volumes.* Orality and Literacy in the Greek and Roman World. 2001. ISBN 90 04 12049 1
219. MacLeod, L. *Dolos and Dike in Sophokles' Elektra.* 2001. ISBN 90 04 11898 5
220. McKinley, K.L. *Reading the Ovidian Heroine.* "Metamorphoses" Commentaries 1100-1618. 2001. ISBN 90 04 11796 2
221. Reeson, J. *Ovid* Heroides *11, 13 and 14.* A Commentary. 2001. ISBN 90 04 12140 4
222. Fried, M.N. & S. Unguru. *Apollonius of Perga's Conica:* Text, Context, Subtext. 2001. ISBN 90 04 11977 9
223. Livingstone, N. *A Commentary on Isocrates' Busiris.* 2001. ISBN 90 04 12143 9
224. Levene, D.S. & D.P. Nelis. *Clio and the Poets.* Augustan Poetry and the Traditions of Ancient Historiography. 2001. ISBN 90 04 11782 2
225. Wooten, C.W. *The Orator in Action and Theory in Greece and Rome.* 2001. ISBN 90 04 12213 3
226. Galán Vioque, G. *Martial, Book VII. A Commentary.* 2001. ISBN 90 04 12338 5
227. Lefèvre, E. *Die Unfähigkeit sich zu erkennen: Sophokles' Tragödien.* 2001. ISBN 90 04 12322 9
228. Scheidel, W. *Death on the Nile.* Disease and the Demography of Roman Egypt. 2001. ISBN 90 04 12323 7